HOME HEALTH NURSING

Nursing Diagnoses & Care Plans

Carol A. Bedrosian, R.N., P.H.N., M.S.N.

APPLETON & LANGE
Norwalk, Connecticut/San Mateo, California

ISBN 0-8385-3842-8

9 780838 538425

90000

93 / 10 9 8 7 6 5 4 3

Prentice-Hall International (UK) Limited, *London*
Prentice-Hall of Australia Pty. Limited, *Sydney*
Prentice-Hall Canada, Inc., *Toronto*
Prentice-Hall Hispanoamericana, S.A., *Mexico*
Prentice-Hall of India Private Limited, *New Delhi*
Prentice-Hall of Japan, Inc., *Tokyo*
Simon & Schuster Asia Pte. Ltd., *Singapore*
Editora Prentice-Hall do Brasil Ltda., *Rio de Janeiro*
Prentice-Hall, *Englewood Cliffs, New Jersey*

Library of Congress Cataloging-in-Publication Data

Bedrosian, Carol A.
 Home health nursing.

 Bibliography: p.
 1. Nursing care plans. 2. Home nursing—Planning.
3. Home care services. I. Title. [DNLM: 1. Home
Care Services. 2. Home Nursing. 3. Patient Care
Planning. WY 115 B413h]
RT49.B43 1988   362.1′4   88-16788
ISBN 0-8385-3842-8

Production Editor: Bellamy Printz
Designer: Steve Byrum

PRINTED IN THE UNITED STATES OF AMERICA

*This book is dedicated to my mother and father,
and to my brother Wayne.*

■ Contents

■ About the Author

Carol Bedrosian has worked in the field of Home Health in California for the past 10 years; 8 years as Director of Nursing in Home Health, and the past 2 years as a Corporate Director of Home Care Services. She presently works as an independent consultant and lecturer in the fields of gerontology and home health. Bedrosian has also taught for five years as an Assistant Professor of Nursing at California State University.

■ Preface

In this current era of cost containment, hospitalized patients are being discharged as early as possible. Concerns over the ability of the patient to function safely and independently at home, following discharge, are intensified because of tight reimbursement restrictions on home health services. Even though all age groups may be eligible to receive covered home health benefits, the elderly comprise the largest group of clients receiving care by home health agencies. They are at particular risk with these early discharges. Home health nurses are being challenged to plan, coordinate, and deliver a comprehensive health program in the client's place of residence. This program should meet the client's basic needs, as well as provide treatment and appropriate nursing support. Home health care has been shown to be a less expensive alternative to hospital and institutional care. Home health nurses must clearly recognize that the quality of their documentation, with regards to their assessments and interventions, determines whether the client is eligible to receive covered home health benefits.

The home health nursing care plans in this book are intended to provide practical and concise guidelines in assessing the needs of clients in the home. They also assist the home health nurse in developing a plan of care with the collaboration of the physician and other health professionals. The clinical problems and conditions, most frequently occurring in older adults, are the focus of this book.

Each home health care planning guide is organized as follows.

Introduction (Subject Presentation): At the beginning of each home health care planning guide, a definition and general introduction to the pathophysiology of each disorder and a discussion of selected procedures and treatments are presented. This section is intended to provide the home health nurse with a concise review and clarification of a particular disorder, procedure, or treatment. It is not intended to be an in-depth presentation of etiology of disease.

Potential Complications: This section includes a list of potential complications that may occur with each specific condition or treatment that is presented. This list is intended to serve as a reference for the home health nurse when assessing and evaluating the client for significant changes that would necessitate a modification in the plan of treatment or require hospitalization.

Types of Clients/Clinical Conditions Seen by Home Health Agencies: The information presented in this section describes the type of client that may be eligible to receive Medicare covered home health services. This section is only to be used as a guideline since it is only one of the components that need to be considered when determining covered services. Other criteria for Medicare eligibility to receive home health services are: (1) homebound status of the client; (2) providing of a skilled service; (3) care provided must be part-time and intermittent; (4) physician must sign orders for treatment, and (5) services provided are not duplicated by another service.

Related Nursing Diagnosis: Nursing diagnoses is a term used to describe existing or potential health problems that a client with a particular condition may experience. The purpose of this section is to assist the home health nurse in selecting those nursing diagnoses that may be applicable to the client's condition. These nursing diagnoses must be confirmed or ruled out after the home health nurse has observed and evaluated the clinical manifestations and condition of the client. With the exception of the nursing diagnoses "anxiety" and "knowledge deficit," those nursing diagnoses that are not unique to a specific condition, but may apply to any home care client (e.g., spiritual distress), has not been consistently listed, and should be evaluated when developing each plan. In addition, there are many factors (e.g., poor memory, expensive therapy, knowledge deficit) that may contribute to a client's non-compliance to the prescribed treatment and teaching plan. There are also factors (e.g., chronic debilitating diseases, impaired mental status, unavailable support systems) that may affect the ability of the client or caregiver to maintain a safe environment. As a result, the nursing diagnoses "non-compliance" and "home maintenance management, impaired" have not been included and should be considered when developing each plan of care.

The nursing diagnoses are listed in alphabetical order to assist the home health nurse in readily selecting those diagnoses that may be applicable to the client. Diagnoses selected are those that have been developed and approved by the North American Nursing Diagnosis Association (NANDA). Defining characteristics (signs and symptoms) listed for each nursing diagnosis presented are not all-inclusive and must be assessed for the individual client.

Goals: Long and short term goals, specific to the condition or treatment under discussion, have been listed. They are measurable, observable, and serve to assist the home health nurse in evaluating the progress that the client and/or caregiver has achieved. Only those goals that are appropriate for the client should be selected by the home health nurse when developing the plan of care. In addition to using the goals in this book, the home health nurse may want to write additional goals that are specific to the client.

Nursing Actions/Treatments: Nursing actions encompass activities from teaching and counseling to physical care and carrying out prescribed medical treatments. Each of these actions are intended to assist the client in achieving the highest possible level of wellness. To accomplish this goal, the home health nurse must provide services that are well planned, systematic and individualized through the use of nursing process.

Nursing actions listed for each condition, and/or treatment, include specific areas to be observed, assessed, and evaluated by the home health nurse, as well as specific nursing interventions. The suggested areas of instruction are directed either to the client and/or the person(s) involved in care of the client. In some instances, alternative nursing actions may need to be considered and added by the home health nurse.

Rehabilitation Potential: The rehabilitation potential is a statement relative to the client's condition. This potential assesses the capability of the client to attain goals that have been defined, collaboratively by the client or caregiver, home health nurse, physician, and other health professionals. It is written in a fashion that allows the nurse to ascertain the level of predictability to achieve the stated goals. *Excellent, good, fair, guarded,* or *poor,* is the scale used to assist the home health nurse in assessing the client's rehabilitation potential, relative to a full or partial return to a level of functioning.

Excellent: is rated as a client able to independently attain or perform a goal without assistance;

Good: client is able to function with periodic and infrequent supervision;

Fair: ongoing daily assistance needed to obtain goals;

Guarded: condition too unstable to determine rehabilitation potential at this time;

Poor: totally dependent on 24-hour assist if goals are to be met.

Ongoing/Discharge Evaluation of Teaching: The primary purpose of this section is to provide a tool to evaluate, (either on an ongoing basis or at the time of discharge), the effectiveness of previous areas of instruction in achieving the goals that have been defined for the client. The evaluation is designed to become part of the client's record and may be photocopied as needed.

There are several terms used throughout this book whose meaning should be clarified. First, the word *client* is used rather than patient because it provides the connotation of one who is mutually interactive with the home health provider in terms of planning care, participating in own care, and ultimately assuming self-care to the highest level of functioning possible. The term *caregiver* is used to describe significant other(s) who serve as support systems to the client and who may or may not reside with the client.

■ How to Use the Nursing Care Plans

1. Refer to the section on introduction, nursing diagnoses, and nursing actions for review of the specific areas of assessment and interventions, prior to making the first home visit.
2. Collect subjective and objective data from client and/or caregiver on the first home visit to assess the client's current health status and to determine eligibility for Medicare-covered services.
3. Collaborate with the client's physician and other health professionals to review assessment findings and to develop a plan of care.
4. Select nursing diagnoses, goals, and nursing actions, from the home health nursing care plan(s) that are specific to the client's condition and in accordance with the orders received from the physician to develop an individualized plan of care.
5. The goals established for the client change frequently and are to be evaluated on an ongoing basis as well as at the time of discharge using the "Ongoing/Discharge Evaluation Form."

Current therapeutic concepts are presented with the realization that not all modalities of treatment can be fully discussed. Each home health nursing care plan is designed to allow the home health nurse to select those components of the guide that pertain to specific individual client needs. The home health nurse is advised to read the applicable care plan(s) prior to seeing the client and when collaborating with the physician to insure a comprehensive assessment of the client's needs as well as to develop a personalized and individualized plan of care. In addition to the specific nursing actions or treatments discussed, the home health nurse will also want to evaluate the client for home health aid and other health services as may be needed by the client in rehabilitating to the highest possible level of independent functioning.

It should be well understood that all recommendations in these home health nursing care plans must be considered in light of the client's clinical condition. It is expected that any of the medical orders or treatments presented in this home health care book are to be discussed first with the client's physician and orders received prior to giving any care.

The home health nurse should include in the teaching to the client the importance of keeping scheduled physician appointments and the need to see the physician once every 60 days and more often as indicated when receiving covered home health benefits.

It is the author's expectation that the home health nursing care plans presented in this book will serve as a quick reference to the development of an individualized home care program and will assist the nurse in developing a written plan of care in a minimal period of time.

■ Acknowledgments

I would like to express my sincere appreciation to my family and friends for their support and encouragement during the many stages of this book.

I especially want to thank my friends Vernon and Veronica Boolootian for their encouragement and for providing me the environment in which to write, and Bonnie Peterson for the many long hours of typing and assistance in the preparation of this book.

A special thank you goes to Stuart Horton, Editor, for his support, encouragement, and professional advice in helping to make this book a reality; to Marion Kalstein-Welch, Executive Editor, Nursing, for providing the necessary support during the development of this book; and to Bellamy Printz, Production Editor, for her understanding, support, and many hours of expert editorial assistance.

Finally, I gratefully acknowledge Jack E. Wilkinson, M.D., General Surgeon, Fresno, Calif.; Sally E. Martin, R.N., M.S.N., Associate Chief of Nursing Services for Nursing Home Care, V.A. Medical Center, Sepulveda, Calif.; and Carolyn Schmitz, R.N., M.S.N., Director of Nursing for East Bay Health America, Albany, Calif., for the numerous hours spent reviewing this book and sharing of their professional expertise and knowledge.

CARDIOVASCULAR DISORDERS

■ Cardiac Arrhythmias

Pacemaker Implantation

Arrhythmias are abnormal disturbances in cardiac rate and/or rhythm resulting from electrophysiologic alterations in myocardial cells. Based on these alterations, arrhythmias are classified according to: disturbances of impulse formation, of impulse conduction, or a combination of both. The resultant physiologic effects of these disturbances vary according to the cause of the arrhythmia as well as the effectiveness of the compensatory mechanisms of the body in maintaining cardiac output.

There are a variety of factors that predispose to arrhythmic activity, some of which are: tissue hypoxia, electrolyte and acid–base imbalance, coronary artery disease, congenital defects, inflammatory and metabolic disorders of the myocardium, neuroendocrine disturbances, ingestion of cardiac stimulants such as caffeine and medications. Clinical manifestations that are associated with decreased cardiac output secondary to arrhythmias are weakness, chest pain, cold, clammy skin, dizziness, light-headedness, decreased urinary output, and dyspnea.

Depending on the client's age, cardiac condition, and general state of health, a permanent pacemaker may be indicated for treatment of a recurrent or permanent arrhythmia. A pacemaker is an electronic device used to generate and maintain a series of timed electrical stimuli to the heart muscle when disturbances of the impulse formation or impulse conduction system result in compromised cardiac functioning. Depending on the client's clinical situation, the pacemaker used may either be temporary or permanent. A temporary pacemaker is generally used in those clinical conditions that require immediate correction of a transient, symptomatic arrhythmia, whereas a permanent pacemaker may be indicated for treatment of a recurrent or a permanent arrhythmia. An example of the use of a permanent pacemaker is in a client with irreversible cardiac damage and complete block in the cardiac conduction system.

There are various types of pacemakers, but generally pacemakers are classified as either fixed or demand. Fixed pacemakers (which are rarely used) initiate impulses at a constant rate, regardless of the client's rhythm. Demand pacemakers (which are more commonly used) initiate impulses only when the client's heart rate falls below a preset level.

The pacemaker system contains the pulse generator (power source) and the electronic circuitry (pacing circuit and sensing circuit), which is responsible for sending out appropriately timed signals and sensing cardiac activity. The pacemaker can pace the atria, the ventricles, or both by delivering the electrical impulse through a pacing lead(s) to the myocardium. Types of temporary pacemakers include transvenous, transthoracic, and epicardial pacemakers; these are regulated by an external pacemaker device. With a permanent pacemaker the transvenous endocardial approach is more commonly used, and the pulse generator is implanted under the skin, usually in a subcutaneous pocket below the clavicle laterally (anterior upper axilla).

POTENTIAL COMPLICATONS

Cardiac Arrhythmias:
1. Cardiac rate and rhythm disturbances,
2. thromboembolic phenomena associated with pooling of blood secondary to irregular myocardial contractions,
3. cardiac arrest.

Pacemaker Implantation:
1. Pacemaker malfunction (e.g., failure to capture, sense, fire; oversensing, which may occur as a result of battery failure; dislodgement or breakage of the pacemaker catheter wires; loose catheter terminals; electromagnetic interference).
2. S&S of infection of skin over implant site.

TYPES OF CLIENTS/CLINICAL CONDITIONS SEEN BY HOME HEALTH AGENCIES

1. Newly diagnosed with cardiac arrhythmias: initiation of prescribed treatment regimen and inclusive teaching plan for home-care management of cardiac condition, including new medications, diet, need for ongoing evaluation of cardiac functioning in response to prescribed therapy.
2. Changes in ongoing plan of treatment for management of unstable cardiovascular system and complications associated with arrhythmia: need for instruction, supervision, assessment of client's response to new medications and/or treatments and reporting to physician.
3. Recent pacemaker implantation: instruction in pacemaker care and handling of emergency situations, assessment of pacemaker functioning.
4. Changes in prescribed plan of treatment for management of problems and complications associated with pacemaker.

RELATED NURSING DIAGNOSIS

Activity Intolerance

related to:
Decreased cardiac output secondary to arrhythmia

as seen by:
Dyspnea on exertion; weakness and fatigue; abnormal heart rate or BP in response to activity

Anxiety

related to:
1. Arrhythmic condition
2. Pacemaker care
3. Knowledge deficit regarding prescribed treatment regimen

as seen by:
Facial tension; overexcitedness; verbalization of fears and concerns

Bowel Elimination, Alteration in: Constipation

related to:
1. Inadequate dietary fiber and/or fluids in diet
2. Decreased activity levels

as seen by:
Straining at stool; hard, formed stools; decreased frequency and amount from usual pattern

Cardiac Output, Alteration in: Decreased

related to:
A disturbance of impulse formation or impulse conduction of the heart

as seen by:
Dizziness; shortness of breath; fainting, weakness; fatigue, drop in BP below normal for client; irregular pulse; pulse rate less than 60 or greater than 100 beats per minute; palpitations; confusion; chest pain, diminished or absent peripheral pulses

Cardiac Output, Alteration in: Decreased

related to:
Pacemaker malfunction

as seen by:
Light-headedness; confusion; irregular pulse; dizziness; heart rate increase or decrease of more than five beats from preset rate; chest pain; fainting; shortness of breath; hypotension; fatigue; peripheral edema

Gas Exchange, Impaired

related to:
Altered oxygen supply secondary to decreased cardiac output

as seen by:
Dyspnea; fatigue; restlessness; confusion, irritability

Infection, Potential for

related to:
Pacemaker implant site; breakdown of
body's first line of defense

as seen by:
Increased redness and swelling;
hematoma formation; pronounced
tenderness; drainage; tissue
breakdown; fever; elevated WBC
count

Injury, Potential for: Increased Risk of Falls and Injuries

related to:
Decreased cerebral perfusion
secondary to arrhythmia activity or
pacemaker malfunction

as seen by:
Dizziness; syncope; weakness; fatigue;
confusion

Knowledge Deficit (Specify)

related to:
1. Prescribed plan of treatment for
cardiac and pacemaker care
2. Potential complications; S&S to
report to home health nurse or
physician

as seen by:
Lack of information; inadequate
understanding; inability to perform
skills necessary to meet health-care
needs at home

Mobility, Impaired Physical

related to:
1. Activity intolerance
2. Prescribed activity restrictions and
limitations
3. Muscle weakness and stiffness of
shoulder joint on operative side

as seen by:
Weakness and fatigue, reluctance to
move because of fear of injury to
pacemaker; c/o of limited movement
of arm or shoulder on side of
pacemaker implantation; imposed
medical restrictions

Self-Care Deficit: Feeding, Bathing/Hygiene, Dressing/Grooming, Toileting (Specify)

related to:
1. Activity intolerance
2. Impaired physical mobility
3. Prescribed activity restrictions and
limitations

as seen by:
Limited participation in self-care
activities associated with weakness
and fatigue; reluctance to move;
fatigue

Self-Concept, Disturbance in

related to:
Altered body image associated with
  pacemaker implantation

as seen by:
Lack of follow-through; uncooperative
  behavior; depression

Skin Integrity, Impairment of: Actual/Potential

related to:
1. Surgical incision
2. Impaired wound healing secondary
   to infection

as seen by:
Fever, redness, swelling, exudate;
  tenderness; tissue breakdown

Tissue Perfusion, Alteration in: Cerebral

related to:
Decreased cardiac output, secondary to
  arrhythmic activity or pacemaker
  malfunction

as seen by:
Confusion, dizziness, fainting

LONG-TERM GOAL

To maintain optimal cardiac function through controlled rhythm and rate for restoration of balance between oxygen demand and supply.

SHORT-TERM GOALS

The client with an arrhythmia/pacemaker will be able to:

1. Verbalize understanding of normal cardiac conduction, nature of arrhythmia, prescribed treatment, factors that provoke, S&S of new or recurring cardiovascular problems to report to home health nurse or physician.
2. Accurately take pulse and record/state preset pacemaker rate, alterations in rate and rhythm to report to physician.
3. Verbalize understanding of purpose, type, and function of pacemaker.
4. Verbalize knowledge of unacceptable variations and pacemaker failure to report to physician.
5. Verbalize S&S of skin breakdown or infection/demonstrate prescribed skin care.
6. Verbalize importance and identify areas to watch for electromagnetic interference with pacemaker stimuli.
7. Demonstrate purpose and correct use of telephone monitoring device for checking pacemaker functioning.

8. Demonstrate compliance with prescribed diet and dietary restrictions.
9. Demonstrate compliance with prescribed medication therapy/identify side effects.
10. Verbalize importance of not smoking.
11. Demonstrate compliance with prescribed limitations and restrictions with planned rest periods, safety measures with ambulation and daily activities.
12. Demonstrate prescribed ROM exercises of arm and shoulder on side of pacemaker implantation.
13. Verbalize importance of following prescribed bowel regimen, avoiding straining at stool.
14. Verbalize importance of wearing a Medic Alert bracelet with pacemaker information.
15. Demonstrate a positive adjustment to pacemaker.

NURSING ACTIONS/TREATMENTS

1. Assess cardiovascular status/identify complications.
2. Assess vital signs/identify trends (e.g., pulse deficit, hypotension), instruct how to check pulse, how to take for a full minute at rest and record; about importance of preset pacemaker rate remaining constant, alterations in rate and rhythm to report to home health nurse or physician.
3. Instruct about normal cardiac conduction, nature of arrhythmia, factors that provoke arrhythmia, importance of following prescribed treatment regimen, S&S of new or recurring cardiovascular problems to report to home health nurse or physician.
4. Assess and evaluate pacemaker functioning/instruct about purpose and type (e.g., fixed-rate or asynchronous, demand or synchronous, temporary or permanent pacemaker), unacceptable variations and pacemaker malfunctioning to report to home health nurse or physician.
5. Observe and evaluate implantation site daily for S&S of skin breakdown or infection/instruct in prescribed skin care and to avoid restrictive clothing over implant site.
6. Observe/instruct to watch for electromagnetic interference with pacemaker stimuli that can temporarily interfere with usual pacemaker operation (e.g., high-powered radio or television transmitters, some models of microwave ovens).
7. Observe/instruct about having pacemaker checked regularly, purpose and use of prescribed telephone monitoring device.
8. Assess and evaluate nutritional status/instruct about prescribed dietary restrictions (e.g., caffeine, alcohol); increase or decrease in potassium as prescribed.
9. Observe/instruct to take medications as ordered (e.g., antiarrhythmics), purpose and action, side effects, toxicity/evaluate medication effectiveness.

10. Observe/instruct about importance of not smoking.
11. Observe and evaluate for signs of activity intolerance, self-care deficits/instruct to follow prescribed restrictions and limitations with daily activities and sexual functioning, planned rest periods.
12. Observe/instruct prescribed ROM exercises for arm and shoulder on side of pacemaker implantation.
13. Assess bowel elimination pattern/instruct about importance of not straining at stool and prescribed measures to treat or avoid constipation (e.g., increase in dietary fiber and fluids, increased activities as allowed, use of stool softeners and laxatives)/evaluate effectiveness of bowel regimen.
14. Assess risk factors for falls and injuries in daily activities/instruct in safety measures with ambulation and ADL.
15. Assess emotional effects of having a pacemaker; encourage verbalization of feelings/refer to social services as ordered to assist with adjustment to pacemaker and provide information regarding community services (e.g., American Heart Association, Smokenders, International Association of Pacemaker Patients).
16. Observe/instruct to wear Medic Alert bracelet with details of pacemaker information (e.g., type of pacemaker, date of implantation, rate setting, physician's name).

REHABILITATION POTENTIAL

Rehabilitation potential *excellent good fair guarded poor* with control of arrhythmia, for *full partial* return to a previous level of independent functioning.

Client's Name _____

Medical Record # _____

ONGOING/DISCHARGE EVALUATION OF TEACHING

The Client with an Arrhythmia/Pacemaker

Teaching Tools:

Printed materials given: _____

Audiovisual aids used: _____

Return Information/Demonstration/Interpretation by

_____ Client

_____ Caregiver

	OF:	Met	Not Met	Comments
☐	Normal cardiac conduction; nature of client's specific arrhythmia.	_____	_____	_____
☐	Factors that provoke arrhythmias, S&S of complications; actions to take.	_____	_____	_____
☐	Importance of compliance with prescribed treatment regimen.	_____	_____	_____
☐	How to take pulse; preset pacemaker rate; alterations in rate and rhythm to report to physician.	_____	_____	_____
☐	Purpose and type of			

Client's Name _____

Medical Record # _____

pacemaker;
unacceptable
variations and
pacemaker
malfunctioning.   _____   _____   _____

☐ S&S of skin
   breakdown or
   infection of
   pacemaker
   implantation
   site; prescribed
   skin care.   _____   _____   _____

☐ Interference
   with pacemaker
   stimuli by
   electromagnetic
   devices.   _____   _____   _____

☐ Use and
   purpose of
   telephone
   monitoring
   device to check
   pacemaker
   functioning.   _____   _____   _____

☐ Diet and dietary
   restrictions.   _____   _____   _____

☐ Medications
   and
   administration,
   purpose and
   action, side
   effects.   _____   _____   _____

☐ Importance of
   not smoking.   _____   _____   _____

☐ Activity
   restrictions and
   limitations,
   planned rest
   periods.   _____   _____   _____

Client's Name _____

Medical Record # _____

☐ Safety
measures with
ambulation,
daily activities. _____ _____ _____

☐ Exercise of arm
and shoulder
on side of
pacemaker
implantation. _____ _____ _____

☐ Bowel regimen,
importance of
not straining. _____ _____ _____

☐ Medic Alert
bracelet. _____ _____ _____

Signature of Home Health Nurse _____

Date _____

■ Carotid Endarterectomy

Carotid endarterectomy is the surgical removal of atheromatous plaque from the intima of an extracranial carotid artery to increase the flow of blood to the brain and reduce the risk of microemboli and distal occlusion. An incision is made along the anterior border of the sternocleidomastoid muscle, and the obstructing atheromatous plaque is removed. The most important causative factor of carotid occlusion is atherosclerosis, in which the arteries are damaged by the deposition of a lipoid material under the intimal lining of the arterial wall, especially at areas of bifurcation. As the atheromatous plaque enlarges, blood flow decreases and there is an increased risk of thrombus formation and embolization to more distal parts of the artery. This could result in a transient ischemic attack or a cerebral vascular accident.

Those individuals experiencing transient ischemic attacks and reversible ischemic neurologic deficits are more likely to benefit from a carotid endarterectomy. However, the role of a carotid endarterectomy in those clients with a stroke in evolution or with a recent stroke remains controversial among vascular surgeons and neurosurgeons.

POTENTIAL COMPLICATIONS

1. Wound infection,
2. cranial nerve impairment secondary to trauma arising from operative procedure. Cranial nerves at risk include the facial, hypoglossal, glossopharyngeal, vagus and/or accessory nerves,
3. neurologic deficits secondary to thrombus or embolus formation (e.g., TIA, stroke).

TYPES OF CLIENTS/CLINICAL CONDITIONS SEEN BY HOME HEALTH AGENCIES

1. Observation and care of surgical incision; dressing changes of draining wound.
2. Wound infection.
3. Initiation and instruction of prescribed treatment regimen for home-care management of postsurgical carotid endarterectomy client.
4. Changes in ongoing plan of treatment for management of postsurgical complications; need for instruction, supervision, evaluation of client's response to new medications and/or treatments.

RELATED NURSING DIAGNOSIS

Anxiety

related to:
1. Altered body image secondary to postsurgical complications

as seen by:
Feelings of inadequacy; lack of participation in self-care;

2. Concern over ability to perform prescribed wound care

indifference; expressed fears; feelings of apprehension

Bowel Elimination, Alteration in: Constipation

related to:
1. Inadequate dietary fiber and/or fluids in diet
2. Decreased activity levels postsurgery

as seen by:
Straining at stool; hard, formed stool; decreased frequency and amount from usual pattern

Communication, Impaired: Verbal

related to:
Altered speaking ability associated with damage to cranial nerves VII, IX, X, and/or XII

as seen by:
Difficulty swallowing and speaking; hoarseness; asymmetrical movement of vocal cords and soft palate when says "ah"; deviation of tongue toward affected side; facial ptosis

Infection, Potential for

related to:
Incisional area, breakdown of the body's first line of defense

as seen by:
Chills and fever; increased redness and swelling; pain and unusual drainage; elevated WBC count

Knowledge Deficit (Specify)

related to:
1. Inadequate understanding of prescribed plan of treatment for postsurgical carotid endarterectomy
2. Potential complications, S&S to report to home health nurse or physician

as seen by:
Lack of information; inadequate understanding; inability to perform skills necessary to meet health-care needs at home

Skin Integrity, Impairment of: Actual/Potential

related to:
1. Surgical incision
2. Impaired wound healing secondary to infection or inadequate nutritional status

as seen by:
Increased redness, swelling, pain, unusual drainage, elevated temperature

Swallowing, Impaired

related to:
Damage to cranial nerves VII, IX, X,
XII

as seen by:
Difficulty with chewing and
swallowing; loss of gag reflex

LONG-TERM GOAL

To achieve an optimal level of health and satisfying life-style following improved cerebral circulation and stabilization of neurologic status.

SHORT-TERM GOALS

The client with a carotid endarterectomy will be able to:

1. Verbalize nature of disease process, risk factors, and surgical procedure, S&S of complications to report to home health nurse or physician.
2. Demonstrate compliance with prescribed diet and dietary restrictions.
3. Demonstrate compliance with prescribed medication therapy/identify side effects and toxicity.
4. Demonstrate prescribed wound care/verbalize S&S of infection to report to home health nurse or physician.
5. Identify S&S associated with cranial nerve damage and prescribed measures to manage.
6. Demonstrate compliance with prescribed activity levels/verbalize importance of planned rest periods and of avoiding straining or lifting.
7. Verbalize importance of not straining at stool/demonstrate correct use of prescribed stool softeners and/or laxatives.
8. Demonstrate improvement in speech and swallowing difficulties.
9. Demonstrate reduction in level of anxiety.

NURSING ACTIONS/TREATMENTS

1. Assess cardiovascular and neurologic status/identify complications.
2. Assess vital signs/identify trends (e.g., sudden variations in blood pressure, elevated temperature).
3. Instruct in nature of disease process, risk factors, surgical procedure, importance of following prescribed treatment regimen, S&S of complications to report to home health nurse or physician.
4. Assess and evaluate nutritional status/instruct on well-balanced diet, prescribed dietary restrictions (e.g., sodium, saturated fat, and cholesterol), adequate hydration/obtain dietary consultation as needed.

5. Observe/instruct to take medications as ordered, their purpose and action, side effects, toxicity/evaluate medication effectiveness.
6. Assess and evaluate healing of incision area/instruct about prescribed wound-care management, S&S of infection to report to home health nurse or physician.
7. Assess cranial nerve impairment (e.g., S&S resulting from trauma to facial, hypoglossal, glossopharyngeal, vagus, and/or accessory nerves)/instruct about prescribed measures for management of symptoms.
8. Observe and evaluate level of physical tolerance to perform ADL/instruct on performing activities according to tolerance, planned rest periods, avoiding straining or lifting.
9. Assess bowel elimination pattern/instruct about importance of not straining at stool/prescribed measures to treat or avoid constipation (e.g., increase in dietary fiber and fluids, use of stool softners and/or laxatives as ordered, increased activities as allowed)/evaluate effectiveness of bowel regimen.
10. Refer to speech therapy as ordered for evaluation and treatment of communication disorder or dysphagia.
11. Assess level of anxiety/encourage to express feeling/provide emotional support and teaching.

REHABILITATION POTENTIAL

Rehabilitation potential   *excellent   good   fair   guarded   poor*   for a   *full partial*   return to an improved level of independent functioning without evidence of neurologic deficits.

Client's Name _____

Medical Record # _____

ONGOING/DISCHARGE EVALUATION OF TEACHING
The Client Who Has Had an Endarterectomy

Teaching Tools:
Printed material given: _____

Audiovisual aids used: _____

Return Information/Demonstration/Interpretation
_____ Client
_____ Caregiver

OF:	Met	Not Met	Comments
☐ Nature of disease process, risk factors, surgical procedure.	_____	_____	_____
☐ S&S of complications; actions to take.	_____	_____	_____
☐ Importance of compliance with prescribed treatment regimen.	_____	_____	_____
☐ Diet and dietary restrictions.	_____	_____	_____
☐ Medications and administration, purpose and action, side effects, toxicity.	_____	_____	_____
☐ Wound care management, S&S of			

Client's Name _____

Medical Record # _____

	infection to report to home health nurse or physican.	_____	_____	_____
☐	Activities according to tolerance, planned rest periods, avoiding straining or lifting.	_____	_____	_____
☐	Bowel regimen; importance of not straining.	_____	_____	_____
☐	S&S of cranial nerve impairment of nerves VII, IX, X, XI, XII; prescribed measures to manage.	_____	_____	_____

Signature of Home Health Nurse _____

Date _____

■ Chronic Venous Insufficiency

Stasis Ulcer

Chronic venous insufficiency is a circulatory disorder of the lower extremities resulting from destruction of the venous valves and characterized by decreased return of venous blood. Severe impairment of venous blood return and persistently increased venous hydrostatic pressure result in chronic dependent edema of the ankles with tissue induration, bluish brown skin discoloration (from extravasation of blood into the subcutaneous tissues), stasis dermatitis, and subsequent development of stasis ulcers (usually over the medial malleolus) caused by the edema impairing oxygen and nutrient delivery. Postphlebitic and varicose ulcers are found to account for the majority of leg ulcers.

POTENTIAL COMPLICATIONS

1. Stasis ulcers,
2. cellulitis,
3. thrombosis or embolus.

TYPES OF CLIENTS/CLINICAL CONDITIONS SEEN BY HOME HEALTH AGENCIES

1. Newly diagnosed: initiation of prescribed treatment regimen of dressing changes, specialized procedures for treatment and management of stasis ulcer.
2. Impaired healing with associated complications: changes in ongoing plan of treatment requiring continued instruction, supervision, evaluation, and report to home health nurse or physician of response to changes in therapy.
3. Recent hospitalization for radical excision of ulcer and surrounding fibrotic tissue with subsequent skin grafting: need for assessment of healing process and response to treatment regimen.

RELATED NURSING DIAGNOSIS

Anxiety

related to:
1. Disease process
2. Potential complications
3. Becoming disabled
4. Knowledge deficit regarding prescribed treatment regimen

as seen by:
Distress; feelings of inadequacy and helplessness regarding condition and healing of stasis ulcer

Comfort, Alteration in: Pain

related to:
Dependent edema with induration of
subcutaneous tissue associated with
stasis ulcer

as seen by:
Protective or guarding behavior of
affected extremity; communication
of pain and discomfort; feelings of
anxiety

Infection, Potential for

related to:
Stasis ulcer, breakdown of the body's
first line of defense

as seen by:
Increased redness, swelling, unusual
drainage, fever, elevated WBC
count

Injury, Potential for: Increased Risk of Accidental Tissue Injury

related to:
Decreased tactile sensitivity

as seen by:
Decreased sensation in superficial
tissue of affected leg and disregard
for teaching to avoid use of heating
pad and hot-water bottle to feet and
legs; walking barefoot; wearing tight
garters with resultant injury to
tissues

Knowledge Deficit (Specify)

related to:
1. Prescribed plan of treatment
   regarding management of venous
   insufficiency and stasis ulcer
2. Potential complications, S&S to
   report to home health nurse or
   physician

as seen by:
Lack of information; lack of
understanding; inability to perform
necessary skills to meet health-care
needs at home

Mobility, Impaired Physical

related to:
1. Pain or discomfort and weakness of
   lower extremities associated with
   impaired venous circulation

as seen by:
Decreased ability to purposefully move
within home environment; difficulty
in following through with

2. Prescribed activity restrictions

progressive ambulatory activities and exercise program; imposed medical restrictions

Skin Integrity, Impairment of: Actual

related to:
Breakdown of fragile skin areas secondary to impaired venous circulation

as seen by:
Disruption of skin surfaces, disruption of skin layer, inflammation and oozing of ulceration

Self-Care Deficit: Feeding, Bathing/Hygiene, Dressing/Grooming, Toileting (Specify)

related to:
1. Impaired physical mobility
2. Prescribed activity restrictions

as seen by:
Limited participation in self-care activities, associated with pain and discomfort; weakness of lower extremities; imposed medical restrictions

Self-Concept, Disturbance in

related to:
1. Altered body image
2. Changes in life-style
3. Low self-esteem

as seen by:
Increased dependency on others to meet physical and daily needs; lack of follow-through; statements about condition being unable to improve; not taking responsibility for daily self-care needs

Tissue Perfusion, Alteration in: Venous

related to:
Reduced venous blood flow

as seen by:
Chronic edema; induration; discoloration; pain of affected extremity

LONG-TERM GOAL

Reduction of inflammatory process and healing of stasis ulcer.

SHORT-TERM GOALS

The client with chronic venous insufficiency/stasis ulcer will be able to:

1. Verbalize nature of disease process, clinical manifestations, S&S of complications to report to home health nurse or physician.
2. Verbalize importance of optimal nutrition and increased hydration in healing process.
3. Verbalize effect obesity has on venous circulation/demonstrate compliance with prescribed weight reduction diet.
4. Demonstrate compliance with prescribed medication therapy/identify side effects.
5. Demonstrate good skin and measures to improve venous circulation of affected extremity.
6. Verbalize importance of/demonstrate progressive ambulatory activities with balanced rest periods/verbalize hazards of prolonged immobilization.
7. Demonstrate prescribed measures of ulcer care.
8. Demonstrate safety measures to avoid injury of extremity with decreased sensation.
9. Verbalize importance of/identify measures to relieve pressure on skin.
10. Demonstrate prescribed wound care/verbalize S&S of impaired healing of graft and donor sites to report to home health nurse or physician.
11. Demonstrate follow-through with prescribed treatment regimen/positive adaptation to illness.

NURSING ACTIONS/TREATMENTS

1. Assess cardiovascular status/identify circulatory complications.
2. Assess ulcer for color, size, odor, drainage, and amount and surrounding skin for inflammation/instruct about S&S of infection to report to home health nurse or physician.
3. Assess vital signs/identify trends (e.g., elevated temperature).
4. Instruct about nature of disease process, adverse effects of gravity and orthostasis on venous circulation, importance of compliance with prescribed treatment regimen, S&S of complications to report to home health nurse or physician.
5. Assess and evaluate nutritional status/instruct as to importance of optimal nutrition, increased hydration to 2500 to 3500 ml per day as prescribed.
6. Assess/instruct as to importance of prescribed weight reduction diet/weigh and record weekly/evaluate weight loss.
7. Observe/instruct to take medications as ordered; explain purpose and action, side effects/evaluate medication effectiveness.
8. Assess and evaluate skin integrity of edematous extremity, c/o burning pain/in-

struct about good skin care and measures to improve venous circulation (e.g., elevation of affected extremity), hygenic skin care, avoiding trauma, excessive pressure, and vasoconstricting factors (e.g., constrictive clothing, smoking, crossing legs, extremes of temperature).

9. Observe/instruct about progressive ambulatory activities with balanced rest periods and about hazards of prolonged immobilization.
10. Assess and evaluate decreased sensation in affected extremity/instruct in safety measures to avoid tissue injury (e.g., avoid use of hot-water bottle, heating pad; walking barefoot; wearing tight garters).
11. Observe/instruct as to prescribed ulcer care and infection control principles (e.g., topical or oral antibiotics, debriding ointments, cleaning and removal of devitalized tissue, wet to dry dressings, soaks, rationale and use of compression dressings: Unna's boot, elastic stockings)/evaluate healing of ulcer.
12. Observe/instruct as to purpose and measures to relieve pressure on skin (e.g., use of foam rubber, sheepskin, egg-crate mattress, repositioning).
13. Assess and evaluate healing of skin graft and donor site (following radical excision of stasis ulcer and surrounding fibrotic tissue)/perform and instruct about prescribed wound care treatment, S&S of impaired healing to report to home health nurse or physician.
14. Assess feelings of low self-esteem and lack of follow-through with prescribed treatment regimen/encourage verbalization of feelings/provide emotional support/refer to social services to assist with adherence to prescribed treatment regimen and positive adaptation to illness.

REHABILITATION POTENTIAL

Rehabilitation potential *excellent good fair guarded poor* for *full partial* return to an improved level of wellness for maximal independence in ADL.

Client's Name _____

Medical Record # _____

ONGOING/DISCHARGE EVALUATION OF TEACHING

The Client with Chronic Venous Insufficiency/Stasis Ulcer

Teaching Tools:

Printed materials given: _____

Audiovisual aids used: _____

Return Information/Demonstration/Interpretation

_____ Client
_____ Caregiver

	OF:	Met	Not Met	Comments
☐	Nature of disease process, clinical manifestations.	_____	_____	_____
☐	S&S of complications; actions to take.	_____	_____	_____
☐	Importance of compliance with prescribed treatment regimen.	_____	_____	_____
☐	Optimal nutrition; increased hydration, effect on healing process.	_____	_____	_____
☐	Obesity and associated effects on venous circulation.	_____	_____	_____

Client's Name _____

Medical Record # _____

☐ Weight
reduction diet. _____ _____   _____

☐ Medications
and
administration,
purpose and
action, side
effects. _____ _____   _____

☐ Skin care of
edematous
extremity. _____ _____   _____

☐ Measures to
improve venous
circulation to
lower
extremities. _____ _____   _____

☐ Progressive
ambulatory
activities with
balanced rest
periods;
hazards of
prolonged
immobilization. _____ _____   _____

☐ Measures to
avoid tissue
injury of
extremity with
decreased
sensation. _____ _____   _____

☐ Treatment of
stasis ulcers,
infection
control
principles. _____ _____   _____

☐ Measures to
relieve pressure
on skin. _____ _____   _____

Client's Name _____

Medical Record # _____

☐ Wound care
treatment of
skin graft,
donor site; S&S
of impaired
healing to
report to
physician.   _____ _____   _____

Signature of Home Health Nurse _____

Date _____

■ Congestive Heart Failure

Congestive heart failure (CHF) is a combination of signs and symptoms that make up a syndrome characterized by vascular congestion and a cardiac output that is inadequate to meet the metabolic demands of the body. A cardinal feature of CHF is an increase in total body sodium and excess retention of water which occurs as a compensatory response to the decreased cardiac output in this condition. The resultant hypervolemia in turn results in an increase in venous retention, increased cardiac work load, and characteristic findings such as edema and orthopnea. CHF is the end result of many diseases that may be classified in the following major areas: increase in work load (e.g., hypertensive heart disease, metabolic or systemic diseases such as hyper- and hypothyroidism, anemias, systemic infections); alteration in myocardial contractability (e.g., myocardial infarction and arrhythmias, and cardiomyopathics), and intracardiac defects (e.g., valvular and congenital defects). Heart failure can be chronic or acute and may result from dysfunction of the right or left ventricle or a combination of both.

In right-sided heart failure, the right ventricle meets with increased pulmonary vascular resistance resulting from lung diseases such as chronic obstructive pulmonary disease or left-sided heart failure or pulmonary emboli and is characterized by dependent pitting edema, liver engorgement, jugular vein distension, weight gain, weakness, and dizziness. In left-sided heart failure, which occurs after left ventricular damage, the left ventricle is unable to empty completely, causing blood to back up into the lungs. This results in pulmonary hypertension and edema. Clinical manifestations observed may be primarily respiratory and include tachypnea, dyspnea, rales, and cough with pink frothy sputum associated with pulmonary edema. Other clinical manifestations are associated with decreased tissue perfusion and include central nervous system alterations, skeletal muscle weakness, oliguria (decreased renal perfusion), decreased bowel sounds, and cool, pale skin.

Various compensatory mechanisms of the body operate to assist the client to maintain an adequate cardiac output and tissue perfusion. However, if heart failure progresses, cardiac reserve power will be lost and the adaptive mechanisms will fail to reverse heart failure and maintain an adequate cardiac output. This state is known as cardiac decompensation. Unless the client is admitted to the hospital and this clinical state reversed, cardiac arrest and death may follow.

POTENTIAL COMPLICATIONS

1. Pulmonary edema,
2. respiratory infections,
3. thromboembolism,
4. malnutrition,
5. renal failure,
6. cardiogenic shock.

TYPES OF CLIENTS/CLINICAL CONDITIONS SEEN BY HOME HEALTH AGENCIES

1. Newly diagnosed with CHF: initiation of prescribed treatment regimen and inclusive teaching plan for home-care management of cardiac condition.
2. Exacerbation of CHF: prescribed changes in plan of treatment; client instruction and supervision of new treatments; evaluation of response to treatment changes.
3. Recent hospitalization related to unstable cardiovascular status and complications of CHF (e.g., pulmonary edema, respiratory infections): need for assessment of client's response to new medications and/or treatments; need for change.

RELATED NURSING DIAGNOSIS

Activity Intolerance

related to:
1. Imbalance between oxygen demand and supply secondary to decreased cardiac output
2. Inadequate nutritional status

as seen by:
Exertional dyspnea; weakness and fatigue; abnormal changes in BP and heart rate in response to activity; excess anxiety

Anxiety

related to:
1. Recurring S&S of congestive heart failure
2. Changes in life-style
3. Increased dependency on others for care
4. Knowledge deficit regarding prescribed treatment regimen

as seen by:
Fearfulness of not being able to care for self at home; inability to perform ADL without assistance; apprehension regarding new medications and treatments; activity intolerance

Bowel Elimination, Alteration in: Constipation

related to:
1. Inadequate fluids and/or dietary fiber
2. Decreased mobility because of activity intolerance, prescribed activity limitations
3. Medication toxicity

as seen by:
Straining at stool; hard, formed stools; changes in usual bowel pattern elimination

Cardiac Output, Alteration in: Decreased

related to:
Failure of the heart to pump
   effectively

as seen by:
Fatigue; dyspnea; irregular pulse;
   irregular respirations; rales; cool,
   pale skin; jugular vein distension;
   changes in mental status, chest pain;
   diminished or absent peripheral
   pulses

Fluid Volume, Alteration in: Excess

related to:
Increase in total body sodium and
   excess retention of water

as seen by:
Edema, weight gain, shortness of
   breath, dyspnea, pulmonary
   congestion, change in mental status;
   restlessness and anxiety

Grieving

related to:
Altered body functioning and life-style
   changes

as seen by:
Apathetic behavior; alterations in
   eating habits and activity levels;
   anger

Infection, Potential for

related to:
Inadequate oxygen transport and
   debilitated condition, secondary to
   CHF and inadequate nutritional
   status

as seen by:
Change in characteristics of sputum;
   increase in cough; anorexia;
   abnormal breath sounds; elevated
   temperature

Injury, Potential for: Increased Risk of Falls and Injuries

related to:
Hypoxia secondary to decreased
   cardiac output

as seen by:
Weakness, dizziness, syncope,
   confusion

Knowledge Deficit (Specify)

related to:
1. Inadequate understanding of disease
   process and related S&S

as seen by:
Lack of information; inadequate
   understanding; inability to perform

2. Prescribed treatment for management of cardiac condition
3. Potential complications, S&S to report to home health nurse or physician

skills necessary to meet health-care needs at home

Mobility, Impaired Physical

related to:
Tissue hypoxia

as seen by:
Decreased muscle strength; decreased endurance; weakness and fatigue

Nutrition, Alteration in: Less than Body Requirements

related to:
1. Decreased oral intake secondary to: Anorexia, weakness and fatigue
2. Impaired transport and absorption of nutrients secondary to alteration in tissue perfusion and edema within bowel wall

as seen by:
Weight loss; activity intolerance; pale conjunctiva and mucous membranes

Oral Mucous Membrane, Alteration in

related to:
Dehydration of oral mucous membrane secondary to oxygen therapy

as seen by:
Oral pain or discomfort; thirst; coated tongue; halitosis

Respiratory Function, Alteration in

Airway Clearance, Ineffective

related to:
1. Fluid accumulation in the lungs associated with pulmonary edema
2. Ineffective mobilization of secretions secondary to decreased energy or fatigue

as seen by:
Dyspnea, rales, ineffective cough

Breathing Pattern, Ineffective

related to:
Fluid accumulation in the lungs

as seen by:
Exertional dyspnea; shortness of

secondary to pulmonary venous congestion

breath; persistent cough, weakness and fatigue; cyanosis

Gas Exchange, Impaired

related to:
1. Ineffective airway clearance and breathing pattern
2. Pulmonary venous congestion

as seen by:
Inability to mobilize secretions; cough; rales, dyspnea, restlessness

Self-Care Deficit: Feeding, Bathing/Hygiene, Dressing/Grooming, Toileting (Specify)

related to:
1. Activity intolerance
2. Impaired mobility
3. Prescribed activity levels within threshold of cardiac limitations

as seen by:
Limited participation in self-care activities associated with weakness and fatigue; exertional dyspnea; imposed medical restrictions

Self-Concept, Disturbance in

related to:
1. Altered body image
2. Life-style changes
3. Low self-esteem

as seen by:
Refusal to participate in self-care; increased dependency on others for daily needs; anger

Skin Integrity, Impairment of: Potential

related to:
1. Poor nutrition
2. Decreased mobility
3. Poor tissue perfusion

as seen by:
Redness over bony areas; S&S of irritation; edema; tissue breakdown

Tissue Perfusion, Alteration in: Systemic

related to:
Decreased cardiac output

as seen by:
Decreased BP; increased pulse rate; fatigue and weakness

LONG-TERM GOAL

To meet the metabolic demands of the body and maintain optimal cardiac function through restoration of balance between oxygen demand and supply.

SHORT-TERM GOALS

The client with congestive heart failure will be able to:

1. Verbalize nature of disease process, causes and contributing factors, S&S of new or recurring problems to report to home health nurse or physician.
2. Accurately take pulse, describe alterations in rate or rhythm to report to physician.
3. Verbalize effect of temperature extremes on cardiac status.
4. Demonstrate compliance with prescribed dietary and fluid restrictions.
5. Demonstrate compliance with prescribed medication therapy/identify side effects and toxicity.
6. Verbalize importance of taking pulse before taking digitalis, when to hold medication and call physician.
7. Verbalize importance of increasing intake of food and fluids high in potassium if taking a potassium-depleting diuretic.
8. Demonstrate compliance with prescribed measures to improve respiratory status and facilitate removal of secretions.
9. Demonstrate compliance with prescribed activities within threshold of cardiac limitations, planned rest periods, energy conservation techniques, safety measures with ambulation and ADL.
10. Demonstrate prescribed measures to care for edematous skin.
11. Verbalize knowledge of S&S of electrolyte imbalance to report to home health nurse or physician.
12. Demonstrate correct use of oxygen therapy, IPPB therapy, vaporizer or humidifier as prescribed.
13. Identify measures to decrease dryness and breakdown of oral mucous membrane when on oxygen therapy.
14. Verbalize purpose of arterial blood gas analysis and other prescribed diagnostic lab work.
15. Report weight gain over parameters set by physician.
16. Verbalize importance of following prescribed bowel regimen, avoiding straining at stool.
17. Verbalize importance of keeping emergency oxygen supply phone numbers by phone.
18. Verbalize feelings of loss related to physical condition/demonstrate effective adaptation to life-style changes to manage daily activities.

NURSING ACTIONS/TREATMENTS

1. Assess cardiovascular and pulmonary status/identify complications.
2. Assess vital signs/identify trends (e.g., hypo- or hypertension, tachycardia,

pulse deficit)/instruct how to take pulse and about alterations in rate and rhythm to report to physician.

3. Instruct about nature of disease, causes and contributing factors, importance of following prescribed treatment regimen, S&S of complications to report to home health nurse or physician.

4. Observe/instruct to avoid temperature extremes, exposure to infections, their effect on cardiac status.

5. Assess and evaluate nutritional status (e.g., decreased oral intake)/instruct about prescribed diet with restrictions (e.g., sodium, fluid amounts, smaller, more frequent meals), importance of resting before meals.

6. Observe/instruct about taking medications as ordered, purpose and action, side effects, and toxicity/evaluate medication effectiveness.

7. Observe/instruct about taking resting pulse rate for 1 minute prior to taking digitalis, notifying physician if pulse rate is lower than 60, above 120 beats per minute, or more irregular than usual before taking medication.

8. Assess/instruct about importance of increasing intake of foods and fluids high in potassium if taking a potassium-depleting diuretic.

9. Assess and evaluate for S&S of alterations in respiratory function (e.g., type, frequency, productivity of cough, color and character of sputum, exertional dyspnea, orthopnea, paroxysmal nocturnal dyspnea)/instruct about measures to alleviate and facilitate removal of pulmonary secretions (e.g., body positioning, alignment, respiratory therapy, prescribed medications).

10. Observe and evaluate for signs of activity intolerance/instruct about activities within threshold of cardiac limitations, energy conservation techniques, planned rest periods, avoiding strenuous exercise.

11. Assess risk factors for falls, injuries with daily activities/instruct regarding safety measures with ambulation and ADL.

12. Assess and evaluate location, extent, severity of edema/instruct about good skin care, optimal nutritional status, increased mobility, S&S of breakdown to report to home health nurse or physician.

13. Assess/instruct S&S of electrolyte imbalance to report to home health nurse or physician (e.g., tremors, muscular weakness, nausea, change in mental status).

14. Observe/instruct about prescribed oxygen therapy: delivery system (e.g., oxygen concentrator, liquid oxygen, oxygen tank), flow rate, duration and frequency, breathing device (e.g., nasal cannula, face mask)/care of equipment, safety principles (e.g., danger of smoking near oxygen system)/evaluate effectiveness of oxygen therapy.

15. Observe/instruct about prescribed IPPB therapy: use and care of equipment, aerosol medications, pressure and oxygen concentration, duration and frequency of treatment/obtain respiratory consultation as needed.

16. Observe/instruct about use and purpose of vaporizer or humidifier.

17. Assess and evaluate oral mucous membrane for dryness and breakdown when on oxygen therapy/instruct about good oral hygiene and adequate hydration.

18. Monitor/instruct purpose of arterial blood gas analysis and other diagnostic lab work as ordered by physician.
19. Assess and evaluate weight gain/instruct to weigh daily and record as ordered/report weight gain over parameters set by physician.
20. Assess bowel elimination pattern/instruct about importance of not straining at stool and prescribed measures to treat or avoid constipation (e.g., increase in fluids and dietary fiber, use of stool softeners, laxatives, increased activities as allowed)/evaluate effectiveness of bowel regimen.
21. Assess ability to accept condition with prescribed limitations, including sexual activity (e.g., S&S of depression and/or grieving, disturbance in self-concept)/assist with establishing daily goals/provide emotional support/refer to social services as ordered to provide counseling to assist to adjustment to illness and provide information regarding community services (e.g., American Heart Association, homemaker chore services, Meals on Wheels).
22. Refer to rehabilitative services as ordered for assistance with energy conservation techniques or prescribed cardiac rehabilitation program.
23. Observe/instruct about importance of keeping emergency and oxygen supply phone numbers by phone.

REHABILITATION POTENTAL

Rehabilitation potential *excellent good fair guarded poor* for *partial full* return to an independent level of functioning consistent with physical limitations of cardiac condition.

Client's Name _____

Medical Record # _____

ONGOING/DISCHARGE EVALUATION OF TEACHING
The Client with Congestive Heart Failure

Teaching Tools
Printed materials given: _____

Audiovisual aids used: _____

Return Information/Demonstration/Interpretation
_____ Client
_____ Caregiver

OF:	Met	Not Met	Comments
☐ Nature of disease process, causes and contributing factors.	_____	_____	_____
☐ S&S of complications; actions to take.	_____	_____	_____
☐ Importance of compliance with prescribed treatment regimen.	_____	_____	_____
☐ How to take pulse; alterations in rate and rhythm to report to physician.	_____	_____	_____
☐ Effect of temperature extremes on cardiac status.	_____	_____	_____

Client's Name _____

Medical Record # _____

☐ Importance of avoiding exposure to infections. _____ _____   _____

☐ Predisposing factors to decreased oral intake, measures to correct. _____ _____   _____

☐ Diet and dietary restrictions. _____ _____   _____

☐ Medications and administration, purpose and action, side effects, toxicity. _____ _____   _____

☐ Foods and fluids high in potassium. _____ _____   _____

☐ S&S of altered respiratory functioning, measures to alleviate and facilitate removal of pulmonary secretions. _____ _____   _____

☐ Activities and exercises within threshold of cardiac limitations; energy conservation techniques. _____ _____   _____

Client's Name _____

Medical Record # _____

☐ Risk factors for falls and injuries in home; safety measures with ambulation and daily activities.   _____   _____   _____

☐ Skin care of edematous area; S&S of irritation and breakdown to report to home health nurse or physician.   _____   _____   _____

☐ S&S of electrolyte imbalance to report to home health nurse or physician.   _____   _____   _____

☐ Oxygen therapy; safety principles.   _____   _____   _____

☐ IPPB therapy.   _____   _____   _____

☐ Vaporizer or humidifier.   _____   _____   _____

☐ Measures to decrease dryness and promote healing of oral mucous membrane when on oxygen therapy.   _____   _____   _____

☐ Recording of daily weight; importance of reporting

Client's Name _____

Medical Record # _____

excessive
weight gain to
physician.   _____ _____   _____

☐ Bowel regimen,
importance of
not straining.   _____ _____   _____

☐ Purpose of
prescribed
diagnostic lab
work.   _____ _____   _____

☐ Emergency and
oxygen supply
phone numbers
kept by phone.   _____ _____   _____

Signature of Home Health Nurse _____

Date _____

■ Coronary Artery Bypass Graft Surgery

Coronary artery bypass graft (CABG) is a surgical procedure performed to improve blood flow and oxygenation to ischemic areas through revasculization of the myocardium.

With coronary artery bypass graft surgery a section of a blood vessel (usually a segment of the saphenous vein or internal mammarian artery) circumvents the occluded area to supply blood to the ischemic region of the myocardium. The exact surgical procedure depends on the client's condition and the number of arteries being bypassed. The most common procedure, aortocoronary bypass, involves grafting a section of blood vessel proximally to the ascending aorta and distally to the coronary artery, beyond the occluded area.

POTENTIAL COMPLICATIONS

1. Infection of incisional wound and graft sites,
2. arrhythmia,
3. CHF,
4. anemia,
5. postpericardiotomy syndrome,
6. reocclusion,
7. suture rupture,
8. postoperative depression,
9. pericardial effusion.

TYPES OF CLIENTS/CLINICAL CONDITIONS SEEN BY HOME HEALTH AGENCIES

1. Observation and care of surgical wound; dressing changes of draining wound.
2. Postsurgical complications related to coronary bypass graft including infection of incisional or graft sites: need for assessment of client's response to new medications, treatments, need for change.
3. Prescribed home cardiac rehabilitation program: observation of response to program and/or need for change in therapy.

RELATED NURSING DIAGNOSIS

Activity Intolerance

related to:
1. Postsurgical pain and discomfort
2. Fear of harming self

as seen by:
Reluctance to move and participate in graded exercise and activity program; weakness and fatigue

Anxiety

related to:
1. Prescribed activity restrictions
2. Alterations in life-style
3. Knowledge deficit regarding prescribed treatment regimen

as seen by:
Anger; asking many questions; feelings of inadequacy and helplessness postsurgery

Bowel Elimination, Alteration in: Constipation

related to:
1. Inadequate dietary fiber and/or fluids
2. Decreased activity levels

as seen by:
Straining at stool; hard, formed stools; decreased frequency and amount from usual pattern

Breathing Pattern, Ineffective

related to:
1. Surgical incisions
2. Decreased energy or fatigue

as seen by:
Splinted or guarded respirations; altered depth of respiation; c/o painful respiration; altered chest excursion; shortness of breath; exertional dyspnea; verbal report of fatigue

Comfort, Alteration in: Pain

related to:
Surgical incisions

as seen by:
Splinted, guarded respirations; decreased physical activities; c/o pain

Coping, Ineffective Individual

related to:
1. Alterations in life-style
2. Fear of postsurgical complications

as seen by:
Lack of participation in treatment plan; worry; irritability; verbalization of inability to cope

Infection, Potential for

related to:
Incisional areas, breakdown of the

as seen by:
Chills and fever; increased redness and

body's first line of defense

swelling; pain and unusual drainage; elevated WBC count

Knowledge Deficit (Specify)

related to:
1. Prescribed treatment regimen related to cardiac rehabilitation
2. Potential complications, S&S to report to home health nurse or physician

as seen by:
Verbalization of lack of information; inadequate understanding; inability to perform skills necessary to meet health-care needs at home

Mobility, Impaired Physical

related to:
1. Decreased muscle strength and endurance postsurgery
2. Prescribed activity restrictions
3. Pain or discomfort
4. Activity intolerance

as seen by:
Reluctance to move and participate in daily activities; c/o pain with movement; weakness and fatigue; imposed medical restrictions

Self-Care Deficit: Feeding, Bathing/Hygiene, Dressing/Grooming, Toileting (Specify)

related to:
1. Impaired physical mobility
2. Activity intolerance
3. Prescribed activity restrictions

as seen by:
Decreased participation in self-care activities associated with weakness and fatigue; postsurgical pain or discomfort; medically imposed restrictions

Self-Concept, Disturbance in

related to:
1. Body image
2. Alterations in life-style and role performances

as seen by:
Refusal to acknowledge changes in life-style and prescribed restrictions and limitations; expressed anger; depression

Skin Integrity, Impairment of: Actual/Potential

related to:
1. Surgical incisions

as seen by:
Increased redness; swelling; pain;

2. Impaired healing secondary to infection and inadequate nutritional status

unusual drainage; elevated temperature

LONG-TERM GOAL

To achieve an optimal level of health and a productive and satisfying life-style free of complications and psychological distress.

SHORT-TERM GOALS

After a coronary artery bypass graft surgery, the client will be able to:

1. Verbalize nature of coronary artery disease, risk factors, nature and type of surgery, S&S of complications to report to home health nurse or physician.
2. Demonstrate how to take pulse/describe alterations in rate or rhythm to report to physician.
3. Verbalize prescribed measures in pain management.
4. Verbalize clinical manifestations of angina pectoris, precipitating factors to avoid, S&S to report to home health nurse or physician.
5. Verbalize importance of reporting excessive weight gain to physician.
6. Demonstrate compliance with prescribed diet and dietary restrictions.
7. Demonstrate compliance with prescribed medication therapy/identify side effects, toxicity.
8. Verbalize importance of taking pulse before taking digitalis, when to hold medication and call physician.
9. Verbalize purpose of prescribed diagnostic lab work.
10. Demonstrate compliance/verbalize importance of graded exercises and activities, allowances and limitations within limits of cardiac status, planned rest periods, S&S of fatigue, shortness of breath, and nausea to report to home health nurse or physician.
11. Demonstrate prescribed wound care management/identify S&S of infection to report to home health nurse or physician.
12. Verbalize purpose/demonstrate correct use and application of antiembolic stockings.
13. Verbalize importance of not straining at stool and prescribed measures to improve bowel functioning.
14. Demonstrate reduction in level of anxiety, effective use of coping mechanisms and a positive adaptation to alteration in body image and life style-changes.

NURSING ACTIONS/TREATMENTS

1. Assess cardiovascular and respiratory status/identify complications.
2. Assess vital signs/identify trends (e.g., pulse deficit, hyper- or hypotension, elevated temperature)/instruct how to take and record pulse, about alterations in rate and rhythm to report to physician.
3. Instruct as to nature of disease process, risk factors (e.g., obesity, stress, smoking, diet high in saturated fats and cholesterol, inactivity), nature and type of cardiac surgery, importance of compliance with prescribed treatment regimen, S&S of complications report to home health nurse or physician.
4. Assess and evaluate area and level of pain/instruct about prescribed pain management measures postsurgery.
5. Assess and evaluate clinical manifestations associated with angina pectoris, circumstances under which it occurs/instruct to modify activities, avoid temperature extremes, emotional stress, nicotine/report to physician.
6. Assess and evaluate weight gain/instruct to weigh and record daily as ordered/report weight gain of more than two pounds a day or more than five pounds a week and/or swelling in ankles or around incisions.
7. Assess and evaluate nutritional status/instruct about well-balanced diet with prescribed fluid and dietary restrictions (e.g., sodium, saturated fats and cholesterol, calories, caffeine)/obtain dietary consultation as needed.
8. Observe/instruct to take medications as ordered, purpose and action, side effects, toxicity/evaluate medication effectiveness.
9. Monitor/instruct about purpose of prescribed lab work.
10. Observe/instruct to take resting pulse rate for 1 minute before taking digitalis and notify physician if pulse rate is below 60, above 120 beats per minute, or more irregular than usual before taking medication.
11. Observe and evaluate level of physical tolerance to perform self-care activities and ADL (e.g., weakness and fatigue, exertional dyspnea, excess anxiety)/instruct about prescribed graded exercises and activities, allowances and limitations within limits of cardiac status, planned rest periods, S&S of fatigue, shortness of breath, nausea to report to physician.
12. Observe and evaluate healing of incisional area/instruct about prescribed wound care management, S&S of infection to report to home health nurse or physician.
13. Observe/instruct as to purpose and correct use and application of antiembolic stockings.
14. Assess bowel elimination pattern/instruct about importance of not straining at stool and prescribed measures to treat or avoid constipation (e.g., increase in prescribed dietary fiber and fluids, increased activities as allowed, use of prescribed stool softeners, laxatives)/evaluate effectiveness of bowel regimen.
15. Assess level of anxiety and ineffective coping mechanisms, disturbances in self-concept/provide emotional support/assist with establishing daily goals/

refer to social services as ordered to provide information regarding community services to assist with cardiac rehabilitation (e.g., local chapter of Mended Hearts Association, American Heart Association, counseling services).

16. Assess alterations in functional skills, decreased endurance/refer to rehabilitative services as ordered to establish and instruct in home cardiac rehabilitation program.

REHABILITATION POTENTIAL

Rehabilitation potential   *excellent   good   fair   guarded   poor*   for   *full partial*   return to an improved quality of life and functioning consistent with physical limitations of cardiac condition.

Client's Name _____

Medical Record # _____

ONGOING/DISCHARGE EVALUATION OF TEACHING

The Client with a Coronary Artery Bypass

Teaching Tools:

Printed materials given: _____

Audiovisual aids used: _____

Return Information/Demonstration/Interpretation

_____ Client

_____ Caregiver

	OF:	Met	Not Met	Comments
☐	Nature of disease process, risk factors, nature and type of cardiac surgery.	_____	_____	_____
☐	Importance of compliance with prescribed treatment regimen.	_____	_____	_____
☐	S&S of complications; actions to take.	_____	_____	_____
☐	Pain management measures postsurgery.	_____	_____	_____
☐	How to take and record pulse; alterations in rate or rhythm to report to physician.	_____	_____	_____

Client's Name _____

Medical Record # _____

☐   Clinical manifestations of angina pectoris, precipitating factors to avoid, S&S to report to physician.   _____   _____   _____

☐   Recording of daily weight; importance of reporting excessive weight gain to physician.   _____   _____   _____

☐   Well-balanced diet; prescribed fluid and dietary restrictions.   _____   _____   _____

☐   Medications and administration purpose and action, side effects, toxicity.   _____   _____   _____

☐   Purpose of prescribed lab work.   _____   _____   _____

☐   Graded exercises and activities, allowances and limitations within limits of cardiac status planned rest periods.   _____   _____   _____

Client's Name _____

Medical Record # _____

☐ Wound care
   management.   _____ _____   _____

☐ Purpose and
   application of
   antiembolic
   stockings.   _____ _____   _____

☐ Effect of
   straining at
   stool on cardiac
   status;
   prescribed
   measures to
   improve bowel
   functioning.   _____ _____   _____

Signature of Home Health Nurse _____

Date _____

■ Coronary Artery Disease:

Angina Pectoris/Myocardial Infarction

Coronary artery disease (CAD) is the term given to a number of abnormal conditions that produce occlusion of the coronary arteries and interference with the flow of blood to the myocardium. The most common cause of CAD, producing myocardial ischemia, is atherosclerosis. This condition accounts for more than 90 percent of the cases and results from lipoprotein abnormalities, arterial wall injury, and platelet dysfunction.

The following are risk factors for atherosclerosis: hypertension, diabetes, hereditary hyperlipoproteinemia, smoking, obesity, and a diet high in saturated fats, cholesterol, and carbohydrates. CAD is characterized by a thickening of the arterial wall with a fatty fibrous plaque, which narrows the lumen of the coronary vessel, resulting in increased resistance to blood flow.

The widely accepted theory which explains the development of atherosclerosis is that of vessel wall injury. The vessel wall is injured by factors such as excessive pressure caused by hypertension, inhaled chemicals from cigarette smoke, etc. The injury allows platelets to aggregate, and substances such as cholesterol containing low density lipoproteins (LDL) to accumulate within the layers of the blood vessel. These factors stimulate the proliferation of smooth muscle cells in the blood vessels which causes encroachment upon the lumen of the blood vessel, resulting in ischemia.

Myocardial ischemia and myocardial infarction are the most common disorders affecting the cardiac muscle. Myocardial ischemia occurs when the myocardial need for oxygen is greater than the capacity of the diseased coronary arteries to supply the oxygen. This results in the classic symptom of angina. Angina occurs whenever the demand on the heart is increased, as with physical exertion or emotional stress, and results in myocardial hypoxia and chest pain that lasts an average of 3 minutes. These ischemic attacks usually subside with nitrates and rest and when the imbalance between oxygen demand and supply is corrected. Other causes of diminished coronary artery blood flow may be coronary artery vasospasm, tachyarrythmias, thrombus formation, embolism, and congenital deficits in the coronary vascular system.

Myocardial infarction (MI) occurs when an occlusion of a coronary artery, causing diminished coronary artery blood flow for over 30 to 45 minutes, results in myocardial ischemia and necrosis. Occlusion may occur as a result of atherosclerosis, thromboembolism, or coronary artery spasm. The necrotic, or infarcted, area of the myocardium produces impaired contractility and pumping efficiency in the affected area of the heart muscle. Disorders of conduction and of rhythm may also occur. MI usually occurs in the left ventricle. The onset of MI is characterized by mild discomfort to severe substernal chest pain that may radiate to the left arm, jaw, or neck with resulting dyspnea, diaphoresis, clammy skin, pallor, and anxiousness. Usual signs are tachycardia, hypotension, low-grade fever, arrhythmias.

Prognosis is dependent on the degree of heart damage and the ability of collateral circulation to bypass the occluded area and the effectiveness of the compensatory mechanisms in maintaining cellular homeostasis.

POTENTIAL COMPLICATIONS

1. Arrhythmias,
2. congestive heart failure,
3. thromboembolism,
4. Dressler's syndrome (post-MI syndrome),
5. cardiogenic shock,
6. ventricular aneurysm or rupture,
7. sudden death.

TYPES OF CLIENTS/CLINICAL CONDITIONS SEEN BY HOME HEALTH AGENCIES

1. Persistent or recurrent chest pain; instruction and evaluation of client's response to newly ordered or changing medications; reporting significant changes in cardiac status to physician.
2. Recent MI: discharged home with inclusive teaching program regarding prescribed post-MI rehabilitation and treatment regimen.
3. Post-MI client with an unstable cardiovascular status, requiring changes in prescribed medications and treatment regimen: need for instruction and assessment of response to therapy changes.
4. Discharged home after hospitalization for post-MI complications.

RELATED NURSING DIAGNOSIS

Activity Intolerance

related to:
Imbalance between oxygen supply and
  demand

as seen by:
Fatigue; weakness; abnormal heart and
  respiratory rate and BP in response
  to activity; exertional dyspnea; chest
  pain

Anxiety

related to:
1. Increase in anginal attacks with
   partial relief from nitrates and rest
2. Altered body image and life-style
   changes
3. Fear of recurrent "heart attack"
   and death
4. Knowledge deficit regarding
   prescribed home-care treatment
   regimen

as seen by:
Increased facial tension and
  apprehension; expressed fearfulness
  regarding heart condition and effect
  on life; increased questioning of
  managing at home post-MI

Bowel Elimination, Alteration in: Constipation

related to:
1. Prescribed activity restrictions
2. Inadequate dietary fiber and fluid intake

as seen by:
Straining at stool; frequency and amount less than usual pattern

Breathing Pattern, Ineffective

related to:
1. Chest pain
2. Decreased energy or fatigue

as seen by:
Exertional dyspnea; shortness of breath; altered depth of respiration; verbal report of fatigue

Cardiac Output, Alterations in: Decreased

related to:
Decreased myocardial contractility and altered conductivity secondary to myocardial damage

as seen by:
Weakness and fatigue; irregular heart rate; dizziness; restlessness; chest pain; changes in mental status

Comfort, Alteration in: Pain

related to:
Myocardial ischemia

as seen by:
c/o Restlessness; chest pain; apprehension; guarding behavior; diaphoresis; BP and pulse rate changes; increased or decreased respiratory rate

Gas Exchange, Impaired

related to:
Altered oxygen supply secondary to
1. Decreased cardiac output
2. Ineffective breathing patterns

as seen by:

Dyspnea; irritability; restlessness; cough; rales; pink, frothy sputum

Grieving

related to:
"Heart attack" and alteration in body image and life-style changes

as seen by:
Alterations in activity level; verbalization of distress over cardiac condition and effect on life; anger

Knowledge Deficit (Specify)

related to:
1. Disease process and related S&S
2. Prescribed plan of treatment for management of cardiac condition
3. Potential complications and S&S to report to home health nurse or physician

as seen by:
Verbalization of lack of information, inadequate understanding; inability to perform skills necessary to meet health-care needs at home

Injury, Potential for: Increased Risk of Falls and Injuries

related to:
1. Generalized weakness posthospitalization
2. Dizziness
3. Changes in mental status

as seen by:
Unsteady gait, weakness and fatigue; changes in alertness

Mobility, Impaired Physical

related to:
1. Activity intolerance
2. Chest pain
3. Prescribed activity restrictions

as seen by:
Weakness and fatigue; decreased endurance; reluctance to attempt movement; medically imposed restrictions

Oral Mucous Membrane, Alteration in

related to:
Dehydration of oral mucous membrane secondary to oxygen therapy

as seen by:
Oral pain or discomfort; thirst; coated tongue; halitosis

Self-Care Deficit: Feeding, Bathing/Hygiene, Dressing/Grooming, Toileting (Specify)

related to:
1. Activity intolerance
2. Impaired physical mobility
3. Prescribed activity restrictions

as seen by:
Reluctance to participate in daily activities and meet self-care needs, associated with weakness and fatigue; chest pain; exertional dyspnea

Self-Concept, Disturbance in

related to:
1. Altered body image
2. Life-style changes
3. Low self-esteem
4. Changes in role performance

as seen by:
Withdrawn behavior; refusal to participate in self-care; feelings of helplessness; crying; anger; inability to accept positive reinforcement; changes in role responsibility in family

LONG-TERM GOAL

To meet the metabolic demands of the body and maintain optimal cardiac function through restoration of balance between oxygen demand and supply.

SHORT-TERM GOALS

The client with coronary artery disease: angina pectoris/myocardial infarction will be able to:

1. Verbalize nature of disease process, risk factors, S&S of new or recurring complications to report to home health nurse or physician.
2. Take pulse rate/describe alterations in rate or rhythm to report to physician.
3. Verbalize importance of well-balanced diet with prescribed dietary restrictions.
4. Demonstrate compliance with prescribed medication therapy/identify complications, toxicity.
5. Verbalize importance of taking pulse before taking digitalis, when to hold medication and call physician.
6. Verbalize/demonstrate compliance with prescribed anticoagulant therapy, safety precautions with use, adverse reactions to report to physician.
7. Verbalize purpose of prescribed blood work.
8. Verbalize factors that precipitate angina/identify measures to relieve chest pain or require calling physician if pain persists.
9. Verbalize characteristics of MI and angina pectoris and actions to take with each/verbalize S&S to report to home health nurse or physician.
10. Demonstrate compliance with graded exercise program and activities/verbalize allowances and restrictions within the threshold of cardiac limitations, and of planned rest periods.
11. Demonstrate correct use of prescribed oxygen therapy/identify safety principles with use.
12. Verbalize understanding/identify measures to decrease dryness and breakdown of oral mucous membrane when on oxygen therapy.

13. Verbalize purpose/demonstrate correct use and application of antiembolic stocking.
14. Verbalize importance of not straining at stool and of prescribed measures to improve bowel functioning.
15. Verbalize importance of/wear Medic Alert bracelet.
16. Verbalize how to summon help in an emergency situation.
17. Exhibit decreased level of anxiety and apprehension with positive adaptation to cardiac condition.

NURSING ACTIONS/TREATMENTS

1. Assess cardiovascular status/identify complications.
2. Assess vital signs/identify trends (e.g., hypo- or hypertension, pulse deficit)/instruct how to take and record pulse and about alterations in rate and rhythm to report to physician.
3. Instruct about nature of disease process (e.g., CAD, angina pectoris, MI), risk factors (e.g., obsesity, smoking, stress, diet high in saturated fat and cholesterol, inactivity), importance of compliance with prescribed treatment regimen, S&S of complications to report to physician.
4. Assess and evaluate nutritional status/instruct about prescribed diet with restrictions (e.g., sodium, saturated fats and cholesterol, calories, caffeine)/obtain dietary consultation as needed.
5. Observe/instruct about taking medications as ordered, purpose and action, side effects, toxicity/evaluate medication effectiveness.
6. Observe/instruct to take resting pulse for 1 minute before taking digitalis and to notify physician if pulse rate is below 60 or above 120 beats per minute or more irregular than usual before taking medication.
7. Assess/instruct about anticoagulant therapy, safety precautions to reduce risk of bleeding (e.g., avoid straining at stool; hard-bristled toothbrushes; aspirin or aspirin-containing products), adverse reactions to report to physician (e.g., bleeding, including bruises and petechial, hematuria, tarry stools)/educate regarding measures to control any bleeding (e.g., apply firm manual pressure for 10 minutes).
8. Monitor/instruct about purpose of prescribed blood work (e.g., coagulation times, digitalis levels, arterial blood gas analysis, cardiac enzyme levels to screen for evidence of progression of MI and need to rehospitalize).
9. Assess and evaluate clinical manifestations associated with angina pectoris, circumstances under which it occurs, factors that may precipitate it (e.g., specific activities; temperature extremes; emotional stress; nicotine)/instruct to modify activities, rest and take prescribed nitrates, call physician if pain persists.
10. Assess/instruct about patterns of chest pain (e.g., angina compaired to MI), actions to take with each, S&S to report to home health nurse or physician.

11. Observe and evaluate level of physical tolerance to perform self-care activities and ADL (e.g., angina, exertional dyspnea, fatigue, excess anxiety)/instruct about graded exercises and activities, allowances and restrictions within threshold of cardiac limitations/planned rest periods.
12. Observe/instruct about prescribed oxygen therapy: delivery method, flow rate, duration, care of equipment, safety principles with use (e.g., danger of smoking near oxygen system), care of equipment, obtain respiratory consultation as needed/evaluate effectiveness of oxygen therapy.
13. Assess and evaluate oral mucous membrane for dryness and breakdown when on oxygen therapy/instruct about good oral hygiene and adequate hydration.
14. Assess bowel elimination patterns/instruct about importance of not straining at stool and prescribed measures to treat or avoid constipation (e.g., stool softeners/laxatives, increased dietary fiber, adequate hydration)/evaluate effectiveness of bowel regimen.
15. Observe/instruct about importance of wearing Medic Alert bracelet with information on medical condition and anticoagulant medication.
16. Assess and evaluate alterations in functional skills, self-care deficits/refer to rehabilitative services as ordered to instruct in prescribed graded cardiac exercise program and energy conservation techniques.
17. Assess/instruct how to summon help in an emergency situation (e.g., dialing 911).
18. Assess anxiety and apprehension associated with altered body image and changes in life-style/encourage to verbalize concerns about sexual activity to condition/refer to social services to assist with adjustment to illness and provide information regarding community services for assistance with cardiac rehabilitation (e.g., American Heart Association; Smokenders; counseling services).

REHABILITATION POTENTIAL

Rehabilitation potential *excellent good fair guarded poor* for *full partial* return to an independent level of functioning consistent with physical limitations of cardiac condition.

Client's Name _____

Medical Record # _____

ONGOING/DISCHARGE EVALUATION OF TEACHING

The Client with Coronary Disease: Angina Pectoris/Myocardial Infarction

Teaching Tools:

Printed materials given: _____

Audiovisual aids used: _____

Return Information/Demonstration/Interpretation

_____ Client

_____ Caregiver

OF:	Met	Not Met	Comments
☐ Nature of disease process, risk factors.	_____	_____	_____
☐ S&S of complications, actions to take.	_____	_____	_____
☐ Importance of compliance with prescribed treatment regimen.	_____	_____	_____
☐ How to take pulse, alterations in rate or rhythm to report to physician.	_____	_____	_____
☐ Well-balanced diet; prescribed dietary restrictions.	_____	_____	_____

Client's Name _____

Medical Record # _____

☐ Medications and administration, purpose and action, side effects, toxicity. _____ _____ _____

☐ Anticoagulant therapy; precautions to reduce risk of bleeding, adverse reactions to report to physician; measures for control of bleeding. _____ _____ _____

☐ Purpose of periodic blood work to monitor coagulation time and of other diagnostic lab tests. _____ _____ _____

☐ Precipitating factors of angina pectoris; measures to relieve chest pain, when to call physician. _____ _____ _____

☐ Characteristics of MI and angina pectoris; actions to take with each; S&S to report to home health nurse or physician. _____ _____ _____

Client's Name _____

Medical Record # _____

☐ Graded exercise program and activities; allowances and restrictions within threshold of cardiac limitations; planned rest periods. _____ _____ _____

☐ Oxygen therapy, safety principles with use. _____ _____ _____

☐ Measures to decrease dryness and breakdown of oral mucous membrane when on oxygen therapy. _____ _____ _____

☐ Effect of straining at stool on cardiac status; prescribed measures to improve bowel functioning. _____ _____ _____

☐ Medic Alert bracelet. _____ _____ _____

☐ How to summon help in an emergency situation. _____ _____ _____

Client's Name _____

Medical Record # _____

Signature of Home Health Nurse _____

Date _____

■ Hypertension

Hypertension, in age groups of 50 years or younger, is defined as a sustained elevation of arterial blood pressure, with the systolic pressure greater than 140 mmHg and/or the diastolic pressure greater than 90 mmHg. In the elderly, hypertension is the major risk factor for stroke, coronary artery disease, and heart failure and is defined as a systolic pressure of 160 mmHg (or greater) and/or a diastolic pressure of 95 mmHg (or greater). Risk factors include obesity, stress, excessive sodium retention, hyperlipidemia, genetic predisposition, and smoking.

Hypertension occurs as two major types: essential or idiopathic, which accounts for the most common type of hypertensive disorder (90 to 95 percent of the cases) with unknown etiology and secondary hypertension, which accounts for 5 to 10 percent of all areas of hypertension. Some of the known causes of secondary hypertension are adrenal disorders (pheochromocytoma, primary hyperaldosteronism, Cushing's syndrome), renal parenchymal diseases (acute or chronic glomerulonephritis or pyelonephritis), thyroidtoxicosis, or renovascular hypertension.

Complex control mechanisms that maintain a balance between cardiac output and peripheral vascular resistance are responsible for ensuring adequate perfusion to all organ systems of the body. Major renal and neural mechanisms responsible for blood pressure control include the vasoconstrictor center of the medulla, the cerebral cortex (subject to emotion, tension, and anxiety), baroreceptors, chemoreceptors, peripheral sensory receptors, and catecholamines. The major renal factors include the renin–angiotensin–aldosterone system, antidiuretic hormone, and sodium and water regulatory activities of the kidney. Blood pressure therefore reflects the response to all these control mechanisms. A disturbance in one mechanism may cause inappropriate vascular constriction, predisposing to hypertension.

Hypertension is a chronic disease that is often asymptomatic until pathologic changes occur in vital organs in response to vascular damage. These pathologic changes are a result of sustained diastolic pressure elevations, with resultant increase in fluid pressure against the vascular walls. This results in constriction and damage to the endothelium of the small vessels, while large vessels harden and narrow, resulting in diminished perfusion. In response, the blood pressure rises even higher as the body attempts to maintain perfusion. The clinical manifestations are associated with the extent and location of blood vessel deterioration, which eventually may cause progressive dysfunction of the following target organs: brain, eyes, heart, kidneys, and lungs. For example, the effect of hypertension on the heart eventually results in increased cardiac work load, left ventricular hypertrophy, progressing to congestive heart failure, and finally pulmonary edema.

Hypertension is classified according to the degree of severity, depending on the diastolic pressure, as follows: Class I (mild: 90 to 104 mmHg); Class II (moderate: 105 to 115 mmHg); Class III (severe: above 115 mmHg). Accelerated or malignant hypertension is a severe, rapid sustained elevation with a diastolic blood pressure greater than 120 mmHg and a concurrent Grade III to IV retinopathy (papilledema).

POTENTIAL COMPLICATIONS

Dependent on severity and extent of target organ damage, e.g.,

Brain:
1. Progressive encephalopathy,
2. cerebrovascular accident.

Heart:
1. Angina pectoris,
2. myocardial infarction,
3. congestive heart failure.

Kidney:
1. Uremia and kidney failure.

Eyes:
1. Retinopathy,
2. blindness.

Blood vessels:
1. Aneurysm,
2. atherosclerosis.

TYPES OF CLIENTS/CLINICAL CONDITIONS SEEN BY HOME HEALTH AGENCIES

1. Newly diagnosed with hypertension: initiation of prescribed treatment regimen and inclusive teaching plan.
2. Progression of hypertensive condition and complications: prescribed changes in current plan of treatment, client instruction and supervision of new medications and treatments, evaluation of response to therapy changes.
3. Long-term hypertensive client presenting with uncontrolled BP and instability of condition: Orders include ongoing observation assessment of BP and condition to assist physician with evaluation for change in prescribed treatment regimen or need for hospitalization.

RELATED NURSING DIAGNOSES

Activity Intolerance

related to:	as seen by:
Decreased tissue oxygenation secondary to diminished perfusion	Fatigue; weakness; exertional dyspnea associated with lack of follow-through with progressive activity program; abnormal heart rate or BP

Anxiety

related to:
1. Elevated BP and fear of complications
2. Need for lifelong treatment
3. Knowledge deficit related to prescribed treatment regimen

as seen by:
Expressed concern regarding BP elevations; overeating; verbalization of fears of possible disability and related complications; asking numerous questions regarding medication therapy and effectiveness of controlling BP

Bowel Elimination, Alteration in: Constipation

related to:
1. Alteration in tissue perfusion to the bowel
2. Inadequate fluids and/or dietary fiber
3. Decreased activities resulting from activity intolerance and prescribed limitations
4. Medication toxicity

as seen by:
Straining at stool; hard, formed stools; changes in usual pattern of bowel elimination; c/o feeling of pressure or fullness in abdomen or rectum

Comfort, Alteration in: Headache

related to:
Increased intracranial pressure secondary to severe increase in BP

as seen by:
Rubbing head, c/o headache; dizziness

Coping, Ineffective Individual

related to:
1. Hypertensive condition
2. Body image problem with need for lifelong treatment and supervision of prescribed medications
3. Inadequate relaxation techniques

as seen by:
Lack of follow-through with prescribed medications and diet therapy; verbalized anxiety and feelings of hopelessness; overeating

Fluid Volume, Alteration in: Excess

related to:
Excess sodium and water retention

as seen by:
Edema; weight gain; elevated BP

Injury, Potential for: Increased Risk of Falls and Injuries

related to:
1. Visual disturbance related to vascular changes of the retina
2. Postural hypotension associated with diuretic therapy

as seen by:
Blurred vision; impaired visual acuity; scotoma; dizziness and light-headedness with changes in position

Knowledge Deficit (Specify)

related to:
1. Disease process
2. Prescribed plan of treatment for hypertensive condition
3. Potential complications and S&S to report to home health nurse or physician

as seen by:
Verbalization of lack of information; inadequate understanding; inability to perform skills necessary to meet health-care needs at home

Nutrition, Alteration in: More than Body Requirements

related to:
Excess intake

as seen by:
Weight 10 percent above that desirable for height, body build, and age; eating in response to anxiety

Self-Care Deficit: Feeding, Bathing/Hygiene, Dressing/Grooming, Toileting (Specify)

related to:
1. Activity intolerance
2. Prescribed activity restrictions
3. Visual impairments
4. Discomfort

as seen by:
Decreased participation in self-care activities associated with weakness and fatigue; visual changes and headache; imposed medical restrictions

Sensory-Perceptual Alteration: Visual

related to:
Visual disturbances associated with vascular changes of the retina

as seen by:
Blurred vision; impaired visual acuity; scotoma

Tissue Perfusion, Alteration in: Systemic

related to:
Increased peripheral vascular resistance

as seen by:
Restlessness; chest pain; dyspnea tachycardia; further increase in BP; diminished or absent peripheral pulses; confusion, constipation

LONG-TERM GOAL

To minimize vascular damage with resultant pathologic changes in vital organs through compliance with lifelong treatment regimen.

SHORT-TERM GOALS

The client with hypertension will be able to:

1. Verbalize understanding of type of hypertension and progression of disease, effect on body, risk factors, S&S of complications to report to home health nurse or physician.
2. Accurately take and record blood pressure and pulse and know what alterations to report to physician.
3. Verbalize importance of compliance with prescribed diet and dietary restrictions.
4. Verbalize taxing effect of excessive weight on cardiovascular system/demonstrate compliance with prescribed weight reduction diet.
5. Demonstrate compliance with prescribed medication therapy/identify side effects.
6. Demonstrate measures to minimize effects of postural hypotension associated with diurectic therapy and safety measures with ambulation and activities.
7. Verbalize importance of increasing foods and fluids high in potassium if taking a potassium-depleting diuretic.
8. Verbalize effect of consistent progressive exercise program with balanced rest periods on lowering of hypertension and its effect on improving tissue perfusion.
9. Verbalize prescribed measures to promote good bowel functioning and effect of straining on blood pressure.
10. Demonstrate safety measures with ambulation and daily activities with relationship to visual disturbances.
11. Demonstrate modifications in life-style to effectively decrease level of stress and anxiety/verbalize effect on hypertensive condition.

NURSING ACTIONS/TREATMENTS

1. Assess cardiovascular and neurologic status/identify complications.
2. Assess vital signs/identify trends (e.g., hypo- or hypertension).
3. Observe/instruct how to take and record blood pressure and pulse and alterations to report to physician.
4. Instruct about type of hypertension, progression of disease, effects on the body, risk factors (e.g., obesity, inactivity, smoking, emotional stress, diet high in saturated fats and cholesterol), importance of compliance with prescribed treatment regimen, and S&S of complications to report to home health nurse or physician.
5. Assess and evaluate nutritional status/instruct about prescribed well-balanced diet and dietary restrictions (e.g., sodium, calories, caffeine, alcohol, low saturated fat, and low cholesterol).
6. Instruct about prescribed weight reduction diet and taxing effect of excessive weight on cardiovascular system.
7. Observe/instruct to take medications as ordered (e.g., antihypertensives, diuretics), purpose and action, side effects, toxicity/evaluate medication effectiveness.
8. Observe and evaluate for dizziness or light-headedness while on diuretic therapy/instruct to rise slowly from supine or sitting position to minimize effects of postural hypotension/educate on safety factors with ambulation and daily activities.
9. Assess/instruct about importance of increasing intake of foods and fluids high in potassium if taking a potassium-depleting diuretic.
10. Assess and evaluate response to daily stressors/instruct to modify stressful lifestyle and activities and about effect on hypertensive condition.
11. Observe and evaluate ability to perform self-care activities/instruct on energy conservation techniques, regular progressive activity and exercise program with balanced rest periods, their effect on lowering hypertension and improving tissue perfusion.
12. Assess bowel elimination pattern/educate as to importance of avoiding straining, its effect on blood pressure/instruct about prescribed means to treat or avoid constipation (e.g., increase in dietary fiber and fluids, use of stool softeners and laxatives, and increased activities as allowed)/evaluate effectiveness of bowel regimen.
13. Assess and evaluate visual disturbances associated with vascular changes of retina/instruct about safety measures with ambulation and daily activities to reduce risk of falls and injuries and to report to physician if vision worsens.
14. Assess coping responses, level of anxiety, stress factors/refer to social services as ordered to provide information regarding needed community services (e.g., American Heart Association, support groups to stop smoking, alcohol rehabilitation, weight control and stress management programs).

REHABILITATION POTENTIAL

Rehabilitation potential *excellent good fair guarded poor* for *full partial* return of effective blood pressure control and independence in managing self-care and ADL.

Client's Name _____

Medical Record # _____

ONGOING/DISCHARGE EVALUATION OF TEACHING
The Client with Hypertension

Teaching Tools:
Printed materials given: _____

Audiovisual aids used: _____

Return Information/Demonstration/Interpretation
_____ Client
_____ Caregiver

OF:	Met	Not Met	Comments
☐ Type of hypertension; progression of disease process; risk factors.	_____	_____	_____
☐ S&S of complications; actions to take.	_____	_____	_____
☐ Importance of compliance with prescribed treatment regimen.	_____	_____	_____
☐ Home monitoring and recording of blood pressure and pulse; what alterations to report to physician.	_____	_____	_____
☐ Diet and dietary restrictions.	_____	_____	_____

Client's Name _____

Medical Record # _____

☐ Weight
reduction diet;
effects of
excessive
weight on
cardiovascular
system. _____ _____   _____

☐ Medications
and
administration,
purpose and
action, side
effects, toxicity. _____ _____   _____

☐ Diuretic
therapy;
measures to
minimize
effects of
postural
hypotension;
safety factors
with
ambulation and
daily activities. _____ _____   _____

☐ Foods and
fluids high in
potassium. _____ _____   _____

☐ Effects of daily
stressors on
life-style and
hypertensive
condition;
measures to
reduce. _____ _____   _____

☐ Consistent,
progressive
activities and
exercise
program,
balanced rest
periods; effect

Client's Name _____

Medical Record # _____

on lowering
blood pressure.   _____   _____   _____

☐   Effect of
straining at
stool on
hypertension;
measures to
promote good
bowel
functioning.   _____   _____   _____

☐   Long-term
effects of
hypertension
on retinal
vessels; safety
factors with
ambulation and
daily activities
in relation to
visual
disturbances.   _____   _____   _____

Signature of Home Health Nurse _____

Date _____

■ Thrombophlebitis

Thrombophlebitis is a condition that can affect either the superficial or deep veins and is characterized by inflammation of the venous wall with thrombus formation. Factors that predispose to the development of thrombophlebitis include: (1) venous stasis, or pooling of blood, in the venous vessels, which can occur in clients on prolonged bed rest or with impaired mobility status or in those with varicose veins or heart failure; (2) injury to the endothelial lining of the vein, which may result from the irritating effects of intravenous injections or trauma to the vessel walls with subsequent inflammation and congestion, as may occur with fractures and dislocations; (3) hypercoagulability of blood with thrombus formation, which may occur in conditions with an increased platelet count or elevated viscosity of blood, such as in dehydration, malignant disease, and certain blood disorders (e.g., polycythemia).

The signs and symptoms characteristic of thrombophlebitis include the presence of a tender, palpable cord of the involved superficial vein, with erythema and increased warmth of the adjacent skin. In deep-vein thrombosis, signs and symptoms include aching or cramping in the calf secondary to dorsiflexion of the foot and/or walking (Homan's sign); a swollen, pale, cold extremity secondary to obstructed venous flow; and an increase in the circumference of the affected calf or thigh. Characteristic signs of inflammation that accompany thrombophlebitis are fever, leukocytosis, and an elevated erythrocyte sedimentation rate.

POTENTIAL COMPLICATIONS

1. Embolism,
2. chronic venous insufficiency (postphlebitic ulcers),
3. spontaneous bleeding associated with anticoagulant therapy.

TYPES OF CLIENTS/CLINICAL CONDITIONS SEEN BY HOME HEALTH AGENCIES

1. Initiation of prescribed treatment regimen for instruction and supervision of anticoagulant therapy and inclusive teaching plan for home-care management of thrombophlebitis
2. Periodic blood studies to assess for stabilization of client's prothrombin times with established parameters of drug dosage.
3. Initiation of and instruction in new medications and treatments for management of condition at home after recent hospitalization for treatment of complications, evaluation of response to therapy.

RELATED NURSING DIAGNOSIS

Anxiety

related to:
1. Pain and tenderness of affected extremity
2. Fear of dislodgement of thrombus (embolus)
3. Knowledge deficit regarding prescribed treatment regimen

as seen by:
Apprehension; reluctance to move; verbalization of fear and dislodging thrombus; asking numerous questions regarding condition and treatment regimen

Comfort, Alteration in: Pain

related to:
Obstruction of vessel lumen secondary to vein inflammation and impaired venous blood flow

as seen by:
Guarding of affected area; c/o pain in affected extremity; facial mask of pain

Knowledge Deficit (Specify)

related to:
1. Inadequate understanding of disease process and related S&S
2. Prescribed plan of treatment for management of thrombophlebitis
3. Potential complications and S&S to report to home health nurse or physician

as seen by:
Verbalization of lack of information; inadequate understanding; inability to perform skills necessary to meet health-care needs at home

Mobility, Impaired Physical

related to:
1. Prescribed activity restrictions
2. Pain
3. Fear of dislodging thrombus

as seen by:
Imposed medical restrictions; guarding of affected area; reluctance to move

Self-Care Deficit: Feeding, Bathing/Hygiene, Dressing/Grooming, Toileting (Specify)

related to:
1. Impaired mobility status
2. Prescribed activity restrictions

as seen by:
Decreased participation in self-care activities associated with imposed medical restrictions; pain; reluctance to move

Skin Integrity, Impairment of: Potential

related to:
1. Restricted, limited activity
2. Edema of affected extremity

as seen by:
Reddened or irritated areas over bony
prominences; tissue breakdown over
affected extremity

Tissue Perfusion, Alteration in: Peripheral

related to:
Reduced venous blood flow in affected
extremity secondary to occlusion
from thrombus formation

as seen by:
Swelling and increased warmth around
inflamed area; tenderness and pain
in affected extremity; redness along
course of vein; positive Homan's
sign

LONG-TERM GOAL

To reduce the inflammatory process of the venous wall and lower risk of clot
formation.

SHORT-TERM GOALS

The client with thrombophlebitis will be able to:

1. Verbalize nature of disease process, clinical manifestations, risk factors for
   thrombus formation, new or recurring problems to report to physician.
2. Identify prescribed measures to promote venous blood flow.
3. Verbalize importance/demonstrate compliance with prescribed diet and dietary
   restrictions and hydration of 2500 to 3000 ml per day.
4. Demonstrate compliance with prescribed medication therapy/identify side
   effects.
5. Demonstrate compliance with prescribed anticoagulant therapy, safety precautions with use, and adverse reactions to report to physician.
6. Verbalize purpose of prescribed blood studies for coagulation times and other
   diagnostic lab work.
7. Demonstrate compliance with prescribed activities, progressive ambulation and
   exercise program/verbalize hazards of prolonged immobility.
8. Identify measures to protect affected extremity and increase in S&S of thrombophlebitis to report to home health nurse or physician.

9. Demonstrate prescribed skin care of affected extremity.
10. Verbalize importance/wear Medic Alert bracelet.
11. Demonstrate reduction in level of anxiety to effectively manage daily activities and treatment regimen.

NURSING ACTIONS/TREATMENTS

1. Assess cardiovascular and pulmonary status and affected extremity for impaired venous blood flow (e.g., change in color, temperature, increase in size compared to unaffected extremity, tenderness and pain, positive Homan's sign)/identify complications.
2. Instruct on nature of disease process, clinical manifestations, risk factors for thrombus formation (e.g., cardiac disease, vasoconstricting factors such as crossing legs, constrictive clothing, smoking, prolonged sitting or standing, obesity, immobility, temperature extremes).
3. Instruct about importance of compliance with prescribed treatment regimen, new or recurring S&S to report to home health nurse or physician.
4. Observe/instruct on prescribed measures to promote venous blood flow (e.g., elevation of affected extremity with proper positioning, proper use and application of antiemoblic stockings, avoiding vasoconstricting factors).
5. Assess and evaluate nutritional status/instruct about well-balanced diet with prescribed dietary restrictions (e.g., low in saturated fat) and increased hydration to 2500 to 3000 ml per day to help decrease blood viscosity.
6. Observe/instruct about taking analgesics and other medications as ordered, purpose and action, side effects/evaluate medication effectiveness.
7. Observe/instruct about prescribed anticoagulant therapy, safety precautions to reduce risk of bleeding (e.g., avoid aspirin and aspirin-containing products and hard-bristled toothbrushes), adverse reactions to report to physician (e.g., bruising and petechiae, tarry stools, hematuria, nosebleeds)/educate regarding measures to control any bleeding (e.g., apply manual pressure for 10 minutes).
8. Monitor/instruct on purpose of lab studies for blood coagulation times and other prescribed diagnostic lab work as ordered.
9. Observe/instruct about prescribed activities, progressive ambulation and regular exercise program, leg and foot exercises, self-care activities, hazards of prolonged immobility.
10. Assess/instruct to avoid trauma, excessive pressure, temperature extremes to extremities, importance of not rubbing painful extremity, daily measuring and recording circumference of affected and unaffected extremity, reporting increase in S&S of thrombophlebitis, failure to respond to therapy.
11. Assess and evaluate skin integrity of edematous extremity, c/o burning, aching pain/instruct about hygenic skin care, measures to avoid trauma and excessive pressure.

12. Observe/instruct to wear a Medic Alert bracelet with information on medical condition and anticoagulant medication.
13. Assess level of anxiety associated with medical condition/encourage verbalization of feelings and concerns/provide emotional support.

REHABILITATION POTENTIAL

Rehabilitation potential *excellent good fair guarded poor* for resolution of thrombophlebitis and *full partial* return to an independent level of functioning to manage ADL.

Client's Name _____

Medical Record # _____

ONGOING/DISCHARGE EVALUATION OF TEACHING
The Client with Thrombophlebitis

Teaching Tools:
Printed materials given: _____

Audiovisual aids used: _____

Return Information/Demonstration/Interpretation
_____ Client
_____ Caregiver

OF:	Met	Not Met	Comments
☐ Nature of disease process; clinical manifestations.	_____	_____	_____
☐ S&S of complications; actions to take.	_____	_____	_____
☐ Importance of compliance with prescribed treatment regimen.	_____	_____	_____
☐ Risk factors for thrombus formation.	_____	_____	_____
☐ Measures to promote venous blood flow to affected extremity including proper use and application of antiembolism stockings.	_____	_____	_____

Client's Name _____

Medical Record # _____

☐ Diet and dietary restrictions. _____ _____ _____

☐ Importance of increased hydration. _____ _____ _____

☐ Medications and administration, purpose and action, side effects. _____ _____ _____

☐ Anticoagulant therapy; precautions to reduce risk of bleeding; adverse reactions to report to physician; measures to control any bleeding. _____ _____ _____

☐ Purpose of periodic blood work to monitor coagulation times and of other diagnostic lab tests. _____ _____ _____

☐ Progressive ambulation and regular exercise program; leg and foot exercises; self-care activities. _____ _____ _____

☐ Hazards of prolonged immobility. _____ _____ _____

Client's Name _____

Medical Record # _____

☐ Measures to
protect
extremity.   _____   _____   _____

☐ Skin care of
edematous
extremity.   _____   _____   _____

☐ Measuring and
recording
circumference
of affected and
unaffected
extremity;
increase in S&S
of thrombo-
phlebitis to
report to
physician.   _____   _____   _____

☐ Importance of
wearing Medic
Alert bracelet.   _____   _____   _____

Signature of Home Health Nurse _____

Date _____

RESPIRATORY DISORDERS

■ Chronic Obstructive Pulmonary Disease

Chronic obstructive pulmonary disease (COPD) is a progressive, chronic condition consisting of a group of pulmonary diseases characterized by increased resistance to air flow, air trapping, and hypoxemia. The three diseases that often make up the condition known as COPD are chronic bronchitis, pulmonary emphysema, and bronchial asthma; less common disorders are bronchiectasis and cystic fibrosis. Clients often present with some combination of these disorders, although each of the disorders can cause COPD by itself.

In chronic bronchitis the tissue of the bronchioles is irritated, for example, by cigarette smoke, resulting in hypertrophy of the mucus-producing cells, with an associated inflammation of bronchial mucosa. This results in an excessive production of mucus, associated cough, and resultant progressive destruction and dilation of the bronchioles. This clinical picture of inflammation and edema of the bronchi, along with increased mucus production, results in obstruction to air flow and inadequate ventilation and diffusion of gases. Cigarette smoking and severe air pollution are the most common causative factors of chronic bronchitis.

Emphysema is characterized by overinflation and destruction of the bronchioles and alveolar ducts and sacs, resulting in loss of elastic recoil and the trapping of air in the alveoli during expiration. Chronic emphysema is usually caused by other diseases such as long-standing bronchitis. However, it can develop in response to predisposing factors such as long-term inhalation of cigarette smoke and other pulmonary irritants.

Asthma is characterized by bronchospasm, tissue swelling, and the production of a sticky, tenacious mucus that is difficult to expectorate. As a result, the mucus and bronchospasm blocks the small airway passages, obstructing air flow, primarily during expiration. Asthma occurs in two forms: extrinsic (atopic), caused by specific allergens, and intrinsic (nonatopic), caused by infections. Other factors may also aggravate intrinsic asthma attacks (e.g., temperature and humidity changes, emotional stress). Chronic and sustained asthmatic attacks can develop into irreversible smooth-muscle hypertrophy and permanent narrowing of respiratory passageways characteristic of COPD.

Primary clinical manifestations of COPD are anxiousness, exertional dyspnea, a slowing of expiratory flow, chronic cough, and expectoration.

POTENTIAL COMPLICATIONS

1. Respiratory infections,
2. respiratory distress or failure,
3. cor pulmonale,
4. congestive heart failure,
5. arrhythmias,
6. malnutrition,
7. depression.

TYPES OF CLIENTS/CLINICAL CONDITIONS SEEN BY HOME HEALTH AGENCIES

1. Recent hospitalization with acute exacerbation of COPD.
2. Unstable respiratory status, respiratory distress: prescribed changes in current plan of treatment; instruction, supervision, and evaluation of response to changes in prescribed treatment regimen.
3. Initiation of prescribed inhalation therapy: IPPB; oxygen therapy; arterial blood gas analysis.

RELATED NURSING DIAGNOSIS

Activity Intolerance

related to:
1. Imbalance between oxygen supply and demand
2. Inadequate nutritional status

as seen by:
Verbal report of weakness and fatigue; exertional dyspnea; abnormal heart rate and BP in response to activity; decreased oral intake of food and fluids

Anxiety

related to:
1. Debilitated condition
2. Breathlessness
3. Changes in life-style
4. Exacerbation of disease process
5. Knowledge deficit regarding prescribed treatment regimen

as seen by:
Restlessness; c/o inability to breathe; increased heart and respiratory rate; fear of suffocation; feelings of uncertainty or helplessness

Bowel Elimination, Alteration in: Constipation

related to:
1. Decreased activity levels
2. Inadequate dietary fiber and fluids

as seen by:
Change in bowel elimination pattern, frequency and amount less than usual; straining at stool

Comfort, Alteration in: Pain

related to:
Chronic tissue hypoxia

as seen by:
C/o chest pain aggravated by activities; c/o headache

Grieving

related to:
1. Loss of normal respiratory functioning
2. Changes in life-style

as seen by:
Guilt; anger; depression; alteration in activity levels; changes in eating habits

Infection, Potential for

related to:
1. Debilitated condition
2. Retained secretions
3. Inadequate nutritional status
4. Respiratory treatments, use of equipment

as seen by:
Fever; chills; weakness and fatigue; anorexia; S&S of respiratory infection; nausea and vomiting

Injury, Potential for: Increased Risk of Falls and Injuries

related to:
1. Decreased mental alertness and acuity secondary to cerebral hypoxia
2. Impaired mobility status

as seen by:
Confusion; disorientation; altered sense of balance; weakness and fatigue; dizziness

Knowledge Deficit (Specify)

related to:
1. Disease process, related S&S
2. Potential complications, S&S to report to home health nurse or physician
3. Prescribed plan of treatment for respiratory disorder

as seen by:
Verbalization of lack of information; inadequate understanding; inability to perform skills necessary to meet health-care needs at home

Mobility, Impaired Physical

related to:
Tissue hypoxia

as seen by:
Decreased muscle strength; unsteady gait; decreased endurance; weakness and fatigue

Nutrition, Alteration in: Less than Body Requirements

related to:
1. Anorexia
2. Dyspnea and fatigue

as seen by:
Body weight 20 percent or more below normal for height, weight, and age;

3. Increased sputum production
4. Increased metabolic needs secondary to increased work in breathing

repeated inadequate food intake; weakness; inadequate caloric intake in relationship to metabolic needs of body; alteration in ability to taste

Nutrition, Alteration in: More than Body Requirements

related to:
Excessive intake of food and fluids

as seen by:
Weight 10 percent or more above desired weight for body build, height, and age; overeating in response to anxiety; difficulty with breathing; weakness and fatigue

Oral Mucous Membrane, Alteration in

related to:
1. Dry mucous membrane secondary to use of oxygen therapy
2. Mouth breathing
3. Poor oral hygiene
4. Decreased fluid intake

as seen by:
Dry mouth; coated tongue; c/o oral pain or discomfort; halitosis; inadequate fluid intake

Respiratory Function, Alteration in

Airway Clearance, Ineffective

related to:
1. Increased resistance to air flow secondary to bronochospasm
2. Obstruction of airway with mucus
3. Tissue destruction with airway collapse
4. Decreased energy and fatigue
5. Difficulty in mobilization of secretions

as seen by:
Tachypnea; dyspnea; ineffective cough; rales, rhonchi; wheezes; stridor; persistent cough, effective or ineffective, with or without sputum; changes in rate and depth of respirations

Breathing Pattern, Ineffective

related to:
1. Hypoventilation secondary to diminished respiratory drive
2. Compensatory hyperventilation with hypoxemia or hypercapnia

as seen by:
Adventitious breath sounds; shallow, rapid respirations; abnormally reduced rate and depth of respiration; decreased ventilation

3. Anxiety
4. Carbon dioxide narcosis
5. Decreased energy or fatigue

with carbon dioxide narcosis; exertional dyspnea; shortness of breath; abnormal arterial blood gases; cough; pursed lip breathing; anxiety; use of accessory muscles for breathing; weakness and restlessness

Gas Exchange, Impaired

related to:
1. Altered oxygen-carrying capacity of the blood secondary to ineffective breathing patterns
2. Trapped air in bronchioles and alveoli

as seen by:
Dyspnea; tachypnea; fatigue; confusion; restlessness; dizziness; decreased ventilation with carbon dioxide narcosis; irritability; headache; cyanosis; abnormal arterial blood gases; increased depth and rate of respirations; increase in BP.

Self-Care Deficit: Feeding, Bathing/Hygiene, Dressing/Grooming, Toileting (Specify)

related to:
1. Activity intolerance
2. Impaired mobility

as seen by:
Decreased participation in self-care activities associated with weakness and fatigue; decreased endurance; chest pain; dyspnea on exertion

Sleep Pattern Disturbance

related to:
1. Breathing difficulties
2. Coughing and increased sputum production
3. Anxiety

as seen by:
Lethargy; disorientation; c/o feeling tired; frequent yawning

Self-Concept, Disturbance in

related to:
1. Altered body image
2. Changes in life-style
3. Lowered self-esteem

as seen by:
Refusing to recognize physical limitations; increased dependency on others for meeting personal needs; lack of follow-through with treatments; signs of grieving

Tissue Perfusion, Alteration in

related to:	**as seen by:**
Impaired ability of the lungs to adequately exchange oxygen and carbon dioxide	Dyspnea, tachypnea; weakness and fatigue

LONG-TERM GOAL

To improve tissue oxygenation and preserve present pulmonary function and activity levels.

SHORT-TERM GOALS

The client with COPD will be able to:

1. Verbalize nature of disease process, precipitating factors to avoid, S&S of complications, actions to take.
2. Verbalize importance of prescribed diet, dietary restrictions, and increased hydration.
3. Identify causative factors of decreased oral intake/demonstrate prescribed measures to improve.
4. Weigh weekly/record/report excessive weight loss or gain to home health nurse or physician.
5. Verbalize effect of obesity on breathing/demonstrate compliance with prescribed caloric restrictions.
6. Demonstrate compliance with prescribed medication therapy/identify side effects.
7. Verbalize effect of constipation and abdominal distension on breathing/demonstrate prescribed measures to improve bowel functioning.
8. Verbalize importance/demonstrate compliance with graded exercise program, balanced rest and activity levels.
9. Demonstrate compliance with prescribed chest physiotherapy, breathing techniques, and exercises.
10. Demonstrate correct use of prescribed oxygen therapy, IPPB therapy, chest physiotherapy, vaporizer or humidifier/identify safety principles with use.
11. Verbalize understanding/identify measures to decrease dryness and breakdown of oral mucous membrane when on oxygen therapy.
12. Verbalize importance of prescribed lab work.
13. Demonstrate increased participation in self-care activities within limitations of condition through use of energy conservation and work simplification techniques.

14. Identify risk factors for falls and injuries/demonstrate safety factors with ambulation and daily activities.
15. Verbalize importance/wear Medic Alert bracelet.
16. Verbalize importance of keeping emergency and oxygen supply numbers by phone.
17. Verbalize feelings about altered body image, changes in life-style, increase in dependency on others/demonstrate effective measures to gain control of anxiety-provoking situations.

NURSING ACTIONS/TREATMENTS

1. Assess cardiovascular, respiratory status/identify complications.
2. Assess vital signs/identify trends (e.g., elevated temperature, tachycardia, increased respiratory rate, increase in BP).
3. Instruct about nature of disease, precipitating factors to avoid (e.g., bronchopulmonary irritants, allergens, stress, exposure to respiratory infections), importance of compliance with prescribed treatment regimen, S&S of complications to report to home health nurse or physician.
4. Assess and evaluate nutritional status/instruct about well-balanced diet with prescribed dietary restrictions (e.g., avoiding very hot or cold foods, gas-forming foods that cause abdominal distension) and increasing fluids to 2000 to 3000 ml per day as prescribed.
5. Assess and evaluate factors predisposing to decreased oral intake (e.g., anorexia, fatigue, dyspnea)/instruct to take small, frequent meals, prescribed high-caloric-high protein supplements as ordered/obtain dietary consultation as needed.
6. Observe and evaluate weight loss/instruct to weigh weekly or more often as indicated/record/report excessive weight loss or gain to home health nurse or physician.
7. Assess obesity problem/instruct about effect on breathing, prescribed calorie-restricted diet/weigh weekly and record/evaluate effectiveness of weight control diet.
8. Observe/instruct about taking medications as ordered, action and purpose, side effects/evaluate medication effectiveness.
9. Assess problem with constipation/instruct as to effect of abdominal distension on breathing, use of prescribed laxatives and stool softeners, foods high in dietary fiber, importance of adequate hydration and activities to bowel functioning/evaluate effectiveness of bowel regimen.
10. Observe/instruct about prescribed graded exercise program with balanced rest and activity levels.
11. Observe/instruct about prescribed chest physiotherapy, breathing techniques, supplementary exercises/evaluate respiratory functioning.
12. Observe/instruct about prescribed oxygen therapy: delivery system (e.g., oxy-

gen concentrator, liquid oxygen, oxygen tank), flow rate, duration and frequency breathing device (e.g., nasal cannula, oxygen mask), care of equipment, safety principles with use (e.g., danger of smoking near oxygen system, increasing of liter flow, and carbon dioxide narcosis)/evaluate effectiveness of oxygen therapy.

13. Observe/instruct about prescribed IPPB therapy: use and care of equipment, aerosol medications, pressure and oxygen concentration, duration and frequency of treatment/obtain respiratory consultation as needed.

14. Observe/instruct about prescribed use and purpose of vaporizer or humidifier.

15. Assess and evaluate oral mucous membrane for irritation and breakdown/instruct as to measures to decrease dryness (e.g., good oral hygiene, adequate hydration, breathing through nose).

16. Monitor/instruct as to purpose of prescribed lab work for arterial blood gas analysis and other diagnostic lab work.

17. Observe and evaluate level of physical tolerance to perform self-care activities, ADL (e.g., exertional dyspnea, fatigue, excess anxiety)/instruct about progressive functional activities within limitations of condition/refer to occupational therapy as ordered (e.g., instruction in work simplification and energy conservation techniques, breathing and endurance exercises).

18. Assess for increased risk factors for falls and injuries/instruct as to safety factors with ambulation and daily activities.

19. Observe/instruct about importance of wearing a Medic Alert bracelet with information of condition, treatments.

20. Observe/instruct importance of keeping emergency and oxygen supply phone numbers by phone.

21. Assess stress-provoking factors (grieving process, disturbance in self-concept)/instruct about gaining control of anxiety-provoking situations, relaxation techniques and establishing daily goals/refer to social services, as ordered, for counseling and providing of information regarding community resources to assist with adjustment to respiratory condition (e.g., American Lung Association, Emphysema Anonymous, Meals on Wheels, transportation services, homemaker chore application).

REHABILITATION POTENTIAL

Rehabilitation potential *excellent good fair guarded poor* for *full partial* return to an improved level of breathing function and activity level.

Client's Name _____

Medical Record #_____

ONGOING/DISCHARGE EVALUATION OF TEACHING
The Client with Chronic Obstructive Pulmonary Disease

Teaching Tools:
Printed materials given: _____

Audiovisual aids used: _____

Return Information/Demonstration/Interpretation
_____ Client
_____ Caregiver

OF:	Met	Not Met	Comments
☐ Nature of disease process; precipitating factors to avoid.	_____	_____	_____
☐ ˙ S&S of complications; actions to take.	_____	_____	_____
☐ Importance of compliance with prescribed treatment regimen.	_____	_____	_____
☐ Oxygen therapy.	_____	_____	_____
☐ IPPB therapy.	_____	_____	_____
☐ Chest physiotherapy.	_____	_____	_____
☐ Vaporizer or humidifier.	_____	_____	_____
☐ Purpose of prescribed lab			

Client's Name _____

Medical Record # _____

work; arterial blood gas analysis. _____ _____ _____

☐ Safety principles to observe with respiratory treatments. _____ _____ _____

☐ Measures to decrease dryness and breakdown of oral mucous membrane when on oxygen therapy. _____ _____ _____

☐ Diet and restrictions; dietary principles; increased fluids. _____ _____ _____

☐ Measures to improve decreased oral intake. _____ _____ _____

☐ Reporting excessive weight loss or gain to physician. _____ _____ _____

☐ Weight reduction diet. _____ _____ _____

☐ Medications and administration; purpose and action; side effects. _____ _____ _____

Client's Name _____

Medical Record # _____

☐ Effect of constipation and abdominal distension on breathing; prescribed measures to improve bowel activity. _____ _____ _____

☐ Graded exercise program; balanced rest and activity levels. _____ _____ _____

☐ Risk factors for falls and injuries; safety factors with ambulation and daily activities. _____ _____ _____

☐ Medic Alert bracelet. _____ _____ _____

☐ Emergency and oxygen supply numbers kept by phone. _____ _____ _____

Signature of Home Health Nurse _____

Date _____

■ Fracture of Ribs and Sternum with Associated Respiratory Involvement

Fractures of ribs and sternum are often seen in the elderly client because of instabilty of gait and falls. The disability resulting from a fall may be associated with restricted painful breathing and ambulation, loss of self-confidence and fear of falling again, and/or increased dependency on others for activities of daily living. Several pathologic conditions, such as Parkinson's disease, peripheral neuropathies, sensory and motor deficits, and osteoporosis occurring as a complication of steroid therapy may be predisposing factors that contribute to instability and falling. Rib fractures are also caused by trauma resulting from crushing injuries, forceful blows, or strain from violent coughing.

Tenderness and slight edema over the fracture site, crepitus, and pain that increases with deep breathing and movement are symptoms associated with rib fractures. Persistent chest pains, which are present even at rest, are found with sternal fractures. Decreased respiratory excursions associated with painful breathing may lead to hypoventilation, with decreased aeration of lungs, inability to cough up secretions, and a predisposition to pneumonia.

POTENTIAL COMPLICATIONS

1. Atelectasis,
2. pneumonia,
3. pneumonitis,
4. respiratory distress,
5. pneumothorax.

TYPES OF CLIENTS/CLINICAL CONDITIONS SEEN BY HOME HEALTH AGENCIES

1. Recent fracture of ribs with alterations in respiratory functioning and impaired mobility status.
2. Pulmonary complications: prescribed changes in plan of treatment, client instruction and supervision of new treatments, evaluation and report to physician of response to treatment changes.

RELATED NURSING DIAGNOSIS

Activity Intolerance

related to:
Imbalance between oxygen demand
and supply, secondary to painful,
shallow respirations

as seen by:
Weakness and fatigue; increased
respiratory and pulse rate

Anxiety

related to:
1. Splinted, painful respirations
2. Inability to manage activities of
daily living

as seen by:
Increased helplessness; apprehension;
pain with movement

Comfort, Alteration in: Pain

related to:
Fractured ribs and sternum

as seen by:
Painful respirations; splinting or
guarding of injured area; facial
expression of pain

Infection, Potential for

related to:
1. Decreased mobility status
2. Alteration in respiratory functioning

as seen by:
Fever and chills; cough with sputum
production; abnormal breath sounds;
shortness of breath

Knowledge Deficit (Specify)

related to:
1. Prescribed plan of treatment for
management of fractures and
related respiratory involvement
2. Potential complications, S&S to
report to home health nurse or
physician

as seen by:
Verbalization of lack of knowledge
and inadequate understanding of
prescribed treatment regimen for
management of respiratory condition

Mobility, Impaired Physical

related to:
1. Pain and discomfort

as seen by:
Reluctance to move; limited range of

2. Prescribed activity restrictions

motion resulting from fracture; imposed medical restrictions

Respiratory Function, Alteration in

Airway Clearance, Ineffective

related to:
Difficulty in mobilization of secretions associated with painful respirations

as seen by:
Shallow respirations; increased respiratory rate; ineffective cough and sputum production

Breathing Patterns, Ineffective

related to:
Pain and discomfort

as seen by:
Altered chest excursion and depth of respiration; splinted or guarded respirations

Gas Exchange, Impaired

related to:
Altered oxygen supply secondary to accumulation of tracheobronchial secretions

as seen by:
Inability to move secretions because of pain with coughing

Self-Care Deficit: Feeding, Bathing/Hygiene, Dressing/Grooming, Toileting (Specify)

related to:
1. Activity intolerance
2. Impaired mobility status
3. Prescribed activity restrictions

as seen by:
Decreased participation in self-care activities associated with pain, weakness and fatigue; imposed medical restrictions

Sleep Pattern Disturbance

related to:
Pain and discomfort resulting from fracture

as seen by:
Inability to assume comfortable sleep position; painful breathing; restlessness

LONG-TERM GOAL

To improve respiratory functioning and minimize complications associated with decreased respiratory excursions and related hypoventilation.

SHORT-TERM GOALS

The client with fractured ribs and sternum will be able to:

1. Identify S&S of respiratory complications and actions to take.
2. Identify risk factors for falls and injuries/identify safety principles with ambulation and daily activities in home environment.
3. Verbalize importance of well-balanced diet and increased hydration to respiratory status.
4. Demonstrate compliance with prescribed medication therapy/identify side effects.
5. Demonstrate splinting of chest and correct use of rib support.
6. Verbalize importance/demonstrate progressive ambulatory activities, ROM exercises, planned rest periods, pain management measures with ADL.
7. Verbalize importance of avoiding exposure to respiratory infections.
8. Demonstrate increased participation in self-care activities within prescribed limitations.

NURSING ACTIONS/TREATMENTS

1. Assess cardiopulmonary status/identify complications.
2. Assess vital signs/identify trends (e.g., elevated temperature, increased respiratory and pulse rate).
3. Assess causative factor of fracture/instruct about risk factors for falls and injuries, safety principles with ambulation and activities, importance of compliance with prescribed treatment regimen, S&S of complications to report to home health nurse or physician.
4. Assess and evaluate nutritional status/instruct on importance of eating balanced meals, increased fluids of 2000 to 3000 ml per day as prescribed.
5. Observe/instruct to take medications as ordered, about safe use of analgesics, purpose and action, side effects/evaluate medication effectiveness.
6. Assess and evaluate degree of pain/instruct about splinting of chest, use of prescribed rib support, importance of position changes and cough and deep breathing exercises every 2 to 4 hours.
7. Observe/instruct about importance of progressive ambulatory activities and range of motion exercises of extremities as ordered with planned rest periods/educate about pain management measures with ADL (e.g., relaxation breathing, prescribed medication therapy).

8. Observe/instruct on importance of avoiding exposure to respiratory infections.
9. Observe and evaluate level of physical tolerance to perform self-care, ADL/refer to occupational therapy as ordered to instruct in energy conservation and work simplification techniques.

REHABILITATION POTENTIAL

Rehabilitation potential *excellent good fair guarded poor* for *full partial* return to an independent level of functioning and improved respiratory functioning.

Client's Name _____

Medical Record # _____

ONGOING/DISCHARGE EVALUATION OF TEACHING

The Client with Fractured Ribs and Sternum

Teaching Tools:

Printed materials given: _____

Audiovisual aids used: _____

Return Information/Demonstration/Interpretation

_____ Client
_____ Caregiver

OF:	Met	Not Met	Comments
☐ Risk factors of falls and injuries in home environment; safety principles with ambulation and activities.	_____	_____	_____
☐ S&S of respiratory complications; actions to take.	_____	_____	_____
☐ Importance of compliance with prescribed treatment regimen.	_____	_____	_____
☐ Well balanced diet; increased fluids.	_____	_____	_____
☐ Medications and administration, purpose and			

Client's Name _____

Medical Record #_____

action, side
effects. _____ _____ _____

☐ Splinting of
chest; use of
rib support. _____ _____ _____

☐ Pain
management
measures. _____ _____ _____

☐ Progressive
ambulatory
activities; ROM
exercises;
planned rest
periods. _____ _____ _____

☐ Importance of
avoiding
exposure to
respiratory
infections. _____ _____ _____

☐ Energy
conservation
and work
simplification
techniques. _____ _____ _____

Signature of Home Health Nurse _____

Date _____

■ Pneumonia

Pneumonia is an acute inflammation of lung parenchyma with the pathology and pattern of response dependent on the causative agent. Some major types of pneumonia may be caused by bacteria, viruses, or fungi but may also result from environmental irritants or from aspiration of foreign material.

Bacterial pneumonias are characterized by a partial consolidation of lung tissue. This is due to the filling of alveoli with an inflammatory exudate in response to the infection. The pneumococcal bacterium is the most common cause of bacterial pneumonia. Viral or mycoplasmal pneumonias are characterized by edema between the alveoli with an infiltrate in the alveolar walls. Exudate is not found in the alveoli and there is no consolidation. Pneumonias caused by a fungus or *Mycobacterium tuberculosis* are characterized by the formation of granulomas, which may become caseous and ulcerate, causing the formation of a cavity.

Some predisposing factors to bacterial and viral pneumonias are atelectasis, respiratory diseases and infections, alcoholism, thoracic injuries, tracheostomy, and chronic debilitating illnesses. Examples of factors predisposing to aspiration pneumonia are debilitation in aged clients, an impaired gag reflex, and nasogastric tube feedings. Clinical manifestations include chills, high fever, diaphoresis, chest pain, cough and sputum production (rust-colored sputum characteristic with a pneumococcal infection, "red currant jelly" sputum characteristic of *Klebsiella* pneumonia).

POTENTIAL COMPLICATIONS

1. Delayed resolution,
2. atelectasis,
3. unstable respiratory condition or respiratory distress,
4. congestive heart failure,
5. cardiac arrhythmias,
6. thrombophlebitis,
7. pleural effusion.

TYPES OF CLIENTS/CLINICAL CONDITIONS SEEN BY HOME HEALTH AGENCIES

1. Unstable respiratory status (e.g., temperature elevations, chills, shortness of breath, cough, chest pain).
2. Initiation and instruction of new medications and treatments for management of condition at home after recent hospitalization for treatment of complications.
3. Initiation of and instruction in antimicrobial therapy.
4. Initiation of and instruction in prescribed inhalation therapy (e.g., oxygen therapy); arterial blood gas analysis.
5. Initiation and instruction in chest physiotherapy.

RELATED NURSING DIAGNOSIS

Activity Intolerance

related to:
Imbalance between oxygen demand
and supply secondary to alteration in
respiratory functioning

as seen by:
Fatigue and weakness; abnormal heart
and respiratory rate or blood
pressure in response to activity;
exertional dyspnea or discomfort

Anxiety

related to:
1. Disease process
2. Debilitated condition
3. Dyspnea
4. Pleuritic pain
5. Knowledge deficit regarding
   prescribed treatment regimen

as seen by:
Apprehension regarding disease
process; restlessness; increased pulse
and respiratory rate; frequent
questioning regarding condition and
prescribed treatments

Comfort, Alteration in: Pain

related to:
1. Pleuritic pain secondary to
   inflammatory process of lungs
2. Coughing

as seen by:
Guarding or splinting of chest;
grimace; incessant, short painful
coughing

Fluid Volume Deficit

related to:
1. Decreased fluid intake
2. Insensible fluid losses secondary to
   profuse diaphoresis,
   hyperventilation, and increased
   pulmonary secretions

as seen by:
Poor skin turgor; hypotension; rapid,
shallow respirations; rapid, weak
pulse; weight loss; dry mucous
membranes; output less than intake

Knowledge Deficit (Specify)

related to:
1. Disease process, and related S&S
2. Inadequate understanding of
   prescribed plan of treatment for
   management of pneumonia

as seen by:
Verbalization of lack of information;
inadequate understanding; inability
to perform skills necessary to meet
health-care needs at home

3. Potential complications and S&S to report to home health nurse or physician

Mobility, Impaired Physical

related to:
1. Tissue hypoxia
2. Pleuritic pain
3. Prescribed activity restrictions

as seen by:
Decreased endurance; muscular weakness and fatigue; splinting of chest with movement; imposed medical restrictions

Nutrition, Alteration in: Less than Body Requirements

related to:
1. Decreased oral intake
2. Increased metabolic needs with infection

as seen by:
Anorexia; weight loss; caloric intake decreased; weakness and fatigue

Oral Mucous Membrane, Alteration in

related to:
1. Dry mucous membrane secondary to prescribed use of oxygen therapy
2. Increased insensible fluid losses
3. Decreased fluid intake
4. Mouth breathing

as seen by:
Dry mouth; coated tongue; c/o oral pain and discomfort; halitosis; not increasing fluids as prescribed

Respiratory Function, Alteration in

Airway Clearance, Ineffective

related to:
Difficulty in mobilization of secretions associated with increased viscosity of mucus

as seen by:
Dyspnea; ineffective cough and expectoration of sputum; abnormal breath sounds; cyanosis; tachypnea

Breathing Pattern, Ineffective

related to:
1. Fatigue and decreased energy levels
2. Pleuritic pain

as seen by:
Hypoventilation; abnormal blood gases; altered chest excursion; exertional dyspnea; splinting or guarding of chest

Gas Exchange, Impaired

related to:
1. Ineffective airway clearance and breathing patterns
2. Nonventilated consolidated areas of lung

as seen by:
Dyspnea; pallor; decreased activity tolerance; disorientation and confusion

Self-Care Deficit: Feeding, Bathing/Hygiene, Dressing/Grooming, Toileting (Specify)

related to:
1. Activity intolerance
2. Impaired mobility secondary to hypoxia, prescribed activity restrictions, and pleuritic pain

as seen by:
Decreased participation in self-care activities associated with fatigue, decreased energy levels, and pain; imposed medical restrictions

Skin Integrity, Impairment of

related to:
1. Immobility
2. Inadequate nutritional status

as seen by:
Reddened or irritated areas over bony prominences; tissue breakdown

Thermoregulation, Ineffective: Pneumonia

related to:
Temperature fluctuation related to disease process

as seen by:
Body temperature above normal range

LONG-TERM GOAL

Return of adequate pulmonary functioning with improved tissue oxygenation through reduction of inflammatory process of lung parenchyma.

SHORT-TERM GOALS

The client with pneumonia will be able to:

1. Verbalize nature of disease process, precipitating factors, S&S of impending respiratory difficulties and complications to report to home health nurse or physician.
2. Demonstrate how to take temperature and read a thermometer.

3. Identify factors contributing to fluid losses and measures to correct.
4. Verbalize measures to reduce pleuritic pain.
5. Verbalize importance of/demonstrate compliance with prescribed diet, increased hydration.
6. Identify causative factors of decreased oral intake/demonstrate prescribed measures to improve.
7. Weigh weekly/record/report excessive weight loss to home health nurse or physician.
8. Demonstrate compliance with prescribed medication therapy/identify side effects.
9. Demonstrate correct use of oxygen therapy, IPPB therapy, chest physiotherapy, vaporizer or humidifer as prescribed/identify safety principles with use.
10. Verbalize understanding/identify measures to decrease dryness and promote healing of oral mucous membrane.
11. Demonstrate increased participation in self-care activities within limitations of condition through use of work-simplification and energy-conservation techniques.
12. Verbalize purpose of prescribed lab work for arterial blood gas analysis and other diagnostic lab tests.
13. Verbalize importance of proper hand-washing technique and disposal of contaminated tissues and supplies.
14. Verbalize importance of keeping emergency and oxygen supply phone numbers by phone.

NURSING ACTIONS/TREATMENTS

1. Assess cardiovascular and respiratory status/identify complications.
2. Assess vital signs/identify trends (e.g., elevated temperature, increased respiratory rate)/instruct how to take temperature and read a thermometer.
3. Instruct as to type of pneumonia, nature of disease process, precipitating factors (e.g., fatigue and chilling, environmental risk factors, exposure to respiratory infections), importance of compliance with prescribed treatment regimen, S&S of complications to report to home health nurse or physician.
4. Assess and evaluate S&S of fluid volume deficit/instruct as to measures to treat fluid losses (e.g., increase fluid intake; treatment of respiratory infection to decrease excessive pulmonary secretions, hyperventilation, and profuse diaphoresis).
5. Assess and evaluate pleuritic pain/instruct about prescribed measures to reduce (e.g., pain medications, cough suppressants, splinting of chest).
6. Assess and evaluate nutritional status/instruct as to importance of well-balanced diet, increased fluids of 2000 to 3000 ml per day as prescribed.
7. Assess and evaluate causative factors of decreased oral intake (e.g., anorexia,

fatigue, dyspnea)/instruct to take small, frequent meals with prescribed high-caloric, high-protein supplements/obtain dietary consultation as needed.

8. Assess and evaluate for weight loss/instruct to weigh weekly, more often as indicated/record/report excessive weight loss to home health nurse or physician.

9. Observe/instruct about taking medications as ordered (e.g., antimicrobial therapy), purpose and action, side effects/evaluate medication effectiveness.

10. Observe/instruct about prescribed physiotherapy, breathing techniques, supplementary exercises.

11. Observe/instruct about prescribed oxygen therapy: delivery system (e.g., oxygen concentrator, liquid oxygen, oxygen tank), flow rate, duration and frequency, breathing device (e.g., nasal cannula, oxygen mask), care of equipment, safety principles (e.g., danger of smoking near oxygen system)/evaluate effectiveness of oxygen therapy.

12. Observe/instruct about principles of IPPB therapy: use and care of equipment, aerosol medications, pressure and oxygen concentration, duration and frequency of treatment/obtain respiratory consultation as needed.

13. Observe/instruct about prescribed use and purpose of vaporizer or humidifier.

14. Observe and evaluate oral mucous membrane for irritation and break-down/instruct about measures to decrease dryness (e.g., good oral hygiene, adequate hydration, breathing through nose).

15. Monitor/instruct as to purpose of lab work for arterial blood gas analysis or other diagnostic lab tests as ordered.

16. Observe/instruct as to importance of proper hand-washing technique, disposal of contaminated tissues, supplies.

17. Observe/instruct importance of keeping emergency and oxygen supply phone numbers by the phone.

18. Observe and evaluate level of physical tolerance to perform ADL (e.g., exertional dyspnea, fatigue, excess anxiety)/instruct about progressive functional activities within limitations of condition/refer to occupational therapist as ordered (e.g., instruction in work simplification and energy conservation techniques, breathing and endurance exercises).

REHABILITATION POTENTIAL

Rehabilitation potential *excellent good fair guarded poor* for *full partial* return to an improved level of respiratory functioning and maximal independence in self-care activities.

Client's Name _____

Medical Record # _____

ONGOING/DISCHARGE EVALUATION OF TEACHING
The Client with Pneumonia

Teaching Tools:
Printed materials given: _____

Audiovisual aids used: _____

Return Information/Demonstration/Interpretation
_____ Client
_____ Caregiver

OF:	Met	Not Met	Comments
☐ Type of pneumonia; nature of disease process; precipitating factors.	_____	_____	_____
☐ S&S of complications; actions to take.	_____	_____	_____
☐ Importance of compliance with prescribed treatment regimen.	_____	_____	_____
☐ How to take a temperature, read a thermometer.	_____	_____	_____
☐ Oxygen therapy.	_____	_____	_____
☐ IPPB therapy.	_____	_____	_____

Client's Name _____

Medical Record #_____

☐ Chest physiotherapy. _____ _____ _____

☐ Breathing techniques; supplementary exercises. _____ _____ _____

☐ Vaporizer or humidifier. _____ _____ _____

☐ Safety principles to observe with respiratory treatments. _____ _____ _____

☐ Purpose of prescribed lab work, blood gas analysis. _____ _____ _____

☐ Measures to decrease dryness and breakdown of oral mucous membrane when on oxygen therapy. _____ _____ _____

☐ Balanced diet and increased fluids. _____ _____ _____

☐ Measures to improve decreased oral intake. _____ _____ _____

☐ Weigh weekly; record; report excessive weight loss to physician. _____ _____ _____

Client's Name _____

Medical Record # _____

☐ Medications
and
administration,
purpose and
action, side
effects.   _____ _____   _____

☐ Measures to
reduce pleuritic
pain.   _____ _____   _____

☐ Measures to
treat fluid
losses.   _____ _____   _____

☐ Proper hand-
washing
technique;
disposal of
contaminated
tissues,
supplies.   _____ _____   _____

☐ Energy-
conservation
and work-
simplification
techniques.   _____ _____   _____

☐ Progressive
functional
activities within
limits of
condition.   _____ _____   _____

☐ Emergency and
oxygen supply
phone numbers
kept by phone.   _____ _____   _____

Signature of Home Health Nurse _____

Date _____

■ Pulmonary Tuberculosis

Tuberculosis is an acute or chronic infection caused by an acid-fast bacillus, *Mycobacterium tuberculosis*. Transmission of tubercle bacilli is generally through inhalation of droplet nuclei but transmission may also occur through the gastrointestinal tract from contaminated milk. After entry into the body, tubercle bacilli usually implant on the alveolar surface of the lungs, where an inflammatory and immune response occurs to form tubercles, which isolate the infecting organism. The bacilli stay dormant and walled off until the body's defenses are lowered, by stress, for example, which allows the bacilli to multiply and reactivate the infection. The center of the tubercle may undergo caseation, a form of necrosis producing a cheeselike substance, which may localize and undergo fibrosis or liquefy and drain necrotic materials, leaving a cavity.

Clinical findings in a primary infection include vague symptoms of weakness and fatigue, anorexia, low-grade fever, and weight loss after a four- to eight-week incubation period. Night sweats, cough, mucopurulent sputum, and chest pain and hemoptysis may be seen as the disease progresses or with reinfection. Dyspnea and orthopnea occur in the late stages of pulmonary tuberculosis.

In the older population the incidence of tuberculosis is increasing and occurs more commonly as a result of reactivation of an earlier infection rather than a new infection.

POTENTIAL COMPLICATIONS

1. Pneumonia,
2. hemorrhage,
3. side effects of antitubercular drug therapy,
4. malnutrition,
5. symptoms of recurrence,
6. empyema,
7. pleural effusion.

TYPES OF CLIENTS/CLINICAL CONDITIONS SEEN BY HOME HEALTH AGENCIES

1. Newly diagnosed with tuberculosis infection: initiation of prescribed antitubercular therapy, inclusive teaching plan for home-care management of tuberculosis client.
2. Unstable respiratory status with increased activity of disease process and the development of complications: changes in ongoing plan of treatment, need for instruction, supervision, and observation of response to therapy.
3. Recurrence of tuberculosis infection: change in chemotherapy, observation for recurrent symptoms, evaluation of response to therapy, report to physician.

RELATED NURSING DIAGNOSIS

Activity Intolerance

related to:
1. Hypoxia secondary to pulmonary damage
2. Inadequate nutritional status

as seen by:
Weakness; easy fatigability; exertional dyspnea; loss of appetite

Anxiety

related to:
1. Diagnosis of TB and effect on quality of life
2. Hemoptysis and chest pain
3. Knowledge deficit regarding disease process and prescribed treatment regimen

as seen by:
Increased questioning regarding condition and treatment; apprehension of effect of TB diagnosis on quality of life and role relationships; fear of disability and death

Comfort, Alteration in: Pain

related to:
1. Chest pains related to muscle strain with excessive coughing and expectoration
2. Pleuritic pain secondary to inflammatory process of lungs

as seen by:
Splinting of chest with coughing; verbalization of pain; grimace

Coping, Ineffective Individual

related to:
1. Inability to accept diagnosis of tuberculosis
2. Stigma attached to disease

as seen by:
Frustration and despair; depression; alienation; anger; withdrawal from relationships

Fluid Volume Deficit

related to:
1. Inadequate intake
2. Vomiting
3. Insensible fluid losses secondary to profuse diaphoresis (''night sweats''), hyperventilation, and increased pulmonary secretions

as seen by:
Concentrated urine; decreased intake of oral fluids; weakness; increased pulse rate; poor skin turgor

Grieving

related to:
Changes in body functioning and life-style

as seen by:
Anger; lack of follow-through with daily activities; withdrawal; depression

Knowledge Deficit (Specify)

related to:
1. Disease process, related S&S
2. Prescribed home-care plan of treatment for management of tuberculosis
3. Potential complications, S&S to report to home health nurse or physician

as seen by:
Verbalization of lack of information; inadequate understanding; inability to perform skills necessary to meet health-care needs at home

Nutrition, Alteration in: Less than Body Requirements

related to:
1. Decreased oral intake
2. Increased metabolic needs

as seen by:
Anorexia; inadequate caloric intake; weight loss or weight below normal

Respiratory Function, Alteration in

Airway Clearance, Ineffective

related to:
Difficulty in expectoration of mucopurulent sputum

as seen by:
Productive cough; dyspnea; adventitious breath sounds

Breathing Pattern, Ineffective

related to:
1. Decreased energy or fatigue
2. Pleuritic pain

as seen by:
Exertional dyspnea; cough; shortness of breath; altered chest excursion; splinting of chest

Gas Exchange, Impaired

related to:
1. Altered oxygen supply associated with ineffective airway clearance and breathing pattern

as seen by:
Dyspnea; restlessness; irritability; decreased activity tolerance

2. Disruption of alveolar ventilation
   and diffusion secondary to
   destruction of alveoli

Self-Care Deficit: Feeding, Bathing/Hygiene, Dressing/Grooming, Toileting (Specify)

related to:
Activity intolerance

as seen by:
Decreased participation in self-care
activities associated with fatigue;
weakness; decreased energy levels

Self-Concept, Disturbance in

related to:
1. Altered body image
2. Changes in life-style, role
   performances
3. Lowered self-esteem

as seen by:
Not taking responsibility for self-care;
lack of follow-through with
prescribed therapy; signs of grieving

Thermoregulation, Ineffective: Tuberculosis

related to:
Temperature fluctuation associated
with disease process

as seen by:
Body temperature above normal range

LONG-TERM GOAL

To control progression and reactivation of tubercular process with no evidence of
untoward symptoms or complications.

SHORT-TERM GOALS

The client with pulmonary tuberculosis will be able to:

1. Verbalize understanding of nature of disease, current status of disease, S&S of
   complications to report to home health nurse or physician.
2. Demonstrate how to take a temperature and read a thermometer.
3. Verbalize prescribed measures to reduce pleuritic pain and discomfort from
   muscle strain.
4. Verbalize importance of eating balanced meals high in carbohydrates and proteins and importance of increased hydration.

5. Identify predisposing factors to decreased oral intake/demonstrate prescribed measures to improve.
6. Identify factors contributing to fluid loss and measures to correct.
7. Weigh weekly/record/report excessive weight loss to physician.
8. Demonstrate compliance with prescribed long-term medication therapy/identify side effects, toxicity.
9. Demonstrate increased participation in self-care activities within limits of present condition, balanced with rest periods.
10. Demonstrate specific measures of infection control.
11. Verbalize purpose of prescribed lab work.
12. Demonstrate adequate adaptive response to altered body image and changes in life-style to effectively cope with disease process and long-term treatment regimen.

NURSING ACTIONS/TREATMENTS

1. Assess pulmonary status/identify clinical manifestations of tuberculosis infection and complications.
2. Assess vital signs/identify trends (elevated temperature, increased pulse and respiratory rate)/instruct how to take a temperature and read a thermometer.
3. Instruct as to nature of disease process, current status of disease, S&S of complications to report to home health nurse or physician/importance of following prescribed long-term treatment regimen.
4. Assess and evaluate level of fatigue and chest pain related to muscle strain with coughing, pleurisy/instruct as to measures to reduce (e.g., prescribed medications, splinting of chest).
5. Assess and evaluate nutritional status/instruct importance of balanced diet high in carbohydrates and protein, increased fluids of 2000 to 3000 ml per day as prescribed/obtain dietary consultation as needed.
6. Assess and evaluate factors predisposing to decreased oral intake/instruct to eat small frequent meals, prescribed high-caloric, high-protein supplements.
7. Assess and evaluate for S&S of fluid volume deficit/instruct as to measures to treat fluid losses (e.g., increase fluid intake, treatment of respiratory infection to decrease excessive pulmonary secretions, hyperventilation, profuse diaphoresis).
8. Observe and evaluate for weight loss/instruct to weigh weekly, more often as indicated/record/report excessive weight loss to physician.
9. Observe/instruct as to importance of taking medications as ordered, continuous, uninterrupted taking of antitubercular agents (e.g., ethambutol, isoniazid (INH), rifampin, streptomycin), purpose and action side effects, toxicity/evaluate medication effectiveness.
10. Observe and evaluate level of physical tolerance to perform self-care activities/ADL (e.g., exertional dyspnea, fatigue, excess anxiety)/instruct about

progressive functional activities within individual limits of condition with planned rest periods.

11. Observe/instruct about specific measures of infection control (e.g., transmission through droplet nuclei, respiratory isolation precautions, good hygiene and hand-washing practices).

12. Monitor/instruct as to purpose of sputum specimens for cultures, other diagnostic lab work as ordered.

13. Assess frustration and despair related to altered body image and changes in lifestyle/provide emotional support and encourage verbalization of feelings/refer to social services as ordered for counseling and assisting through grieving process and adaptation to treatment regimen and to provide information of community resources to assist with home management (e.g., American Lung Association, Meals on Wheels, transportation services, attendant services).

14. Report to Department of Health for follow-up on family and contacts.

REHABILITATION POTENTIAL

Rehabilitation potential *excellent good fair guarded poor* for *full partial* recovery from tuberculosis with controlled progression of infection for return to an increased level of activity and independence.

Client's Name _____

Medical Record #_____

ONGOING/DISCHARGE EVALUATION OF TEACHING
The Client with Pulmonary Tuberculosis

Teaching Tools:
Printed materials given: _____

Audiovisual aids used: _____

Return Information/Demonstration/Interpretation
_____ Client
_____ Caregiver

OF:	Met	Not Met	Comments
☐ Nature of disease process; current status of disease.	_____	_____	_____
☐ S&S of complications; actions to take.	_____	_____	_____
☐ Importance of compliance with prescribed long-term treatment regimen.	_____	_____	_____
☐ How to take temperature and read a thermometer.	_____	_____	_____
☐ Measures to relieve pleuritic pain, fatigue and muscle strain related to coughing.	_____	_____	_____

Client's Name _____

Medical Record #_____

☐ Well-balanced diet high in carbohydrates and protein, increased fluids. _____ _____ _____

☐ Predisposing factors to decreased oral intake, measures to correct. _____ _____ _____

☐ Measures to treat fluid losses. _____ _____ _____

☐ Weigh weekly; record; report excessive weight loss to physician. _____ _____ _____

☐ Medications and administration, purpose and action, side effects, toxicity. _____ _____ _____

☐ Progressive functional activities within limits of condition, balanced rest periods. _____ _____ _____

☐ Measures of infection control. _____ _____ _____

☐ Understand need for and purpose of

Client's Name _____

Medical Record # _____

sputum
specimens and
other diagnostic
work.   _____   _____   _____

_____

Signature of Home Health Nurse _____

Date _____

■ Tracheostomy/ Laryngectomy

Tracheostomy is a surgically created external opening into the trachea through which respiration takes place. After the surgical procedure, a tracheostomy tube is then inserted to permit access to the airway. This procedure may be temporary or permanent, depending on the client's condition and purpose for the tracheostomy.

A laryngectomy is the surgical removal of part or all of the larynx, most commonly performed for the treatment of laryngeal cancer. Only the diseased portion of the larynx or vocal cord is removed in a partial laryngectomy. In a total laryngectomy the larynx, thyroid cartilage, epiglottis, hyoid bone, cricoid cartilage, and two or more rings of the trachea are removed.

This care plan focuses on the adult client discharged home with a permanent tracheostomy after a total laryngectomy for treatment of cancer.

POTENTIAL COMPLICATIONS

1. Wound infection,
2. tracheostomy stenosis,
3. peristomal skin irritation or breakdown,
4. respiratory infection,
5. airway obstruction secondary to secretions, food, dislodged tracheostomy tube,
6. tracheal ulceration, necrosis, tracheoesophageal fistula,
7. respiratory distress.

TYPES OF CLIENTS/CLINICAL CONDITIONS SEEN BY HOME HEALTH AGENCIES

1. Observation and care of surgical incision, dressings.
2. Wound infection.
3. Tracheostomy and stomal care, instructions.
4. Suctioning.
5. Tube feeding (if ordered).
6. Speech rehabilitation.

RELATED NURSING DIAGNOSIS

Airway Clearance, Ineffective

related to:
1. Dislodgement of the tracheostomy tube

as seen by:
Persistent choking; difficulty swallowing; noisy, moist

2. Obstruction of tracheostomy tube
   from thick secretions
3. Aspiration of food, fluids

respirations; increased pulse and
respiratory rate

Anxiety

related to:
1. Altered body image associated with
   loss of ability to communicate
   verbally
2. Breathing through neck
3. Knowledge deficit regarding
   prescribed treatment regimen

as seen by:
Frustration and distress when
   attempting to make self understood;
   feelings of apprehension;
   verbalization of uncertainty and
   fears of managing tracheostomy at
   home

Communication, Impaired Verbal

related to:
1. Surgical removal of part or all of
   larynx
2. Tracheostomy

as seen by:
Inability to make self understood
   through verbal communication

Coping, Ineffective Individual

related to:
1. Altered appearance
2. Loss of ability to communicate
   verbally

as seen by:
Frustration; depression; anxiety;
   irritability; inability to meet personal
   needs

Grieving

related to:
1. Changes in body appearance,
   functioning
2. Changes in life-style

as seen by:
Crying; changes in eating and sleep
   habits; anger; inability to follow
   through with daily activities

Infection, Potential for

related to:
1. Breakdown of the body's first line
   of defense secondary to surgical
   incision
2. Irritation and breakdown of
   peristomal skin

as seen by:
Increased pain; tenderness; swelling;
   unusual drainage; chills and fever;
   weakness and fatigue; abnormal
   breath sounds

3. Aspiration of secretions, food, and fluids
4. Lack of protection to respiratory system secondary to air not passing through nasal passages: trauma or infection

Injury, Potential for: Tissue Trauma to Trachea/Respiratory System

related to:
1. Improper suctioning technique
2. Trauma to respiratory system secondary to air not passing through nasal passages

as seen by:
Presence of blood in secretions aspirated during suctioning; S&S of tracheal irritation, ulceration, infection

Knowledge Deficit (Specify)

related to:
1. Inadequate understanding of prescribed plan of treatment for management of tracheostomy tube and stoma
2. Potential complications, S&S to report to home health nurse or physician

as seen by:
Expressed concern about lack of knowledge; inadequate understanding; inability to perform skills necessary to meet health-care needs at home

Nutrition, Alteration in: Less than Body Requirements

related to:
1. Difficulty swallowing
2. Anorexia
3. Prescribed dietary modifications
4. Depression

as seen by:
Loss of weight; decreased oral intake as a result of altered sense of taste and smell; dislike of foods prescribed; alterations in eating patterns with grieving; inflammation of mucous membranes

Oral Mucous Membrane, Alteration in

related to:
1. Infrequent and inadequate oral hygiene
2. Decreased fluid intake

as seen by:
Dry mouth; coated tongue; c/o oral pain and discomfort; halitosis

Self-Concept, Disturbance in

related to:
1. Altered body image associated with: loss of ability to produce crying and laughing sounds, whistle, sing, blow nose; loss of sense of taste and smell, breathing through nose
2. Life-style changes associated with loss of ability to communicate verbally and with breathing through neck

as seen by:
Withdrawn behavior; increased dependency on others; sense of helplessness; embarassment associated with altered appearance and eating difficulties

Skin Integrity, Impairment of: Actual/Potential

related to:
1. Surgical incision, tracheostomy
2. Impaired healing of incisional area secondary to infection
3. Excoriation or breakdown of skin around stoma associated with continued contact from exudate or secretions

as seen by:
Redness, edema, unusual drainage around incisional area; increased tenderness, irritation; breakdown; elevated temperature

LONG-TERM GOAL

To maintain a patent airway for adequate respiratory functioning and achieve and use an effective communication system.

SHORT-TERM GOALS

The client with a tracheostomy/laryngectomy will be able to:

1. Verbalize purpose and indication for tracheostomy/laryngectomy, demonstrate compliance to prescribed speech rehabilitation program.
2. Verbalize S&S of complications to report to home health nurse or physician.
3. Verbalize importance of eating well-balanced meals, importance of increased hydration.
4. Identify predisposing factors to anorexia, measures to improve.
5. Demonstrate compliance with prescribed medication therapy/identify side effects.

6. Demonstrate prescribed care of stoma and skin care of neck, dressing changes.
7. Demonstrate correct oral and tracheal suctioning procedure.
8. Verbalize knowledge of good oral hygiene.
9. Demonstrate correct procedure for tracheostomy care.
10. Demonstrate correct use of prescribed medical equipment and supplies/verbalize importance of notifying electric company regarding the need for emergency power if dependent on suction machine.
11. Demonstrate compliance with prescribed respiratory therapy.
12. Demonstrate increased ambulation and participation in ADL, balanced rest periods.
13. Verbalize importance of avoiding exposure to infections, not smoking.
14. Verbalize importance of/wear Medic Alert bracelet.
15. Adapt to altered body image and changes in life-style to effectively manage and cope with tracheostomy.

NURSING ACTIONS/TREATMENTS

1. Assess cardiopulmonary status/identify complications.
2. Assess vital signs/identify trends (e.g., elevated temperature, tachycardia, increased respiratory rate).
3. Instruct on purpose and indication for tracheostomy/larygectomy, prescribed speech therapy rehabilitation program (e.g., instruct on laryngeal speech, artificial larynx, esophageal speech, various mechanical aids).
4. Instruct about importance of compliance with prescribed medical regimen, untoward S&S to report to home health nurse or physician.
5. Assess and evaluate nutritional status/instruct about balanced diet with prescribed fluid intake of 2000 to 3000 ml per day.
6. Assess anorexia associated with altered sense of smell and taste (e.g., air not passing through the nose to olfactory organs), difficulty swallowing, prescribed dietary modifications/instruct that there will be some degree of return of taste and smell, measures to stimulate (e.g., use of spices and sweetners), prescribed foods to facilitate swallowing.
7. Observe/instruct about taking medications as ordered, purpose and action, side effects/evaluate medication effectiveness.
8. Assess/instruct as to prescribed stomal and skin care of neck dressing changes, S&S of skin irritation or breakdown to report to home health nurse or physician.
9. Observe/instruct about purpose and procedure of oral and tracheal suctioning.
10. Observe and evaluate for dry mucous membrane and malodorus breath of oral cavity/instruct about good oral hygiene.
11. Observe/instruct about frequency and procedure for sterile tracheostomy care (e.g., aseptic technique, care of inner cannula, changing tracheostomy ties, cuffing, self-insertion of inner and/or outer tracheostomy tubes as prescribed),

handling of emergency situations (e.g., list emergency numbers by phone; emergency tracheostomy kit).

12. Observe/instruct about prescribed use and purpose of porous covering over stoma, measures to avoid aspiration of water and foreign materials.

13. Observe/instruct about correct use of prescribed medical equipment and supplies (e.g., suction machine, humidifier, nebulizer, tracheostomy tubes)/notify electric company of need for emergency power if dependent on suction machine.

14. Observe/instruct about prescribed respiratory therapy (e.g., chest physiotherapy, inhalation treatment)/obtain respiratory consultation as needed/evaluate respiratory functioning.

15. Observe/instruct about progressive ambulation and ADL to tolerance with balanced rest periods.

16. Observe/instruct as to importance of avoiding exposure to infections, not smoking.

17. Observe/instruct about importance of wearing Medic Alert bracelet stating "tracheostomy/neck breather."

18. Assess anxiety/identify stage of grieving associated with altered body image, changes in life-style/provide emotional support/encourage verbalization of feelings/refer to social services as ordered to assist through grieving process and provide information regarding community services to assist with support and adaptation to condition (e.g., Lost Cord Club, American Cancer Society, International Association of Laryngectomes).

REHABILITATION POTENTIAL

Rehabilitation potential *excellent good fair guarded poor* for *full partial* return to an improved level of respiratory functioning and effective speech to manage self-care and daily activities.

Client's Name _____

Medical Record # _____

ONGOING/DISCHARGE EVALUATON OF TEACHING

The Client with a Tracheostomy/Laryngectomy

Teaching Tools:

Printed materials given: _____

Audiovisual aids used: _____

Return Information/Demonstration/Interpretation

_____ Client

_____ Caregiver

OF:	Met	Not Met	Comments
☐ Purpose and indication for tracheostomy/ laryngectomy.	_____	_____	_____
☐ S&S of complications; actions to take.	_____	_____	_____
☐ Importance of compliance with prescribed treatment regimen.	_____	_____	_____
☐ Well-balanced diet, increased fluids.	_____	_____	_____
☐ Predisposing factors to anorexia; measures to correct.	_____	_____	_____
☐ Medications and administration,			

Client's Name _____

Medical Record # _____

purpose and
action, side
effects.   _____   _____   _____

☐ Tracheostomy
  care, frequency
  and procedure.   _____   _____   _____

☐ Stomal and skin
  care of neck;
  dressing
  changes.   _____   _____   _____

☐ Suction
  machine.   _____   _____   _____

☐ Humidifier.   _____   _____   _____

☐ Nebulizer.   _____   _____   _____

☐ Purpose and
  procedure for
  oral and
  tracheal
  suctioning.   _____   _____   _____

☐ Chest
  physiotherapy.   _____   _____   _____

☐ Inhalation
  treatments.   _____   _____   _____

☐ Progressive
  ambulation
  activities and
  ADL to
  tolerance with
  balanced rest
  periods.   _____   _____   _____

☐ Measures to
  promote good
  oral hygiene.   _____   _____   _____

☐ Avoiding
  exposure to

Client's Name _____

Medical Record # _____

infections, not
smoking.   _____   _____   _____

☐ Wear a Medic
Alert bracelet.   _____   _____   _____

☐ Handling of
emergency
situations.   _____   _____   _____

☐ Communication
techniques and
aids (e.g.,
laryngeal
speech, artificial
larynx, various
mechanical
aids).   _____   _____   _____

Signature of Home Health Nurse _____

Date _____

NEUROLOGIC DISORDERS

■ Alzheimer's Disease

Alzheimer's disease is an irreversible, progressive dementia that is characterized by neurofibrillary tangles, neuritic plaques, and granulovascular degeneration found throughout the cerebral cortex, especially in the frontal, parietal, and temporal lobes. The cause and cure of Alzheimer's disease is unknown but many theories and various therapies are under investigation. This disease has been found to progress in stages, with the first symptoms involving forgetfulness, inability to concentrate, and deterioration in personal appearance and hygiene. In the later stages are found extensive memory loss, deterioration in cognitive abilities and resultant psychosocial problems, speech and motor dysfunction (including urinary and fecal incontinence), and the need for total assistance with personal care and hygiene.

The care of a client with Alzheimer's disease presents a challenge to the family providing care as well as to the home health nurse in educating the family. Each stage of the disease, with its associated functional and cognitive losses, results in a continued deterioration in the client's condition and need for ongoing changes in the plan of treatment.

POTENTIAL COMPLICATIONS

1. Aspiration pneumonia,
2. malnutrition,
3. respiratory infections,
4. seizures,
5. decubitus ulcers,
6. injuries associated with inadvertently hurting self secondary to deteriorating condition (e.g., incoordinated body movements, deterioration in cognitive abilities),
7. depression.

TYPES OF CLIENTS/CLINICAL CONDITIONS SEEN BY HOME HEALTH AGENCIES

1. Newly diagnosed with Alzheimer's disease: initiation of prescribed treatment regimen and inclusive teaching plan for home-care management of a progressive degenerative disease.
2. Impairment or loss of functional skills needed to perform and daily self-care activities (e.g., mobility, dressing, feeding, grooming, and hygiene).
3. Progressive of disease process with associated deterioration in cognitive and motor functioning, development of complications: resultant changes in prescribed plan of treatment, need for instruction and supervision of caregiver, evaluation and report to physician of response to treatment changes.

RELATED NURSING DIAGNOSIS

Anxiety

related to:
1. Awareness, in early stages of the disease, things are "not quite right"
2. Impaired memory
3. Inability to concentrate

as seen by:
Verbalization that something is wrong; overexcitedness; rattled behavior; distress

Bowel Elimination, Alteration in: Constipation

related to:
1. Decreased mobility
2. Inadequate fluid and dietary fiber intake
3. Lack of awareness of need to defecate

as seen by:
Motor deficits; dehydration; malnutrition; reduced appetite; abdominal distension; confusion and disorientation, lethargy

Bowel Elimination, Alteration in: Incontinence

related to:
1. Inability to get to or find bathroom on time
2. Unable to recognize the sensation of fullness, indicating the need to defecate
3. Apathy

as seen by:
Involuntary passage of stool; lack of awareness of need to defecate; lack of motivation

Communication, Impaired Verbal

related to:
Progressive difficulty in communication resulting from deterioration in areas of cerebral cortex

as seen by:
Impaired ability to express self verbally; use of behavioral communication; anger and crying in response to simple questions; speech limited to a few words

Coping, Ineffective Individual

related to:
1. Impaired memory
2. Inability to concentrate

as seen by:
Depression and anxiety and awareness in early stages of the disease that

3. Deterioration in personal hygiene

things are "not quite right"; violent behavior

Home Maintenance Management, Impaired

related to:
Difficulty or inability of caregiver to provide full-time care in a safe home environment

as seen by:
Overtaxed caregiver in caring for client with deteriorating cognitive skills, psychosocial problems, and motor deficits

Infection, Potential for

related to:
Increased susceptibility secondary to:
1. Progressive deterioration
2. Physical disablement

as seen by:
S&S of respiratory or urinary tract infections

Injury, Potential for: Increased Risk of Falls and Injuries

related to:
1. Loss of balance and coordination
2. Lack of awareness of environmental hazards in the home

as seen by:
Impaired ability to perform purposeful movements or tasks; clumsy and incoordinated body movements, bumping into furniture

Knowledge Deficit (Specify)

related to:
1. Disease process and related S&S
2. Inadequate understanding of prescribed plan of treatment for Alzheimer's client
3. Potential complications, S&S to report to home health nurse or physician

as seen by:
Verbalization by caregiver of lack of information; inadequate understanding; inability to perform skills necessary to meet health-care needs at home

Nutrition, Alteration in: Less than Body Requirements

related to:
Inadequate oral intake

as seen by:
Forgetfulness; lack of interest in food; difficulty with eating, chewing, and swallowing; weight loss; hyperactivity

Mobility, Impaired Physical

related to:
Deterioration of areas of the cerebral cortex that involve motor functioning

as seen by:
Impairment or loss of coordination to perform purposeful movements or tasks

Oral Mucous Membrane, Alteration in

related to:
Inadequate oral hygiene secondary to resistance of oral care; decreased salivary flow as a result of side effects of drugs

as seen by:
Coated tongue; oral plague; halitosis; oral lesions or ulcers

Self-Care Deficit: Feeding, Bathing/Hygiene, Dressing/Grooming, Toileting (Specify)

related to:
Inability to initiate and perform purposeful movements and tasks

as seen by:
A deterioration in personal hygiene and appearance; difficulty putting clothes on; requiring assistance with bathing

Self-Concept, Disturbance in

related to:
1. Altered body function
2. Lowered self-esteem

as seen by:
Denial of condition; crying; anger; withdrawal from social contacts

Sensory-Perceptual Alteration

related to:
Inability to correctly recognize and interpret sensory stimuli

as seen by:
Disorientation and confusion; change in behavior pattern; difficulty recognizing familiar objects by sight or touch or to recognize sounds or words

Sleep Pattern Disturbance

related to:
1. Excessive wakefulness or agitation
2. Day-night sleep reversal

as seen by:
Disorientation and confusion; agitation; restlessness

Social Isolation

related to:
1. Lack of understanding and fear of disclosure of disease
2. Language decompensation
3. Motor and sensory deficits

as seen by:
Embarrassment to family; recognition by client "things are not quite right" (in early stages of disease) resulting in withdrawal, uncommunicativeness, undesirable behaviors

Swallowing, Impaired

related to:
Motor dysfunction

as seen by:
Coughing; choking; presence of food in mouth with evidence of inability to swallow

Thought Processes, Alteration in

related to:
Loss of memory

as seen by:
Loss of short-term memory; anxiety; altered attention span; decreased ability to grasp ideas

Urinary Elimination Pattern, Alteration in: Incontinence

related to:
Neuropsychological deficits

as seen by:
Failure to recognize the appropriate time or place to urinate, inability to recognize sensation of fullness indicating the need to micturate; inability to get to bathroom quickly enough; apathy

LONG-TERM GOAL

To assist client with Alzheimer's disease to achieve maximal functional ability and productivity while maintaining dignity and self-respect.

SHORT-TERM GOALS

The client with Alzheimer's disease, and/or caregiver, will be able to:

1. Verbalize knowledge of chronic progressive nature of disease, present extent of impairment, importance of compliance with prescribed treatment regimen, S&S of complications to report to home health nurse or physician.

2. Verbalize knowledge of importance of optimal nutritional status, familiar menu, meals served at regularly scheduled times.
3. Verbalize causative factors of decreased oral intake/demonstrate prescribed measures to establish and maintain adequate nutritional status/reduce risk of aspiration and facilitate swallowing.
4. Weigh weekly/record/report excessive weight loss to physician.
5. Verbalize prescribed measures to provide adequate nutritional status to Alzheimer's client who is hyperactive.
6. Demonstrate good oral hygiene measures.
7. Demonstrate compliance in giving medications as ordered/ensure medications are not accessible to client and are consumed when given.
8. Verbalize importance of a safe structured environment, measures to promote well-being.
9. Verbalize importance of regularly scheduled daily exercise and activities within limits of safety and ability of client.
10. Verbalize that tasks of daily living will be accomplished through the following of consistent routines, in a safe, structured environment, programmed to the needs of the client.
11. Verbalize causative factors in altered sleep patterns/demonstrate specific measures to correct.
12. Verbalize prescribed measures to manage problems with constipation.
13. Demonstrate specific measures related to routine, consistent toileting in maintenance of bowel and bladder elimination.
14. Demonstrate follow-through with established home therapy program for management of self-care deficits, functional limitations, problems with dysphagia and ineffective communication patterns.
15. Demonstrate effective coping skills in management of the progressive debilitating effects of Alzheimer's disease and obtain assistance from community resources to help with care.

NURSING ACTIONS/TREATMENTS

1. Assess neurologic status/identify progressive losses in motor, sensory, cognitive functions.
2. Assess vital signs/identify trends (e.g., elevated temperature, increased pulse rate).
3. Assess and evaluate degree of assistance (human or mechanical) needed to aid and protect client.
4. Instruct as to nature of disease, progressive course/present extent of impairment, importance of compliance with prescribed treatment regimen, S&S of complications to report to home health nurse or physician.
5. Observe/instruct as to importance of optimal nutritional status, familiar menus, meals given at regularly scheduled times.

6. Assess/instruct as to causes of decreased oral intake (e.g., unable to manage knife and fork, eating and chewing difficulties, dysphagia), measures to reduce risk of aspiration and facilitate easier swallowing (e.g., give finger foods, semisoft diet, place client in high Fowler's position with head forward with meals and for one half hour following).
7. Assess and evaluate for weight loss, instruct to weigh and record weekly/report excessive weight loss to physician.
8. Assess and evaluate nutritional status of hyperactive client/instruct about prescribed high-caloric diet with between-meal supplements, adequate hydration, avoiding stimulants (e.g., caffeine).
9. Assess and evaluate for resistance to oral hygiene, impairment of oral mucous membrane and gums/instruct about importance of oral health to general comfort and appetite and about alternative measures to provide oral care (e.g., use of swabs with diluted hydrogen peroxide).
10. Observe/instruct about safety measures with medication therapy (e.g., caregiver gives as prescribed, knows purpose and action, side effects, stores medications out of reach/sees that consumed when given)/evaluate medication effectiveness.
11. Instruct caregiver in importance of a safe, structured environment that allows client involvement in ADL (assists in maintaining self-esteem).
12. Observe/instruct as to prescribed program of regularly scheduled activities based on specific needs of client (e.g., reality orientation, resocialization, remotivation, personal hygiene).
13. Observe/instruct about regularly scheduled daily exercises and activities, use of prescribed assistive devices as needed within limits of safety and ability.
14. Observe/instruct measures to promote well-being of client (e.g., safe environment, use of memory aids, avoidance of stressful tasks, measures to avoid inadvertently injuring self as a result of incoordinated body movements).
15. Assess and evaluate causative factors of altered rest patterns/instruct about specific measures to promote sleep (e.g., exercise and activities during the day).
16. Assess constipation problems/instruct about prescribed increase in dietary fiber and fluids, activities/evaluate effectiveness of bowel regimen.
17. Assess and evaluate alterations in elimination patterns/instruct about bowel and bladder elimination program, through routine consistent toileting, for management of incontinence.
18. Observe and evaluate alterations in self-care activities, functional skills, dysphagia, speech deficits/refer to rehabilitative services as ordered to provide instruction and establish home program in handling of chewing and swallowing difficulties, maintaining effective communication patterns, daily exercises to maintain muscle strength and joint motion, management of gait and balance problems to protect from physical injury.
19. Assess psychosocial problems, sexual behavior that violates social norms, sexual needs, violent behavior/instruct about daily goals and plan of action in

care of client/refer to social services as ordered to explore alternatives of care, to assist client and caregiver to cope with disease, and to provide information regarding support groups in the community (e.g., Alzheimer's Disease and Related Disorders Association, counseling services, attendant services).

REHABILITATION POTENTIAL

Rehabilitation potential *excellent good fair guarded poor* for *full partial* return to an improved level of productivity and contact with reality; will always need assistance with daily activities and following of prescribed home-care treatment regimen.

Client's Name _____

Medical Record # _____

ONGOING/DISCHARGE EVALUATION OF TEACHING
The Client with Alzheimer's Disease

Teaching Tools:
Printed materials given: _____

Audiovisual aids used: _____

Return Information/Demonstration/Interpretation
_____ Client
_____ Caregiver

	OF:	Met	Not Met	Comments
☐	Nature of progressive course of disease; effect on motor, sensory, and cognitive functions.	_____	_____	_____
☐	S&S of complications; actions to take.	_____	_____	_____
☐	Importance of compliance with prescribed treatment regimen.	_____	_____	_____
☐	Safe, structured environment for client participation in ADL.	_____	_____	_____
☐	Weigh weekly; record; report excessive			

Client's Name ⎯⎯⎯⎯⎯⎯⎯⎯⎯⎯⎯⎯⎯⎯⎯⎯

Medical Record # ⎯⎯⎯⎯⎯⎯⎯⎯⎯⎯⎯⎯⎯⎯

weight loss to
physician. ⎯⎯⎯ ⎯⎯⎯ ⎯⎯⎯⎯⎯⎯⎯⎯⎯⎯⎯⎯⎯

☐ Well-balanced
diet of familiar
menus, given at
regularly
scheduled
times. ⎯⎯⎯ ⎯⎯⎯ ⎯⎯⎯⎯⎯⎯⎯⎯⎯⎯⎯⎯⎯

☐ Measures to
improve
decreased oral
intake. ⎯⎯⎯ ⎯⎯⎯ ⎯⎯⎯⎯⎯⎯⎯⎯⎯⎯⎯⎯⎯

☐ Measures to
avoid aspiration
and facilitate
swallowing. ⎯⎯⎯ ⎯⎯⎯ ⎯⎯⎯⎯⎯⎯⎯⎯⎯⎯⎯⎯⎯

☐ High-caloric
diet, between-
meal
supplements,
adequate
hydration, no
stimulants for
hyperactive
client. ⎯⎯⎯ ⎯⎯⎯ ⎯⎯⎯⎯⎯⎯⎯⎯⎯⎯⎯⎯⎯

☐ Medications
and
administration,
purpose and
action, side
effects, use of
safety
principles with
administration. ⎯⎯⎯ ⎯⎯⎯ ⎯⎯⎯⎯⎯⎯⎯⎯⎯⎯⎯⎯⎯

☐ Oral hygiene
measures. ⎯⎯⎯ ⎯⎯⎯ ⎯⎯⎯⎯⎯⎯⎯⎯⎯⎯⎯⎯⎯

☐ Importance of
establishing
regularly

Client's Name _____

Medical Record #_____

scheduled daily
exercises and
activities; use
of prescribed
assistive
devices within
limits of safety
and ability.   _____   _____   _____

☐ Reality
   orientation.   _____   _____   _____

☐ Resocialization.   _____   _____   _____

☐ Remotivation.   _____   _____   _____

☐ Measures to
   promote well-
   being of client:
   safe
   environment,
   use of memory
   aids, avoidance
   of stressful
   tasks, measures
   to avoid
   inadvertently
   injuring self.   _____   _____   _____

☐ Measures to
   avoid
   constipation
   and promote
   good bowel
   functioning.   _____   _____   _____

☐ Bowel and
   bladder
   program.   _____   _____   _____

☐ Measures to
   promote sleep.   _____   _____   _____

☐ Measures to
   manage
   ineffective

Client's Name _____

Medical Record # _____

communication
patterns.   _____   _____   _____

_____

Signature of Home Health Nurse _____

Date _____

■ Cerebrovascular Accident

Cerebrovascular accident (CVA) is an impairment in the cerebral circulation resulting in ischemia and neurologic deficits. The severity of damage and associated disturbances in function following a vascular occlusion or hemorrhage will depend on the site of the lesion and adequacy of collateral circulation. There are many factors that may be responsible for impairments in cerebral circulation resulting in a CVA, the most common being atherosclerosis with the formation of a thrombus, an embolism, and hypertensive intracerebral hemorrhage.

CVAs may be grouped in major categories according to their course of activity and extent of neurologic loss:

1. A transient ischemic attack (TIA) results from a temporary interruption of blood flow to focal brain areas, resulting in a short period of impaired neurologic function. A TIA usually lasts a few minutes and clears within 12 to 24 hours. Signs and symptoms are related to the site and degree of occlusion (e.g., hemiparesis, unilateral loss of vision, speech disturbances, staggering or uncoordinated gait).
2. A stroke in evolution is a progressive development of neurologic deficits secondary to increasing cerebral ischemia, which continues to worsen over a few days and may lead to an infarction.
3. A completed stroke results from prolonged ischemia and is characterized by neurologic deficits that are maximal at onset and show little improvement after 1 to 3 days.

POTENTIAL COMPLICATIONS

1. Atelectasis,
2. pneumonia,
3. increasing sensory and motor deficits,
4. seizure activity,
5. spasticity, contractures, injury from falls, etc., related to diminished or impaired mobility status,
6. decubitus ulcers,
7. depression.

TYPES OF CLIENTS/CLINICAL CONDITIONS SEEN BY HOME HEALTH AGENCIES

1. Recent CVA (within last 60 days) with numerous neurologic deficits: initiation of intensive treatment, teaching, rehabilitation program (e.g., bowel and bladder training, therapy services for loss of functional skills and speech deficits).
2. Extension of CVA, or small stroke syndrome, with new or progressive development of existing neurologic deficits and deterioration in motor function.

3. CVA within the past year now presenting with complications: changes in on-going plan of treatment and/or initiation of new treatment interventions, instruction, observation of response to therapy.

RELATED NURSING DIAGNOSIS

Activity Intolerance

related to:
Immobility secondary to paralysis

as seen by:
Fatigue with daily activities; weakness; dyspnea; abnormal heart rate or BP in response to activity

Anxiety

related to:
1. Effects of sensory and motor deficits on the quality of life
2. Knowledge deficit regarding prescribed treatment regimen in psychological and physical rehabilitation

as seen by:
Frustration and despair; irritability; verbalization of fears; increased dependency on others for care

Bowel Elimination, Alteration in: Constipation

related to:
1. Decreased activities secondary to paralysis
2. Inadequate fluids and dietary fiber
3. Impaired ability to communicate need to defecate

as seen by:
Anorexia; frequency and amount of stool, less than usual pattern; hard, formed stools; abdominal distention; failure to respond to urge to defecate

Bowel Elimination, Alteration in: Incontinence

related to:
1. Loss of sphincter control secondary to neuromuscular deficit
2. Altered cognitive and perceptual abilities
3. Impaired ability to communicate need to defecate
4. Impaired ability to ambulate to the bathroom unassisted

as seen by:
Involuntary passage of stool; failure to recognize appropriate time or place to defecate; inability to inform family of need to defecate; need to wait to be assisted to bathroom because of paralysis

Communication, Impaired Verbal

related to:
Aphasia, dysarthria secondary to
   cerebral impairment

as seen by:
Inability to speak; difficulty in
   expressing, understanding, or a
   combination of both; difficulty with
   articulation

Coping, Ineffective Individual

related to:
1. Emotional instability
2. Impaired ability to communicate
   verbally
3. Alterations in body image
   secondary to motor and sensory
   deficits
4. Life-style changes

as seen by:
Irritability; fatigue; lack of follow-
   through with activities;
   communicating inability to cope

Grieving

related to:
1. Altered body image and effect on
   future role performance and life-
   style
2. Having to give up control of self-
   care activities to others

as seen by:
Denial, anger, depression; changes in
   eating habits and sleep patterns

Infection, Potential for

related to:
Increased susceptibility secondary to:
1. Immobility
2. Poor nutritional status
3. Indwelling urinary catheter

as seen by:
S&S of respiratory or urinary tract
   infections

Injury, Potential for: Increased Risk of Falls and Injuries

related to:
1. Visual deficits
2. Spatial-perceptual deficits
3. Decreased awareness of
   environmental hazards in the home

as seen by:
Weakness and fatigue; poor vision;
   impairment or loss of coordination
   to perform purposeful tasks;
   balancing difficulties; reduced

secondary to altered cognitive and perceptual abilities

4. Motor deficits

temperature and/or tactile sensation; altered cognitive and perceptual abilities

Knowledge Deficit (Specify)

related to:
1. Inadequate understanding of cerebrovascular disease
2. Prescribed plan of treatment in management and adjustment to neurologic deficits and psychological rehabilitation
3. Potential complications, S&S to report to home health nurse or physician

as seen by:
Expressed concern for lack of information, inadequate understanding; inability to perform skills necessary to meet health-care needs at home

Mobility, Impaired Physical

related to:
Motor and sensory deficits

as seen by:
Incoordination; unsteady gait; decreased muscle strength, control, and/or endurance; paralysis of extremities

Nutrition, Alteration in: Less than Body Requirements

related to:
1. Dysphagia
2. Impaired ability to feed self
3. Anorexia
4. Inability to acquire food as a result of physical deficits

as seen by:
Weight 20 percent or more below ideal for age, height, and frame; generalized weakness; repeated inadequate food intake; choking during meals; drooling

Powerlessness, Feelings of

related to:
Paralysis and dependency on others to meet needs

as seen by:
Apathy; anger; irritability; passivity; crying; expression of inability to perform self-care and daily activities

Self-Care Deficit, Alteration in: Feeding, Bathing/Hygiene, Dressing/Grooming, Toileting (Specify)

related to:
1. Activity intolerance

as seen by:
Decreased or lack of ability to meet

2. Neuromuscular impairments affecting mobility status
3. Perceptual or cognitive impairments
4. Depression

personal needs associated with weakness and fatigue; decreased endurance; decreased muscle strength; paralysis of extremities; visual disturbances; spatial-perceptual deficits; disorientation or confusion; altered activity level with depression

Self-Concept, Disturbance in

related to:
1. Changes in body image
2. Low self-esteem
3. Life-style and role changes

as seen by:
Signs of grieving; withdrawal from social contacts; self-neglect; change in usual patterns of responsibility

Sensory-Perceptual Alteration

related to:
Inability to correctly recognize and interpret sensory stimuli secondary to neurologic alterations

as seen by:
Disorientation; cognitive alterations; decreased visual acuity; spatial-perceptual deficits

Skin Integrity, Impairment of: Potential

related to:
1. Prolonged bed rest or immobilization
2. Altered nutritional status

as seen by:
Reddened or irritated areas over bony prominences; edema; tissue breakdown

Social Isolation

related to:
Changes in body appearance and body functioning

as seen by:
Lack of communication; withdrawn behavior; expressed feelings of rejection and loss of purpose

Urinary Elimination Pattern, Alteration in: Incontinence

related to:
1. Altered cognitive and perceptual abilities
2. Impaired ability to communicate need to urinate or ambulate to the bathroom.
3. Upper motor neuron lesion with loss of cerebral motor control

as seen by:
Failure to recognize the appropriate time or place to urinate; frequent and uncontrolled micturition

LONG-TERM GOAL

To achieve optimal level of health and functioning through restoring and/or maintaining motor, sensory, and cognitive function affected by vascular lesion in the brain.

SHORT-TERM GOALS

The client with a cerebrovascular accident will be able to:

1. Verbalize nature of disease process, type of CVA, risk factors, importance of compliance with prescribed treatment regimen, S&S of new or recurring problems to report to home health nurse or physician.
2. Demonstrate compliance with prescribed diet, dietary restrictions, adequate hydration.
3. Demonstrate prescribed measures to assist client with problems related to dysphagia, chewing and feeding difficulties.
4. Verbalize purpose of nutritional supplements.
5. Weigh weekly/record/report excessive weight loss to physician.
6. Demonstrate compliance with prescribed medication therapy/identify side effects, toxicity.
7. Verbalize importance/demonstrate compliance with prescribed anticoagulant therapy, safety factors with taking, adverse reactions to report to physician, measures to control any bleeding.
8. Verbalize importance of prescribed blood coagulation studies and other diagnostic lab work.
9. Demonstrate compliance with prescribed exercise program and planned rest periods.
10. Identify risk factors for falls and injuries, safety measures with ambulation and daily activities.
11. Demonstrate progressive ambulation and self-care activities with use of unaffected side and use of ambulatory aids and self-help devices.
12. Demonstrate compliance with prescribed measures in care of immobilized client.
13. Verbalize predisposing factors to constipation, specific measures to improve bowel functioning.
14. Demonstrate compliance with prescribed bowel and bladder program.
15. Demonstrate catheter care and management as prescribed.
16. Demonstrate compliance with speech therapy program for maximized communication skills.
17. Demonstrate compliance with prescribed physical and occupational therapy programs for alterations in functional skills and self-care activities.
18. Demonstrate effective coping mechanisms to adapt to altered body image and changes in life-style.

NURSING ACTIONS/TREATMENTS

1. Assess neurologic status/identify residual deficits in motor, sensory or congitive function.
2. Assess vital signs/identify changes indicating increased intracranial pressure/(e.g., elevation in BP and slowing of pulse) report to physician.
3. Instruct as to nature of disease process, type of CVA, risk factors (e.g., hypertension, diabetes, heart disease, obesity), premonitory symptoms, importance of compliance with prescribed treatment regimen, S&S of complications to report to home health nurse or physician.
4. Assess and evaluate nutritional status/instruct about prescribed diet, dietary restrictions (e.g., sodium, saturated fats), importance of adequate hydration.
5. Assess and evaluate factors contributing to altered nutritional status (e.g., dysphagia, chewing and feeding difficulties associated with motor and sensory deficits, anorexia)/instruct about measures to reduce risk of aspiration (e.g., place client in high Fowler's position with head forward at meals and one half hour after eating, prescribed soft or semi-soft foods), use of self-help devices, measures specific to client to correct anorexia.
6. Assess and evaluate for weight loss/instruct to weigh weekly or more often as needed/record/report excessive weight loss to physician.
7. Observe/instruct as to importance of taking prescribed nutritional supplements.
8. Observe/instruct about taking of medications as ordered, purpose, action, side effects, toxicity/evaluate medication effectiveness.
9. Observe/instruct about prescribed anticoagulant therapy, safety precautions to reduce risk of bleeding (e.g., avoid aspirin or aspirin-containing products, avoid trauma with daily activities, avoid enemas and hard-bristled toothbrushes), adverse reactions to report to physician (e.g., bleeding from nose or gums, bruises and petechiae)/educate regarding measures to control bleeding (e.g., apply firm pressure for 10 minutes).
10. Monitor/instruct as to purpose of prescribed blood coagulation studies and other diagnostic lab work.
11. Observe/instruct as to consistent exercise program, passive range of motion to affected extremities, planned rest periods.
12. Assess and evaluate decreased level of consciousness, visual, spatial-perceptual, and motor function disturbances/instruct as to safety measures with ambulation and daily activities to reduce risk of falls and injuries (e.g., home environment free of hazards, providing assistance to client in daily activities as needed).
13. Observe/instruct as to progressive ambulation and self-care activities with use of unaffected side, use of prescribed ambulatory aids and self-help devices.
14. Observe/instruct as to care of immobilized client (e.g., positioning with changes, alignment of extremities, ROM exercises, skin care, proper use of "elastic stockings").
15. Assess predisposing factors to constipation/instruct about prescribed increase

in fluids and dietary fiber, ability levels, establishing consistent time for defecation, method for dysphagia client to communicate need to defecate, use of prescribed laxatives and stool softeners, avoiding straining at stool/evaluate effectiveness of bowel regimen.

16. Observe/instruct about prescribed bowel and bladder training program for incontinence/evaluate effectiveness of program.

17. Observe/instruct in care and management of indwelling urinary catheter as prescribed.

18. Observe and evaluate alterations in functional skills, self-care activities/refer to rehabilitative services as ordered to establish and instruct in home therapy program (e.g., occupational therapy: energy conservation techniques, sensory stimulation, muscle reeducation, perceptual motor training and eye-hand coordination exercises, self-care training; physical therapy: problems with ambulation, motor control, transfers, use of ambulatory aids, contractures, spasticity).

19. Assess and evaluate impairments in verbal communication/instruct about measures to communicate with client/refer to speech therapy as ordered.

20. Provide psychological and emotional support/instruct on episodes of emotional lability, appropriate coping mechanisms/refer to social services to assist with grieving process associated with feelings of inadequacy and rejection with altered body image/provide information on community services to assist with adjustment to CVA (e.g., local support groups, counseling services, Stroke Club International, the National Institute for Neurological and Communicative Disorder and Stroke, National Easter Seals Society).

REHABILITATION POTENTIAL

Rehabilitation potential *excellent good fair guarded poor* for *full partial* return to an improved level of neurologic functioning to manage ADL.

Client's Name _____

Medical Record # _____

ONGOING/DISCHARGE EVALUATION OF TEACHING

The Client with a Cerebrovascular Accident

Teaching Tools:

Printed materials given: _____

Audiovisual aids used: _____

Return Information/Demonstration/Interpretation

_____ Client

_____ Caregiver

OF:	Met	Not Met	Comments
☐ Nature of disease process; type of CVA; risk factors; premonitory symptoms.	_____	_____	_____
☐ S&S of complications; actions to take.	_____	_____	_____
☐ Importance of compliance with prescribed treatment regimen.	_____	_____	_____
☐ Diet; dietary restrictions; adequate hydration.	_____	_____	_____
☐ Weigh weekly; record; report excessive weight loss to physician.	_____	_____	_____

Client's Name _____

Medical Record #_____

☐ Measures to
manage
problems with:
dysphagia,
chewing
difficulties,
feeding
difficulties.   _____   _____   _____

☐ Measures to
avoid
aspiration.   _____   _____   _____

☐ Nutritional
supplements.   _____   _____   _____

☐ Anticoagulant
therapy; safety
precautions to
avoid bleeding;
adverse
reactions to
report to
physician;
measures to
control any
bleeding.   _____   _____   _____

☐ Purpose of
periodic blood
coagulation
studies and
other diagnostic
lab work.   _____   _____   _____

☐ Medications
and
administration,
purpose and
action, side
effects, toxicity.   _____   _____   _____

☐ Consistent
exercise
program;
passive ROM
exercises to
affected

Client's Name _____

Medical Record #_____

extremities;
planned rest
periods.   _____   _____   _____

☐   Risk factors for
falls and
injuries in
home; safety
measures with
ambulation and
daily activities.   _____   _____   _____

☐   Safe transfer
activities.   _____   _____   _____

☐   Progressive
ambulation and
self-care
activities with
use of
unaffected side.   _____   _____   _____

☐   Energy
conservation
techniques.   _____   _____   _____

☐   Ambulatory
aids; self-help
devices.   _____   _____   _____

☐   Measures to
manage
communication
deficits.   _____   _____   _____

☐   Measures in
care of
immobilized
client.   _____   _____   _____

☐   Measures to
avoid
constipation,
promote good
bowel
functioning.   _____   _____   _____

Client's Name _____

Medical Record # _____

☐   Bowel and
bladder training
program.   _____   _____   _____

☐   Indwelling
urinary
catheter.   _____   _____   _____

Signature of Home Health Nurse _____

Date _____

■ Multiple Sclerosis

Multiple sclerosis is a progressive degenerative disease characterized by patches of demyelination of the white matter of the brain and spinal cord. This is followed by areas of scarring, with plaque formation and interference with transmission of impulses. Multiple sclerosis may be acute or chronic, characterized by unpredictable exacerbations and remissions. Areas of involvement are most often associated with lesions in the pyramidal tracts and posterior columns of the cord, around the ventricles of the brain, in the optic nerves, and in the pons and medulla and cerebellum.

The cause of multiple sclerosis is unknown, but theories suggest a viral infection or an autoimmunologic reaction affecting the nervous system. Because the disease affects various parts of the nervous system, clinical manifestations are related to the areas of involved nerve segments. Early symptoms are usually transitory and include fatigue, numbness and paresthesias, and visual problems such as decreased visual acuity, altered color perception, or blurred vision. As the disease progresses, motor weakness or paralysis of extremities, alteration in coordination and gait, bowel and bladder changes and mood alterations may be seen. Heat exposure exacerbates and cold exposure improves nerve conduction in these patients.

POTENTIAL COMPLICATIONS

1. Atelectasis,
2. pneumonia,
3. motor and sensory deficits,
4. renal calculi,
5. urinary tract infections,
6. decubitus ulcers.

TYPES OF CLIENTS/CLINICAL CONDITIONS SEEN BY HOME HEALTH AGENCIES

1. Newly diagnosed with multiple sclerosis: initiation of prescribed treatment regimen and inclusive teaching plan for home-care management of a progressive degenerative disease.
2. Impairment or loss of functional skills needed to perform ADL, self-care activitites (e.g., mobility, dressing, feeding, grooming and hygiene): establishment of and instruction in prescribed home-rehabilitation program.
3. Exacerbation of disease process with greater areas of neurologic impairment and loss: changes in ongoing plan of treatment, instruction in and supervision of new treatments, observation of response to therapy.
4. Recent hospitalization following complications associated with multiple sclerosis: new or changed home-care orders for management of condition.

RELATED NURSING DIAGNOSIS

Activity Intolerance

related to:
Immobility secondary to motor and
sensory deficits

as seen by:
Weakness and fatigue; abnormal BP,
heart, respiratory rate in response to
activities

Anxiety

related to:
1. Effects of sensory and motor
deficits on the quality of life
2. Altered body image and role
relationships
3. Increased dependency on others for
care
4. Knowledge deficit regarding
prescribed treatment regimen

as seen by:
Increased helplessness and dependency
on family to meet personal needs;
feelings of inadequacy; fear of total
disability; verbalized concerns

Bowel Elimination, Alteration in: Constipation

related to:
1. Spinal cord involvement
2. Decreased activity levels secondary
to loss of motor and sensory
functioning
3. Inadequate nutritional status
4. Side effect of medications

as seen by:
Having to wait after urge to defecate
for assistance to bathroom; straining
at stool; frequent desire to defecate
but without results; abdominal
distension seen with spinal cord
lesion

Bowel Elimination, Alteration in: Incontinence

related to:
Sphincter control disorder secondary to
neuromuscular deficits

as seen by:
Involuntary passage of stool

Breathing Pattern, Ineffective

related to:
1. Decreased energy or fatigue
2. Loss of adequate ventilation
secondary to neuromuscular
impairment

as seen by:
Shortness of breath; dyspnea on
exertion; respiratory depth changes,
verbalized decreased energy or
fatigue

Communication, Impaired Verbal

related to:
Speech disturbances secondary to cerebellar damage

as seen by:
Slow, scanning speech; low-pitched voice

Coping, Ineffective Individual

related to:
1. Progressive loss of functional abilities
2. Altered self-image and/or life-style changes

as seen by:
Inability to meet basic needs; chronic fatigue; general irritability

Grieving

related to:
1. Unpredictable occurrence of remissions and exacerbations
2. Loss of motor and sensory functioning
3. Effects on quality of life

as seen by:
Denial; anger; depression; frustration; despair

Infection, Potential for

related to:
Increased susceptibility secondary to:
1. Indwelling urinary catheter
2. Aspiration
3. Immobility
4. Ineffective breathing patterns

as seen by:
S&S of urinary or respiratory, infections.

Injury, Potential for: Increased Risk of Falls and Injuries

related to:
1. Sensory and visual losses
2. Spastic weakness of extremities
3. Cerebellar ataxia

as seen by:
Diminished perception of temperature, touch, and position sense; visual disturbances; impaired mobility; weakness and fatigue

Knowledge Deficit (Specify)

related to:
1. Disease process, related S&S
2. Inadequate understanding of

as seen by:
Verbalization of lack of information; inadequate understanding; inability

prescribed plan of treatment for multiple sclerosis client

3. Potential complications, S&S to report to home health nurse or physician

to perform skills necessary to meet health-care needs at home

Mobility, Impaired Physical

related to:
1. Activity intolerance
2. Changes in muscular coordination and gait
3. Muscle weakness and spasticity associated with cerebellar and motor nerve tract lesions

as seen by:
Exertional dyspnea; unsteady gait; spasticity; incoordination; intention tremors; paraparesis; weakness of extremities

Nutrition, Alteration in: Less than Body Requirements

related to:
1. Dysphagia
2. Altered ability to feed self

as seen by:
Body weight 20 percent under ideal weight for height, frame, and age; decreased energy levels; chewing and swallowing difficulties; inability to eat unless assisted

Self-Care Deficit: Feeding, Bathing/Hygiene, Dressing/Grooming, Toileting (Specify)

related to:
1. Sensory and motor deficits
2. Activity intolerance
3. Impaired mobility

as seen by:
Decreased or lack of ability to meet daily physical needs, associated with weakness and fatigue; muscle weakness and spasticity; changes in muscular coordination and gait

Self-Concept, Disturbance in

related to:
1. Loss of self-esteem
2. Changes in appearance and body functioning
3. Increased dependency on others to meet physical needs

as seen by:
Signs of grieving; refusal to participate in prescribed treatments and care; unwillingness to discuss limitations; withdrawal

Sensory-Perceptual Alteration

related to:
1. Visual disturbances
2. Sensory loss

as seen by:
Diplopia; blurred vision; nystagmus; impairment in hand-eye coordinated movements with ADL

Skin Integrity, Impairment of: Potential

related to:
1. Immobility
2. Inadequate nutritional status
3. Sensory loss

as seen by:
Reddened, irritated areas over bony prominences; tissue breakdown: injuries sustained by skin (e.g., thermal injury)

Urinary Elimination Pattern, Alteration in: Incontinence or Retention

related to:
1. Weakness of bladder wall musculature
2. Sphincter control disorder secondary to lesions in the corticospinal tract

as seen by:
Inability to control urine; frequency, urgency; bladder distension; overflow incontinence; retention; hesitancy

LONG-TERM GOAL

To shorten exacerbations of the disease process and achieve greater productivity and independence within limitations imposed by neurologic deficits.

SHORT-TERM GOALS

The client with multiple sclerosis will be able to:

1. Verbalize the progressive degenerative nature of disease, factors that precipitate exacerbations, S&S and complications to report to home health nurse or physician.
2. Verbalize importance of well-balanced diet, prescribed high dietary fiber, semisolid foods, fluids of 2000 to 3000 ml per day/demonstrate measures to assist with eating difficulties and avoid aspiration.
3. Weigh weekly/record/report excessive weight loss to physician.

4. Demonstrate compliance with prescribed medication therapy/identify side effects, toxicity.
5. Demonstrate compliance with regular daily exercise program with balanced rest periods, safe ambulatory activities with ambulatory aids, self-help devices, braces and/or splints.
6. Demonstrate increased participation in ADL and self-care activities within limitations of disease and treatment regimen.
7. Demonstrate compliance with prescribed bowel and bladder training program.
8. Verbalize importance of increased fluids for urinary functioning.
9. Demonstrate good skin care measures/verbalize factors predisposing to breakdown.
10. Demonstrate diaphragmatic, pursed-lip breathing exercises.
11. Demonstrate prescribed measures to facilitate emptying of bladder with urinary retention problems.
12. Verbalize prescribed measures to manage problems with constipation.
13. Verbalize complications of prolonged immobility, S&S to report to home health nurse or physician, prescribed measures for treatment, activities to avoid.
14. Demonstrate self-protection measures with sensory impairments to reduce risk of falls and injuries.
15. Verbalize importance of avoiding exposure to infections, S&S of illness to report to home health nurse or physician.
16. Demonstrate prescribed measures to manage visual disturbances.
17. Demonstrate compliance with speech exercises and correct use of prescribed communication devices.
18. Verbalize understanding of episodes of emotional lability, importance of setting of daily goals/demonstrate effective coping mechanisms.
19. Demonstrate effective energy conservation techniques, safe ambulatory and transfer activities.

NURSING ACTIONS/TREATMENTS

1. Assess neurologic and musculoskeletal status: identify deficits in motor, sensory, or cognitive functioning.
2. Assess vital signs, cardiopulmonary status/identify complications.
3. Instruct as to the progressive degenerative nature of disease, factors that precipitate exacerbations (e.g., fatigue, infection, temperature extremes, stress), importance of compliance with prescribed treatment regimen, S&S and complications to report to home health nurse or physician.
4. Assess and evaluate nutritional status (e.g., effect of dysphagia and tremors on eating)/instruct as to well-balanced diet, semi-solid foods, prescribed increase in dietary fiber, fluids of 2000 to 3000 ml per day, measures to assist with eating difficulties/avoiding aspirations.

5. Observe and evaluate weight loss/instruct to weigh weekly or more often as needed/record/report excessive weight loss to physician.

6. Observe/instruct as to taking of medications as ordered (e.g., cholinergics, anticholinergics, corticosteroids, antispasmodics, antidepressants, vitamin B), purpose and action, side effects, toxicity/evaluate medication effectiveness.

7. Assess and evaluate degree of muscle weakness and incoordination/instruct about regular daily exercise program with balanced rest periods, safe transfer activities, ambulatory activities with ambulatory aids, self-help devices, braces and/or splints.

8. Observe/instruct as to ADL and self-care activities within limitations of disease and treatment regimen.

9. Assess alterations in elimination pattern: bowel and bladder incontinence/instruct in prescribed bowel and bladder training program/evaluate effectiveness of program.

10. Assess/instruct about importance of fluid intake of 2000 to 3000 ml per day, effect on urinary functioning (e.g., decreased risk of urinary tract infections and of formation of renal calculi).

11. Observe and evaluate skin condition/instruct about good skin care, predisposing factors to breakdown.

12. Observe/instruct about diaphragmatic, pursed-lip breathing exercises.

13. Assess and evaluate urinary retention problems/instruct about prescribed measures to facilitate emptying of bladder (e.g., intermittent catheterization, self-catheterization, Credé's maneuvers).

14. Assess constipation problems/instruct about prescribed use of suppositories, stool softeners, laxatives, importance of increased activity levels, high-fiber foods, increased fluids/evaluate effectiveness of bowel regimen.

15. Assess and evaluate systems of the body for complications related to prolonged immobility/instruct about S&S to report to home health nurse or physician, prescribed measures to treat, activities to avoid.

16. Assess and evaluate sensory impairments/instruct as to self-protection measures in home environment to avoid skin trauma (e.g., avoiding temperature extremes).

17. Observe/instruct to avoid exposure to infections, S&S of illness to report to home health nurse or physician.

18. Assess and evaluate visual disturbances (diplopia, blurred vision, nystagmus)/instruct about prescribed measures for maximal visual functioning (e.g., wearing an eye patch or frosted lens for diplopia, large-print books).

19. Assess and evaluate dysphagia, communication deficits (e.g., dysarthria, low-pitched voice)/refer to speech therapy as needed to instruct about "swallowing" or "dysphagia training," use of communication devices, speech exercises.

20. Observe and evaluate alterations in functional skills, ambulatory activities/refer to physical and occupational therapy to instruct about energy

conservation techniques, safe ambulatory and transfer activities, correct use of ambulatory aids and self-help devices, braces and/or splints.

21. Assess coping mechanisms/provide psychological and emotional support/instruct regarding episodes of emotional lability, to define goals, answer questions regarding sexual problems/refer to social services as ordered to provide counseling and information regarding needed community resources (e.g., National Multiple Sclerosis Society, counseling services, transportation services, Meals on Wheels).

REHABILITATION POTENTIAL

Rehabilitation potential *excellent good fair guarded poor* for *full partial* achievement of an optimal level of independence and productivity to manage self-care and daily activities.

Client's Name _____

Medical Record # _____

ONGOING/DISCHARGE EVALUATION OF TEACHING
The Client with Multiple Sclerosis

Teaching Tools:
Printed materials given: _____

Audiovisual aids used: _____

Return Information/Demonstration/Interpretation
_____ Client
_____ Caregiver

OF:	Met	Not Met	Comments
☐ Progressive, degenerative nature of disease; effects of demyelination on motor, sensory, and cognitive functioning; factors that precipitate exacerbations.	_____	_____	_____
☐ S&S of complications; actions to take.	_____	_____	_____
☐ Importance of compliance with prescribed treatment regimen.	_____	_____	_____
☐ Well-balanced diet of semisolid foods; increase			

Client's Name _____

Medical Record # _____

in dietary fiber
and fluids. _____ _____ _____

☐ Dysphagia;
measures to
assist with
eating
difficulties and
avoid
aspirations. _____ _____ _____

☐ Weigh weekly;
record; report
excessive
weight loss to
physician. _____ _____ _____

☐ Medications
and
administration,
purpose and
action, side
effects, toxicity. _____ _____ _____

☐ Exercise
program with
balanced rest
periods. _____ _____ _____

☐ Energy
conservation
techniques. _____ _____ _____

☐ Safe transfer
and ambulatory
activities. _____ _____ _____

☐ Ambulatory
aids; self-help
devices; braces
and splints. _____ _____ _____

☐ ADL and self-
care activities
within client's
limitations. _____ _____ _____

Client's Name _____

Medical Record # _____

☐ Bowel and bladder training program. _____ _____ _____

☐ Effect of increased fluids on urinary functioning. _____ _____ _____

☐ Good skin-care measures; factors predisposing to breakdown. _____ _____ _____

☐ Diaphragmatic, pursed-lip breathing exercises. _____ _____ _____

☐ Measures to manage urinary retention problems (e.g., intermittent catheterization, Credé's maneuvers, self-catheterization). _____ _____ _____

☐ Measures to manage constipation problems. _____ _____ _____

☐ Complications of prolonged immobilization; treatment measures; activities to avoid. _____ _____ _____

☐ Self-protection measures with

Client's Name _____

Medical Record #_____

sensory
impairments to
reduce risk of
falls and
injuries.   _____   _____   _____

☐   Measures to
     manage visual
     disturbances.   _____   _____   _____

☐   Measures to
     avoid exposure
     to infections.   _____   _____   _____

☐   Measures to
     manage
     communication
     deficits.   _____   _____   _____

Signature of Home Health Nurse _____

Date _____

■ Parkinson's Disease

Parkinson's disease is a slowly progressive disease that results from a widespread destruction of cells and tracts in the substantia nigra, corpus striatum, and other subcortical structures in the brain concerned with motor function. It is associated with a deficiency of dopamine, a catecholamine that is needed for neurotransmission at the basal ganglia. An imbalance in this neurotransmitter affects the area of the brain responsible for voluntary motion, posture, and support.

Dopamine, an inhibitory neurotransmitter, maintains the balance of hormonal excitation and inhibition controlled by central cortical motor sites. A dopamine deficiency effects automatic movements by depressing the centers controlling peripheral muscle responses. This results in rigidity and spasticity of muscles. Acetycholine, an excitatory neurotransmitter, now has the predominant effect in central and peripheral sites, and is responsible for many of the manifestations seen in the client with Parkinson's disease. Even though it has been established that there is a dopamine deficiency, the causes of this deficiency and of the destruction of cells in the extrapyramidal tract are still unknown.

This progressive motor dysfunction is characterized by five principle signs: (1) Bradykinesia, in which there is a slowing of voluntary movement in starting and carrying out voluntary movements. (2) Poverty of spontaneous activity in which there is a rigidity of facial muscles, resulting in a masklike expression; decreased swallowing, resulting in saliva accumulation and drooling; and the client blinks less often. (3) Tremor at rest, described as "pill-rolling tremors," occurs involuntarily and continously when the person is resting or during stress and stops or decreases with purposeful movement. (4) Loss of postural and righting reflexes results in gait disturbances and poor balance. This is characterized by a shuffling gait with short steps and a continuous movement in the direction in which started (e.g., propulsion, retropulsion, and lateropulsion). In an attempt to remain upright, the client walks with the body bent forward, with knees and elbows slightly bent in a hurried movement to avoid falling. (5) Rigidity in parkinsonism is due to tightly contracted flexor and extensor muscles. When these rigid muscles are stretched, as with passive movement, they give way to small jerking movements called "cogwheel rigidity." "Lead-pipe rigidity" is a smooth rigidity with a catching movement, which is compared to bending a lead pipe and connotes severe immobility. Tasks carried out by a Parkinson's client can be very tiring because of the concentration and attention required to plan voluntary control of each muscle movement.

Clinical manifestations associated with Parkinson's disease are autonomic problems, such as constipation, neurogenic bladder, drooling associated with dysphagia, oily skin, and excessive perspiration, seborrhea, and orthostatic hypotension, sensory complaints of poorly localized aching pain, numbness, and tingling.

Speech difficulties are characterized by a soft, rapid monotonous speech with involuntary repetition of words and phrases or repetition of another person's words or phrases.

Depression frequently occurs in the Parkinson's client and may manifest itself with signs of anorexia, insomnia, and apathy.

POTENTIAL COMPLICATIONS

1. Pneumonia,
2. urinary tract infections,
3. falls and injuries,
4. blepharospasm,
5. oculogyric crises,
6. orthostatic hypotension,
7. gastrointestinal hypomobility and constipation,
8. decubitus ulcers.

TYPES OF CLIENTS/CLINICAL CONDITIONS SEEN BY HOME HEALTH AGENCIES

1. Newly diagnosed with Parkinson's disease: initiation of prescribed treatment regimen and inclusive teaching plan for home management of condition, evaluation of response and tolerance to drug therapy, reporting to physician of need for dosage adjustment.
2. Parkinson's client with the development of complications or adverse reactions to medications: changes in prescribed medications and/or treatments, instruction, observation of response to therapy.
3. Loss of functional skills needed to perform ADL or self-care activities (e.g., mobility, dressing, feeding, grooming, hygiene): need for home therapy program.

RELATED NURSING DIAGNOSIS

Activity Intolerance

related to:
Muscular stiffness and rigidity, tremor, slowness of movement

as seen by:
Weakness, fatigue and frustration because of symptoms; exertional dyspnea

Anxiety

related to:
1. Altered neuromuscular control
2. Decreased coordination and movement affecting ability to manage activities of daily living

as seen by:
Increased helplessness; fearfulness; expressed concern for progressive disability and decreased independence; withdrawal

3. Increasing dependency on others for care
4. Knowledge deficit regarding prescribed treatment regimen
5. Fear of total disability

Bowel Elimination, Alteration in: Constipation

related to:
1. Decreased intestinal motility
2. Weakness in muscles used for defecation
3. Inadequate fluid and dietary fiber intake
4. Decreased activity levels
5. Medication therapy

as seen by:
Straining at stool; abdominal distension; frequency and amount less than usual bowel pattern

Breathing Pattern, Ineffective

related to:
1. Decreased muscle strength
2. Immobility

as seen by:
Dyspnea; shortness of breath; altered chest excursions; respiratory depth changes

Communication, Impaired Verbal

related to:
1. Dysarthria, high-pitched monotone voice secondary to akinesia
2. Palilalia
3. Echolalia

as seen by:
Monotonous and rapid speech, low in volume; involuntary rapid repetition of words or phrases; repetition of another person's words or phrases

Coping, Ineffective Individual

related to:
1. Progressive loss of functional abilities
2. Altered self-image and life-style changes

as seen by:
Lack of interest and apathy; withdrawal; mood disturbance; depression and self-consciousness

Grieving

related to:
1. Actual or perceived loss of motor functioning

as seen by:
Denial; anger; crying; sorrow; regression

2. Progressively debilitating effects of the disease on life-style and role relationships

Knowledge Deficit (Specify)

related to:
1. Disease and related S&S
2. Inadequate understanding of prescribed treatment regimen of client with Parkinson's disease
3. Potential complications, S&S to report to home health nurse or physician

as seen by:
Verbalization of lack of information; inadequate understanding; inability to perform skills necessary to meet health-care needs at home

Infection, Potential for

related to:
Increase susceptibility secondary to:
1. Indwelling urinary catheter
2. Aspiration
3. Ineffective breathing patterns

as seen by:
S&S of urinary or respiratory infections

Injury, Potential for: Increased Risk of Falls and Injuries

related to:
1. Loss of motor functioning
2. Orthostatic hypotension secondary to first few weeks of levodopa therapy
3. Environmental hazards in home
4. Immobility

as seen by:
Gait disturbances; muscle rigidity and tremors of extremities; low BP; immobility

Mobility, Impaired Physical

related to:
Progressive motor dysfunction

as seen by:
Muscle rigidity and tremors of extremities; gait disturbances; postural disturbances; bradykinesia; hypokinesia; contractures

Nutrition, Alteration in: Less than Body Requirements

related to:
Inadequate oral intake secondary to
  tremors and dysphagia

as seen by:
Difficulty chewing and swallowing;
  choking episodes; difficulty or
  inability to feed self; drooling

Oral Mucous Membrane, Alteration in

related to:
Inadequate oral hygiene secondary to
  muscle rigidity and tremors

as seen by:
Coated tongue; halitosis; burning,
  hyperemia, and inflammation of
  gums or mucous membrane; oral
  lesions

Self-Care Deficit: Feeding, Bathing/Hygiene, Dressing/Grooming, Toileting (Specify)

related to:
1. Activity intolerance
2. Impaired physical mobility

as seen by:
Impaired ability to meet physical
  needs, associated with weakness and
  fatigue; exertional dyspnea; muscle
  rigidity and tremors

Self-Concept, Disturbance in

related to:
Feelings of inadequacy and loss of
  self-esteem associated with changes
  in physical appearance and body
  functioning

as seen by:
Increased dependency on others for
  care; depression, withdrawal, refusal
  to participate in care

Skin Integrity, Impairment of

related to:
1. Immobility
2. Inadequate nutritional status
3. Increased skin oiliness and
   perspiration

as seen by:
Redness or irritation over bony
  prominences; edema; disruption of
  skin surface; seborrhea

Social Isolation

related to:
1. Lack of understanding and fear of disclosure of condition
2. Fear of not being accepted

as seen by:
Lack of self-confidence; withdrawal; not communicating

Urinary Elimination Pattern, Alteration in

related to:
Decreased ability of the bladder to contract and expel urine secondary to muscles of the bladder becoming rigid and bradykinetic

as seen by:
Urgency, frequency, hesitancy in starting to void, difficulty in completing voiding, and incomplete voiding with dribbling

LONG-TERM GOALS

To remain as functionally useful and productive as possible through restoring and preserving of motor and sensory functioning.

SHORT-TERM GOALS

The client with Parkinson's disease will be able to:

1. Verbalize nature of chronic progression of disease, S&S of complications to report to home health nurse or physician.
2. Verbalize importance of well-balanced diet, increase in dietary fiber of semi-solid foods, fluids of 2000 to 3000 ml per day/demonstrate use of assistive devices to assist with eating difficulties, activities to avoid aspiration.
3. Verbalize importance of dietary restrictions of protein while on levodopa therapy.
4. Demonstrate use of prescribed nutritional supplements.
5. Demonstrate compliance with prescribed medication therapy.
6. Verbalize S&S of hypotension while on levodopa/demonstrate measures to correct.
7. Weigh weekly/record/report excessive weight loss to physician.
8. Demonstrate compliance with prescribed medication therapy/identify side effects and toxicity.
9. Demonstrate good oral hygiene measures.
10. Demonstrate compliance with prescribed bladder program.
11. Verbalize prescribed measures to manage problems with constipation.

12. Demonstrate good skin care measures/verbalize predisposing factors to breakdown.
13. Demonstrate diaphragmatic, pursed-lip breathing exercises.
14. Verbalize complications of prolonged immobilization, S&S to report to home health nurse or physician, prescribed treatment measures, activities to avoid.
15. Demonstrate safety in home environment with ADL and self-care activities within limitations of disease and treatment regimen.
16. Demonstrate effective energy conservation techniques, safe ambulatory and transfer activities, prescribed exercises, correct use of ambulatory aids, self-help devices/verbalize importance of supportive shoes.
17. Demonstrate correct use of prescribed communication devices, compliance with speech exercises, improvement in swallowing.
18. Demonstrate effective coping mechanisms, measures to handle periods of depression and chronic progression of disease.

NURSING ACTIONS/TREATMENTS

1. Assess neurologic, musculoskeletal status (deficits in motor functioning, degree of muscle rigidity, tremors, bradykinesia)/identify complications.
2. Assess vital signs/identify trends (e.g., elevated temperature, irregular or shallow respirations).
3. Instruct as to nature and chronic progression of disease, S&S (e.g., tremors, increased salivation and drooling, slurred speech), importance of compliance with prescribed treatment regimen, complications to report to physician.
4. Assess and evaluate nutritional status and dysphagia/instruct about planned eating program of small, frequent meals, well-balanced diet, prescribed high-fiber diet, semisolid foods, increased fluids of 3000 ml per day, measures to avoid aspiration, use of assistive devices for eating, avoiding caffeine.
5. Observe/instruct to reduce total amount of protein in diet when on levodopa as prescribed (acts as an antagonist and reduces the clinical effect of the medication).
6. Observe/instruct about use of prescribed nutritional supplements.
7. Assess for weight loss/instruct to weigh weekly and record/report excessive weight loss to physician.
8. Observe/instruct about taking of medications as ordered (e.g., levodopa, levodopa combinations, anticholinergics, antidepressants), purpose and action (noncompliance results in poor control of S&S; vitamin B_6 restriction with levodopa: can reverse effects), side effects, toxicity/evaluate medication effectiveness.
9. Observe for dizziness and light-headedness while on levodopa therapy/instruct about changing position slowly, prescribed use of elastic stockings to minimize effects of postural hypotension.

10. Assess and evaluate for impairment of oral mucous membrane and gums/instruct about importance and measures of good oral hygiene.
11. Observe/instruct about regular, daily activity program with use of assistive devices, passive and active range of motion exercises, ambulation, ADL with balanced rest periods, safe transfer, use of supportive shoes, ambulatory aids, self-help devices as ordered, techniques for unlocking a "fixed position."
12. Assess and evaluate alterations in bladder elimination pattern/instruct about prescribed bladder program.
13. Assess constipation problems/instruct about prescribed use of suppositories, laxatives, stool softeners, prescribed increase in dietary fiber, adequate fluids, activities/establish a bowel routine/evaluate effectiveness of bowel regimen.
14. Assess skin condition for increased oiliness and perspiration/instruct about good skin care, predisposing factors to breakdown.
15. Observe/instruct about diaphragmatic, pursed-lip breathing exercises, S&S of complications to report to home health nurse or physician, prescribed measures to treat.
16. Assess for complications of prolonged immobility, S&S to report to home health nurse or physician, prescribed measures to treat, activities to avoid.
17. Assess/instruct about safety in home environment with ADL and self-care activities within limitations of disease and treatment regimen.
18. Observe and evaluate alterations in functional skills, ambulatory activities/refer to physical therapist and occupational therapist as ordered to instruct in energy conservation techniques, safe ambulation and transfer activities, exercises to increase muscle strength, improve coordination and dexterity, treat muscle rigidity, correct use of ambulatory aids, self-help devices, supportive shoes.
19. Assess dysphagia, communication deficits/refer to speech therapy as ordered to instruct about swallowing or dysphagia training, communication devices, speech exercises.
20. Assess emotional response to disease, depression, ineffective coping mechanisms/provide emotional support and establish realistic goals/refer to social services as ordered to provide counseling and information of support groups in the community (e.g., National Parkinson Foundation, United Parkinson Foundation, American Parkinson's Disease Association).

REHABILITATION POTENTIAL

Rehabilitation potential *excellent good fair guarded poor* for *full partial* achievement of maximal motor and sensory functioning for greater productivity and independence in managing daily activities.

Client's Name _____

Medical Record # _____

ONGOING/DISCHARGE EVALUATION OF TEACHING
The Client with Parkinson's Disease

Teaching Tools:
Printed materials given: _____

Audiovisual aids used: _____

Return Information/Demonstration/Interpretation
_____ Client
_____ Caregiver

OF:	Met	Not Met	Comments
☐ Chronic progression of disease, related S&S.	_____	_____	_____
☐ S&S of complications; actions to take.	_____	_____	_____
☐ Importance of compliance with prescribed treatment regimen.	_____	_____	_____
☐ Well-balanced diet of semisolid foods; increase in dietary fiber, fluids.	_____	_____	_____
☐ Measures to assist with eating difficulties and avoid aspiration.	_____	_____	_____

Client's Name _____

Medical Record # _____

☐ Protein
   restrictions
   when on
   levodopa
   therapy.   _____   _____   _____

☐ Weigh weekly;
   record; report
   excessive
   weight loss to
   physician.   _____   _____   _____

☐ Nutritional
   supplements.   _____   _____   _____

☐ Medications
   and
   administration,
   purpose and
   action, side
   effects.   _____   _____   _____

☐ Measures to
   minimize
   effects of
   orthostatic
   hypotension.   _____   _____   _____

☐ Oral hygiene
   measures.   _____   _____   _____

☐ Exercise
   program
   balanced with
   rest periods.   _____   _____   _____

☐ Techniques for
   unlocking a
   "fixed
   position."   _____   _____   _____

☐ Bladder
   retraining
   program.   _____   _____   _____

Client's Name _____

Medical Record #_____

☐ Measures to
avoid
constipation,
promote good
bowel
functioning. _____ _____ _____

☐ Good skin
measures. _____ _____ _____

☐ Diaphragmatic,
pursed-lip
breathing
exercises. _____ _____ _____

☐ Measures for
management of
complications
related to
prolonged
immobilization;
treatment
measures;
activities to
avoid. _____ _____ _____

☐ Safety
measures with
ADL and self-
care activities. _____ _____ _____

☐ Use of self-help
aids for eating,
dressing,
walking. _____ _____ _____

☐ Measures to
manage
communication
deficits. _____ _____ _____

☐ Energy
conservation
techniques. _____ _____ _____

Signature of Home Health Nurse _____

Date _____

■ Rupture of Intervertebral Disk

Intervertebral disks are flexible fibrocartilage pads between the bodies of vertebrae. The soft, compressible center of each disk is called the nucleus pulposus and is surrounded by a fibrous capsule called the anulus fibrosus. A herniated disk occurs when all or part of the nucleus pulposus ruptures and extrudes through the weakened or torn anulus fibrosus, creating nerve pressure in the spinal canal. In the elderly, degenerative changes in disks may predispose those individuals to similar symptoms, resulting from strain or acute injuries.

Neuromuscular effects include severe muscle spasms and weakness. Also, the pressure exerted on nerve roots by a herniated disk may cause the loss of sensory and/or motor functions in the region of innervation. This may result in later degenerative changes in the involved nerve and weakness and, with continued pressure, atrophy of the affected muscles.

Activities that increase pressure, such as bending, sneezing, and coughing, may cause associated muscle spasm and intensify pain.

The majority of disk lesions occur in the lumbar, lumbosacral, and cervical regions and are generally located proximal to an emerging nerve root.

POTENTIAL COMPLICATIONS

1. Persistent sciatica,
2. sensory and motor deficits,
3. muscle weakness and atrophy,
4. complications of immobility,
5. postural distortion,
6. pain with secondary radiculitis and/or paresthesias.

TYPES OF CLIENTS/CLINICAL CONDITIONS SEEN BY HOME HEALTH AGENCIES

1. Recent ruptured intervertebral disk and associated motor and sensory deficits, acute pain, and immobility: initiation of prescribed treatment regimen and teaching plan for home management of condition, physical therapy program.
2. Exacerbation of herniated disk condition with the development of acute neurologic symptoms: new pain management measures, physical therapy program.

RELATED NURSING DIAGNOSIS

Activity Intolerance

related to:
1. Limited mobility associated with sensory and motor losses
2. Pain

as seen by:
Weakness and fatigue with inability to take care of personal needs and daily activities

Anxiety

related to:
1. Pain and limited mobility
2. Increased dependency on others for care
3. Possible surgery
4. Knowledge deficit regarding prescribed treatment regimen

as seen by:
Crying; increased helplessness, elevated BP; depression

Bowel Elimination, Alteration in: Constipation

related to:
1. Inadequate dietary fiber and fluids
2. Decreased activity levels
3. Neuromuscular impairment

as seen by:
Changes in frequency and pattern of bowel elimination; straining at stool

Comfort, Alteration in

related to:
1. Pain and muscle spasms associated with inflammation at site of injury
2. Stiffness and soreness

as seen by:
Weakness and fatigue; postural distortion; protective behavior to area of pain; body rigidity

Coping, Ineffective Individual

related to:
1. Impaired mobility status
2. Acute pain

as seen by:
Inability to meet physical and daily needs; verbalized inability to cope; general irritability

Injury, Potential for: Increased Risk of Falls and Injuries

related to:
1. Limited mobility secondary to sensory and motor losses
2. Pain and muscle spasms
3. Atrophy of affected muscles

as seen by:
Unsteady gait; limited range of motion, postural distortion; weakness and fatigue

Knowledge Deficit (Specify)

related to:
1. Inadequate understanding of

as seen by:
Verbalization of lack of information;

prescribed plan of treatment for management of herniated disk
2. Potential complications, S&S to report to home health nurse or physician

inadequate understanding; inability to perform skills necessary to meet health-care needs at home

Mobility, Impaired Physical

related to:
1. Activity intolerance
2. Sensory and motor losses
3. Weakness and atrophy of affected muscles
4. Pain and muscle spasms
5. Prescribed activity restrictions with use of back support

as seen by:
Weakness and fatigue; limited movement; impaired muscle strength and control; radiating sciatic pain to leg and foot; imposed medical restrictions

Self-Care Deficit: Feeding, Bathing/Hygiene, Dressing/Grooming, Toileting (Specify)

related to:
1. Activity intolerance
2. Impaired mobility

as seen by:
Inability to take care of personal and daily needs, associated with decreased endurance, limited range of motion, weakness and fatigue when attempting self-care activities

Sensory-Perceptual Alteration

related to:
Sensory loss in the area innervated by the compressed spinal nerve root

as seen by:
Diminished temperature perception; decreased touch sensation; change in usual response to stimuli

Skin Integrity, Impairment of: Potential

related to:
1. Immobilization
2. Improper fit of support, brace, or corset

as seen by:
Reddened areas from pressure of immobility; edema; tissue breakdown; irritation and injury to tissues from incorrect fit of support, brace, or corset

Sleep Pattern Disturbance

related to:
Inability to assume usual comfortable position for sleep because of severe pain

as seen by:
Restlessness; disorientation; c/o feeling tired with decreased energy levels to participate in daily activities

LONG-TERM GOAL

To relieve compression and irritation on spinal nerve roots and reduce inflammation and edema in soft tissues for improvement or return of functional ability.

SHORT-TERM GOALS

The client with a ruptured intervertebral disk will be able to:

1. Verbalize nature of disorder, S&S of nerve root compression, extent of impairment, factors that precipitate.
2. Verbalize S&S of complications.
3. Verbalize importance of well-balanced diet with increased dietary fiber and adequate hydration, effect of excessive weight on spine.
4. Demonstrate compliance with prescribed medication therapy/identify side effects.
5. Verbalize specific measures to avoid constipation and promote good bowel functioning.
6. Verbalize prescribed measures to reduce pain and muscle spasms.
7. Demonstrate correct body alignment, positioning, turning, and transferring techniques.
8. Verbalize importance of/demonstrate correct body mechanics, prescribed back-strengthening exercises and ambulatory activities with use of supports, brace, or corset; planned rest periods; activity restrictions.
9. Verbalize importance of avoiding extremes in temperatures with sensory nerve losses.
10. Verbalize complications related to prolonged immobility, S&S to report to home health nurse or physician, prescribed measures to treat, activities to avoid.
11. Identify factors predisposing to skin breakdown/demonstrate good skin measures.
12. Identify factors predisposing to increased risk of falls and injuries in the home/demonstrate safety measures with daily activities.

NURSING ACTIONS/TREATMENTS

1. Assess neurovascular status: identify sensory and motor deficits, muscle weakness and atrophy, presence and degree of pain.
2. Assess vital signs/identify trends (e.g., rapid pulse rate, BP changes).
3. Instruct nature of disorder, S&S of nerve root compression, extent of impairment, activities that precipitate pain (e.g., coughing, sneezing, bending, and straining).
4. Instruct about importance of compliance with prescribed treatment regimen, S&S of complications to report to home health nurse or physician.
5. Assess and evaluate nutritional status/instruct about well-balanced diet, increased prescribed dietary fiber, adequate hydration, effect of strain on spine with excess weight.
6. Observe/instruct as to medication therapy as ordered (e.g., muscle relaxants, anti-inflammatory agents, analgesics), purpose and action, side effects/evaluate medication effectiveness.
7. Assess for constipation/instruct about prescribed increase in dietary fiber, 2000 to 3000 ml fluids per day, increased activity levels, use of prescribed laxatives and stool softeners, avoiding straining at stool, effect on precipitating muscle spasms/evaluate effectiveness of bowel regimen.
8. Observe/instruct about prescribed measures to relieve pain and muscle spasms (e.g., bed rest with prescribed firm mattress, bed boards, traction with specified weights, moist heat therapy, cold therapy, massage, trancutaneous electrical nerve stimulation [TENS] unit)/evaluate effectiveness of pain management measures.
9. Observe/instruct as to correct body alignment, positioning, turning, transferring techniques.
10. Observe/instruct about correct body mechanics, prescribed back-strengthening exercises and ambulatory program with use of supports, brace, or corset/educate regarding activity restrictions, importance of planned rest periods.
11. Observe/instruct clients with sensory nerve losses to avoid temperature extremes.
12. Assess and evaluate systems of the body for complications related to prolonged immobility/instruct what S&S to report to home health nurse or physician, prescribed measures to treat, activities to avoid.
13. Assess and evaluate skin integrity/instruct about good skin care, predisposing factors to breakdown.
14. Assess for increased risk of falls and injuries in the home/instruct about safety measures with daily activities (e.g., use of prescribed supports and assistive devices, home environment free of hazards)/assist client with daily activities, ambulation as needed.
15. Observe and evaluate alterations in functional skills, ambulatory activities/refer to physical therapy as ordered (e.g., to instruct in use of TENs unit, back-strengthening exercises, traction).

REHABILITATION POTENTIAL

Rehabilitation potential *excellent good fair guarded poor* for *full partial* return to a previous level of care and functional ability to manage daily activities and meet personal needs.

Client's Name _____

Medical Record # _____

ONGOING/DISCHARGE EVALUATION OF TEACHING

The Client with the Ruptured Intervertebral Disk

Teaching Tools:

Printed materials given: _____

Audiovisual aids used: _____

Return Information/Demonstration/Interpretation

_____ Client

_____ Caregiver

OF:	Met	Not Met	Comments
☐ Nature of disorder; S&S of nerve root compression; extent of impairment; activities that precipitate pain.	_____	_____	_____
☐ S&S of complications; actions to take.	_____	_____	_____
☐ Importance of compliance with prescribed treatment regimen.	_____	_____	_____
☐ Well-balanced diet with increased dietary fiber, adequate hydration.	_____	_____	_____
☐ Medications and administration,			

Client's Name _____

Medical Record #_____

purpose and
action, side
effects.   _____ _____   _____

☐ Measures to
avoid
constipation,
promote good
bowel
functioning.   _____ _____   _____

☐ Measures to
relieve pain and
muscle spasms.   _____ _____   _____

☐ Correct body
alignment,
positioning,
turning,
transferring
techniques.   _____ _____   _____

☐ Correct body
mechanics;
ambulatory and
back-
strengthening
exercises with
use of supports,
brace, or corset. _____ _____   _____

☐ Activity
restrictions;
planned rest
periods.   _____ _____   _____

☐ Avoiding
temperature
extremes for
clients with
sensory nerve
losses.   _____ _____   _____

☐ Complications
of prolonged
immobilization;

Client's Name _____

Medical Record # _____

measures to treat; activities to avoid.	_____	_____	_____
☐ Good skin care measures; factors predisposing to breakdown.	_____	_____	_____
☐ Factors predisposing to increased risk of falls and injuries in home; related safety measures.	_____	_____	_____

Signature of Home Health Nurse _____

Date _____

■ Seizure Disorder

Disruption of transmission pathways within the cerebrocortical neurons resulting from abnormal and uncontrolled electrical discharges in the brain results in a transitory disturbance in consciousness, motor, sensory, and autonomic functioning. This disturbance is manifested by convulsive movements or sustained rigidity of peripheral muscles. The triggering mechanisms of seizure activity are not clear, but convulsions have been found to occur in various conditions such as hypoglycemia, epilepsy, brain tumors, infections, head injuries, very high temperatures, uremias, alcohol withdrawal, and electrolyte imbalances. Seizure disorders are described as generalized tonic-clonic, generalized complex partial, or simple partial seizures.

A generalized tonic-clonic or grand mal seizure occurs when hyperexcitability of cerebrocortical neurons extends to the entire brain. This type of seizure is usually preceded by an aura or warning sensation such as an unusual auditory, visual, olfactory, or gustatory and is characterized by a loud cry, loss of consciousness, urinary or fecal incontinence, and biting of tongue. Seizures of this type may last 1 to 10 minutes. Postictal drowsiness can occur and may last for several hours.

Generalized seizures, or petit mal (absence) seizures are of brief duration (5 to 30 seconds) and usually begin with a momentary stare or blank look, blinking or rolling of eyes. Posture is maintained and the individual is able to continue with activities as prior to the seizure. Other seizure types related to petit mal, characterized by a loss of muscle tone with myoclonic jerks and subsequent falling, are called akinetic seizures.

Complex partial seizures are associated with a brief loss of consciousness that may occur with an aura. A common type of this seizure activity is called psychomotor, in which the seizure originates from foci in the temporal lobe, causing purposeful movements that are poorly coordinated and irrelevant to the circumstances (e.g., lip smacking, swallowing, chewing, hand wringing, or picking at objects).

Simple partial seizures, or simple motor seizures, occur from foci in the motor cortex of the frontal lobe or other localized areas, with clinical manifestations related to those function control areas involved. A Jacksonian seizure is a focal motor seizure without loss of consciousness, in which convulsive movements begin in the same group of muscles and extend in an "ordered march." For example, movements may begin in the right thumb, followed by the right hand, arm, and eventually the entire right side. On occasion, a Jacksonian seizure may end in a generalized convulsion with loss of consciousness.

POTENTIAL COMPLICATIONS

1. Respiratory distress,
2. status epilepticus,
3. injuries sustained during a seizure.

TYPES OF CLIENTS/CLINICAL CONDITIONS SEEN BY HOME HEALTH AGENCIES

1. Newly diagnosed with seizure activity: placed on anticonvulsant therapy and teaching program of management of seizure disorder.
2. Client with known seizure disorder experiencing problems with continued seizure activity: prescribed changes in medication therapy, need for assessment and evaluation of effectiveness or further need to regulate medication dosage to client's blood level.

RELATED NURSING DIAGNOSIS

Anxiety

related to:
1. Recurring seizure activity
2. Concern over leading a productive life
3. Knowledge deficit regarding prescribed treatment regimen

as seen by:
Apprehensiveness; uncertainty because of unpredictable nature of seizures; feelings of helplessness and embarrassment

Injury, Potential for: Increased Susceptibility to Injuries

related to:
1. Seizure activity
2. Postictal state
3. Altered level of consciousness

as seen by:
Convulsive movements; postictal drowsiness; confusion; memory loss

Knowledge Deficit (Specify)

related to:
1. Seizure disorder
2. Prescribed plan of treatment
3. Potential complications, S&S to report to home health nurse or physician

as seen by:
Verbalization of lack of information; inadequate understanding in management of seizure disorder

Nutrition, Alteration in: Less than Body Requirements

related to:
Decreased oral intake

as seen by:
S&S of hypoglycemia, with precipitation of a seizure

Oral Mucous Membrane, Alteration in

related to:
Phenytoin concentration in the saliva

as seen by:
Hyperplasia of the gums

Self-Concept, Disturbance in

related to:
1. Altered body image
2. Lowered self-esteem

as seen by:
Not taking responsibility for self-care and/or follow-through with prescribed medication therapy; anxiety; depression; fears regarding level of independence

LONG-TERM GOAL

To pursue normal activities and lead a productive life with control of seizure disorder.

SHORT-TERM GOALS

The client with a seizure disorder will be able to:

1. Verbalize nature of seizure disorder, type of seizure, precipitating factors, S&S of complications to report to home health nurse or physician.
2. Verbalize importance of well-balanced meals at regular times, effect of hypoglycemia in precipitating a seizure/adequate glucose levels to maintain brain's electrical activity.
3. Demonstrate compliance with prescribed medication therapy/identify side effects, toxicity/verbalize risk of overmedication and undermedication.
4. Verbalize effect of phenytoin in saliva on gums, importance of good oral hygiene.
5. Verbalize importance of regularly scheduled exercises, activity modifications for safety with balanced rest periods.
6. Caregiver will recognize, observe, and record seizure activity/identify emergency actions during seizure to take to protect client.
7. Verbalize management principles after seizure activity.
8. Verbalize importance of wearing Medic Alert bracelet.
9. Demonstrate positive adjustment and management of seizure disorder.

NURSING ACTIONS/TREATMENTS

1. Assess neurologic status, frequency of seizures, complications.
2. Assess vital signs/identify trends (e.g., elevated temperature, rapid pulse rate).
3. Instruct as to nature of seizure disorder, type of seizure, precipitating factors (e.g., physical, emotional, environmental stresses), importance of strict compliance with prescribed treatment regimen.
4. Assess and evaluate nutritional status/instruct about well-balanced meals at regular times, importance of adequate glucose levels to maintain brain's electrical activity, S&S of hypoglycemia, effect on precipitating a seizure, actions to take.
5. Observe/instruct about taking medications and following anticonvulsant therapy as ordered, risk of overmedication and undermedication, purpose and action, side effects, toxicity/evaluate medication effectiveness.
6. Assess/instruct about good oral hygiene and effect of phenytoin concentration in salvia on gums.
7. Observe/instruct about regularly scheduled exercise, necessary modification of activities essential for safety, planned rest periods, avoiding fatigue.
8. Instruct caregiver to recognize, observe, and record seizure activity/identify emergency situations, actions to take to protect client.
9. Assess postictal pattern/instruct about management principles.
10. Observe/instruct about importance of wearing Medic Alert bracelet.
11. Assess anxiety, apprehension, altered self-image/encourage to verbalize feelings/provide emotional support/refer to social services as needed to assist with adjustment to condition/provide information regarding community support groups (e.g., Epilepsy Foundation of America, Epilepsy Concern, local support groups).

REHABILITATION POTENTIAL

Rehabilitation potential *excellent good fair guarded poor* for *full partial* return to an independent level of functioning and controlled seizure activity.

Client's Name _____

Medical Record # _____

ONGOING/DISCHARGE EVALUATION OF TEACHING
The Client with a Seizure Disorder

Teaching Tools:
Printed materials given: _____

Audiovisual aids used: _____

Return Information/Demonstration/Interpretation
_____ Client
_____ Caregiver

OF:	Met	Not Met	Comments
☐ Nature of seizure disorder, type of seizure, precipitating factors.	_____	_____	_____
☐ S&S of complications, actions to take.	_____	_____	_____
☐ Importance of strict compliance with prescribed treatment regimen.	_____	_____	_____
☐ Importance of well-balanced diet for normal neuronal function; effect of hypoglycemia in precipitating seizure activity.	_____	_____	_____
☐ Medications and administration, purpose and action, side effects.	_____	_____	_____

Client's Name _____

Medical Record # _____

	OF:	**Met**	**Not Met**	**Comments**
☐	Risk of overmedication and undermedication with anticonvulsant medication.	_____	_____	_____
☐	Effect of phenytoin concentration in saliva on gums; good oral hygiene.	_____	_____	_____
☐	Regularly scheduled exercises; activity modifications for safety; planned rest periods.	_____	_____	_____
☐	Observation and recording of seizure activity by caregiver.	_____	_____	_____
☐	Measures to protect client during a seizure.	_____	_____	_____
☐	Postictal management principles.	_____	_____	_____
☐	Medic Alert bracelet.	_____	_____	_____

Signature of Home Health Nurse _____

Date _____

MUSCULOSKELETAL DISORDERS

■ Amputation: Above or Below the Knee

An amputation is the surgical removal of all or part of a limb. The majority of surgical amputations involve the lower extremities of persons with severe peripheral vascular disease. Other causes that may necessitate amputation are recurrent uncontrolled infections, gangrene, severe trauma, and cancer.

The two basic types of surgical procedures for an amputation are open and closed. The open, or guillotine, amputation is a rarely performed emergency procedure in which the tissues and bone are cut flush and the wound is left open. A second operation is later performed to close the wound and produce a satisfactory stump.

POTENTIAL COMPLICATIONS

1. Excessive bleeding,
2. infection,
3. circulatory deficits,
4. phantom limb pain,
5. contracture deformities,
6. depression,
7. pressure sores.

TYPES OF CLIENTS/CLINICAL CONDITIONS SEEN BY HOME HEALTH AGENCIES

1. Recent amputation: prescribed treatment regimen to include wound site observations and care, dressing changes, specialized instructions regarding stump care, use of prosthesis, establishment of and instruction in home physical therapy program.
2. Client with an amputation, condition of stump now favorable for prosthesis fitting: observation and instruction in care and use of prosthesis required by physical therapist.
3. Recent hospitalization for impaired healing of stump: new orders for dressing changes and stump care.

RELATED NURSING DIAGNOSIS

Activity Intolerance

related to:	as seen by:
1. Prolonged inactivity	Fatigue, dyspnea on exertion;
2. Increased strength required associated with use of prosthesis and assistive devices for ambulation	abnormal cardiac and respiratory response to activity; c/o weakness

Anxiety

related to:
1. Change in body appearance and changes in life-style
2. Knowledge deficit regarding prescribed treatment regimen
3. Fear of disability and loss of independence

as seen by:
Withdrawn behavior; increased helplessness; increased questioning or lack of questioning regarding home rehabilitation program, expressed feelings of inadequacy and dependency on others

Bowel Elimination, Alteration in: Constipation

related to:
1. Decreased mobility status
2. Inadequate intake of dietary fiber and fluids

as seen by:
Straining at stool; changes in frequency and pattern of bowel elimination; hard, formed stools

Comfort, Alteration in

related to:
Postsurgical pain, phantom limb pain

as seen by:
Exhibiting pain behavior (e.g., moaning, crying); c/o pain; little or no movement; protective of stump

Coping, Ineffective

related to:
Loss of body part

as seen by:
Altered affect; hostile or withdrawn behavior; poor grooming; lack of participation in self-care

Grieving

related to:
Loss of body part, effect on life-style and role relationships

as seen by:
Withdrawal from usual relationships; depression; apathetic behavior

Infection, Potential for

related to:
Incisional area secondary to breakdown of body's first line of defense

as seen by:
Pain or tenderness; increased redness and swelling; unusual drainage; tissue breakdown

Injury, Potential for: Increased Risk of Falls and Injuries

related to:
1. Altered mobility status secondary to amputation
2. Improper use of ambulatory assistive devices
3. Improper use and fit of prosthesis
4. Weakness

as seen by:
Unsteady gait and balance; weakness; pain; limited ability to perform ADL; inability to ambulate or transfer without assistance

Knowledge Deficit (Specify)

related to:
1. Prescribed plan of treatment
2. Home rehabilitation program
3. Potential complications S&S to report to home health nurse or physician.

as seen by:
Lack of information; inadequate understanding, inability to perform skills necessary to meet health-care needs at home

Mobility, Impaired Physical

related to:
1. Amputation
2. Improper use or fit of prosthesis
3. Incorrect use of ambulatory assistive devices
4. Prescribed activity restrictions

as seen by:
Inability to move purposefully within home environment; impaired coordination, balance, strength, and endurance; medically imposed restrictions or limitations (e.g., weight-bearing activities)

Self-Care Deficit: Feeding, Bathing/Hygiene, Dressing/Grooming, Toileting (Specify)

related to:
1. Activity intolerance
2. Impaired mobility
3. Apathy or depression
4. Prescribed restrictions

as seen by:
Impaired functional ability; impaired control and functional use of prosthesis; lack of involvement in care, imposed medical restrictions or limitations (e.g., weight-bearing activities)

Self-Concept, Disturbance in

related to:
1. Altered body image
2. Loss of self-esteem
3. Change in role performance

as seen by:
Signs of grieving; unwillingness to look at stump; withdrawal from role responsibilities; lack of participation in home rehabilitation program

Skin Integrity, Impairment of: Actual/Potential

related to:
1. Surgical incision
2. Impaired healing of incisional area secondary to infection, immobility, or inadequate nutritional status
3. Impaired circulation associated with circulatory abnormalities related to disease process

as seen by:
Increasing redness and swelling; altered circulation with prolonged unrelieved pressure; irritation and tissue breakdown; inadequate intake of food and fluids; excessive pressure on incisional area associated with noncompliance with weight-bearing restrictions, improper wrapping of stump, incorrect use of prosthesis

Social Isolation

related to:
1. Loss of body part
2. Loss of self-esteem

as seen by:
Depression; failure to interact with others; nutritional alterations; nonparticipation in rehabilitation program

LONG-TERM GOAL

To restore maximal emotional adaptation and functional ability with minimal limitations on life-style.

SHORT-TERM GOALS

The client with an amputation above or below the knee will be able to:

1. Verbalize nature of disease process or injury, surgical intervention, S&S of complications to report to physician.
2. Demonstrate compliance with prescribed well-balanced diet, high in protein, calcium, vitamin C, and dietary fiber, and adequate hydration.
3. Verbalize cause and management of "phantom limb" sensations.
4. Demonstrate compliance with prescribed medication therapy/identify side effects.
5. Demonstrate compliance with prescribed therapeutic exercises.
6. Verbalize effect of decreased activity level on bowel functioning, prescribed measures to manage constipation problems.
7. Demonstrate prescribed wound care and stump dressing/verbalize importance of weight-bearing restrictions until incisional area is healed.

8. Demonstrate prescribed exercises, care of leg and foot of unaffected extremity, how to check peripheral pulses/identify S&S of altered circulation to report to physician.
9. Demonstrate compliance with daily care of stump as prescribed.
10. Demonstrate prescribed care and use of prosthesis.
11. Demonstrate safe transfer techniques, self-care activities, safe ambulation with the use of prescribed assistive devices/verbalize importance of planned rest periods.
12. Verbalize measures to reduce risks of falls and injuries with ambulation.
13. Verbalize complications of prolonged immobilization, prescribed measures to treat, activities to avoid.
14. Demonstrate effective coping mechanisms in adapting to loss of body part and changes in life-style.

NURSING ACTIONS/TREATMENTS

1. Assess peripheral circulation in remaining extremities, operative site/identify complications.
2. Assess vital signs/identify trends (e.g., elevated temperature, increased pulse rate, BP changes).
3. Instruct as to the nature of disease process or injury, surgical intervention, importance of compliance with prescribed treatment regimen, S&S of complications to report to physician.
4. Assess and evaluate nutritional status/instruct as to prescribed well-balanced diet, high in protein, calcium, vitamin C, and dietary fiber, and adequate hydration.
5. Assess and evaluate for phantom limb sensations/instruct about cause (twitching and spasms of stump muscle), prescribed measures to manage (e.g., use of light intermittent pressure against a firm surface, moist or dry heat, massage of stump)/encourage to keep active.
6. Observe/instruct about taking medications as ordered, purpose and action, side effects/evaluate medication effectiveness.
7. Assess alteration in bowel pattern/instruct about effect of decreased activity levels on bowel functioning, prescribed measures to treat and avoid constipation (e.g., increase in dietary fiber and fluids, increased activity, use of stool softeners and laxatives)/evaluate effectiveness of bowel regimen.
8. Observe/instruct about prescribed therapeutic exercises to strengthen muscles, promote circulation, decrease edema and atrophy of stump.
9. Assess/instruct need for correct body alignment and positioning of stump to avoid contractures (e.g., below-the-knee amputation: Keep knee extended to avoid hamstring contracture. Leg amputation: do not prop stump on a pillow to avoid a hip flexion contracture).
10. Assess and evaluate healing of incisional area/instruct about S&S of infection to report, prescribed wound care and stump dressing (using sterile technique) and weight-bearing restrictions until incision is healed.

11. Assess and evaluate circulation and functional status of unaffected extremity/instruct how to check peripheral pulses, about prescribed exercises and care of leg and foot, avoiding prolonged sitting or standing/S&S of altered circulation to report to home health nurse or physician.
12. Observe/instruct about prescribed care of stump (e.g., washing daily with mild soap and water/drying gently and exposing to air/drying well before bandaging to avoid skin breakdown/avoiding use of powders and creams which may soften or irritate the skin and affect fit of prosthesis/activities as ordered to toughen stump).
13. Assess/instruct about purpose and proper wrapping of stump with elastic bandage or use of stump shrinker (e.g., wrap firmly and evenly, avoid overtightness, rewrap at least 2 times a day and when tension is lost).
14. Observe/instruct about purpose and use of stump sock (e.g., fit, changing daily, not using a worn or damaged sock that could cause skin irritation).
15. Observe/instruct about care, use, and proper fit of prosthesis as prescribed, need for periodic adjustment (as stump heals, it usually shrinks), avoiding use if skin irritated or tissue breakdown/report any skin changes on stump to physician (e.g., blisters, abrasions, rashes).
16. Observe/instruct about safe transfer techniques, self-care activities, safe ambulation with the use of prescribed assistive devices, balanced rest periods.
17. Assess for increased risk of falls and injuries/instruct about safety measures with ambulation and daily activities (e.g., home environment free of hazards, safe ambulation/assist client with activities as needed).
18. Assess and evaluate systems of the body for S&S of complications related to prolonged immobilization/instruct about S&S to report to home health nurse or physician, prescribed measures to treat, activities to avoid.
19. Observe and evaluate mobility status, fit and use of prosthesis/refer to physical therapy as ordered to instruct in prescribed home exercise program, use of assistive devices, use and adjustment to prosthesis.
20. Assess ineffective coping mechanisms and alteration in self-concept/provide emotional support/encourage verbalization of feelings/refer to social services as needed to assist with grieving process, adaptation to altered body image/provide information regarding support groups in the community (e.g., Meals on Wheels; homemaker chore application, community amputee support groups, National Amputation Foundation).

REHABILITATION POTENTIAL

Rehabilitation potential *excellent good fair guarded poor* for *full partial* return to a previous level of independent functioning and positive adaptation to altered body image.

Client's Name _____

Medical Record #_____

ONGOING/DISCHARGE EVALUATION OF TEACHING

The Client with an Amputation: Above or Below the Knee

Teaching Tools:

Printed materials given: _____

Audiovisual aids used: _____

Return Information/Demonstration/Interpretation
_____ Client
_____ Caregiver

OF:	Met	Not Met	Comments
☐ Nature of disease process, injury, surgical intervention	_____	_____	_____
☐ S&S of complications; actions to take.	_____	_____	_____
☐ Importance of compliance with prescribed treatment regimen.	_____	_____	_____
☐ Managment of "phantom limb" sensations.	_____	_____	_____
☐ Medications and administration, purpose and action, side effects.	_____	_____	_____
☐ Importance of well-balanced diet, high in protein, calcium,			

Client's Name _____

Medical Record # _____

OF:	**Met**	**Not Met**	**Comments**
vitamin C, and dietary fiber, adequate hydration.	_____	_____	_____
☐ Effects of decreased activity level on bowel functioning; prescribed measures to manage constipation problems.	_____	_____	_____
☐ Therapeutic exercises.	_____	_____	_____
☐ Correct body alignment and positioning of stump to avoid contractures.	_____	_____	_____
☐ Stump care.	_____	_____	_____
☐ Proper wrapping of stump with elastic bandage.	_____	_____	_____
☐ Use of stump shrinker.	_____	_____	_____
☐ Use of stump sock.	_____	_____	_____
☐ Wound care.	_____	_____	_____

Client's Name _____

Medical Record # _____

OF:	Met	Not Met	Comments
☐ Care of leg and foot of unaffected extremity.	_____	_____	_____
☐ How to check peripheral pulses, S&S of altered circulation to report to home health nurse or physician.	_____	_____	_____
☐ Care and use of prosthesis.	_____	_____	_____
☐ Safe transfer techniques; use of ambulatory assistive devices.	_____	_____	_____
☐ Risk factors for falls and injuries in the home; safety measures with ambulation and daily activities.	_____	_____	_____
☐ Complications of prolonged immobilization; measures to treat; activities to avoid.	_____	_____	_____

Signature of Home Health Nurse _____

Date _____

■ Care of Client in a Cast: Fracture of Upper or Lower Extremity

An interruption in the continuity of a bone is called a fracture or broken bone. A fracture is classified by the bone involved and the nature of the break. For example, a fracture of the right femur with the skin remaining intact is called a closed, or simple, fracture of the right femur, but if there is an associated break in the skin, the fracture would be called an open, or compound, fracture of the right femur. The fracture is further classified according to the line of the fracture. For example, a break straight across the bone is called a transverse fracture; a fracture with several bone fractures is called a comminuted fracture.

Most fractures are a result of a fall or trauma. Fractures may also occur as a result of a weakened bone that fractures with normal activity or after slight injury. These types of fractures may be called pathologic or neoplastic fractures and occur with conditions such as osteoporosis, cancer, or as a complication of steroid therapy.

Casts are the usual treatment for fractures. Casts are made of plaster of paris, fiberglass, or other materials. A cast immobilizes, supports, and protects the injured part during the healing process.

POTENTIAL COMPLICATIONS

1. Impaired circulation,
2. skin irritation and breakdown (near cast edges),
3. infection,
4. pressure sores,
5. fat emoblism
6. delayed union or malunion of the fracture,
7. compartment syndrome.

TYPES OF CLIENTS/CLINICAL CONDITIONS SEEN BY HOME HEALTH AGENCIES

1. Recent fracture, client with cast, decreased mobility status and functional limitations: prescribed treatment regimen includes neurovascular and musculoskeletal assessments, cast care, pain management and rehabilitative therapy program.
2. Complications associated with healing of fracture: change in treatments, medications and therapy; instruction, supervision, report to physician on client's progress and response to therapy changes.

RELATED NURSING DIAGNOSIS

Anxiety

related to:
1. Pain
2. Immobility of body part
3. Increased dependency on others to meet physical needs
4. Knowledge deficit regarding prescribed treatment regimen

as seen by:
Restlessness; irritability; frustration over decreased independence and needing of assistance; increased questioning of treatment orders and home rehabilitation program

Bowel Elimination, Alteration in: Constipation

related to:
1. Decreased mobility status
2. Inadequate dietary fiber and fluids

as seen by:
Frequency and amount of stool less than usual pattern; reports feeling of fullness or unable to move bowels

Comfort, Alteration in: Pain

related to:
Fracture of extremity

as seen by:
Facial mask of pain; guarded movement; muscle spasms; c/o pain

Injury, Potential for: Increased Risk of Falls and Injuries

related to:
Reduced or impaired functional level secondary to fracture, cast, and use of assistive devices for ambulation

as seen by:
Impaired coordination and balance; incorrect use of assistive devices; assistance needed to ambulate; limited ability to perform ADL

Knowledge Deficit (Specify)

related to:
1. Inadequate understanding of prescribed plan of treatment, cast care, rehabilitation program
2. Potential complications, S&S to report to physician.

as seen by:
Verbalization of lack of information; inadequate understanding; inability to perform skills necessary to meet health-care needs at home

Mobility, Impaired Physical

related to:
1. Fracture
2. Incorrect use of ambulatory assistive devices
3. Prescribed activity restrictions

as seen by:
Inability to move purposefully in home environment to independently manage ADL; imposed medical restrictions, weight-bearing restrictions

Self-Care Deficit: Feeding, Bathing/Hygiene, Dressing/Grooming, Toileting (Specify)

related to:
1. Impaired mobility
2. Prescribed activity restrictions

as seen by:
Functional limitations; impaired ability to take care of personal needs without assistance; incorrect use of ambulatory assistive devices; medically imposed restrictions and limitations with activities and weight-bearing activities

Skin Integrity, Impairment of: Potential

related to:
Pressure of cast on tissues

as seen by:
Redness and swelling; tissue irritation and breakdown; drainage; foul odor; c/o pain and/or impaired sensation

LONG-TERM GOAL

To restore structural continuity of the bone and restoration of limb function without complications.

SHORT-TERM GOALS

The client with a fracture of upper or lower extremity in a cast will be able to:

1. Identify causative factor of fracture, safety measures with daily activities.
2. Identify neurovascular changes, impaired mobility, drainage from cast of affected extremity to report to home health nurse or physician.
3. Verbalize importance of prescribed well-balanced diet, high in protein, calcium, vitamin C, and dietary fiber/adequate hydration.

4. Demonstrate compliance with prescribed medication therapy/identify side effects.
5. Verbalize effect of decreased activities on bowel functioning, prescribed measures to manage constipation problems.
6. Demonstrate good skin and cast care/identify areas of breakdown to report to home health nurse or physician.
7. Demonstrate prescribed ambulatory activities with safe and correct use of assistive devices.
8. Verbalize degree of weight bearing.
9. Demonstrate correct positioning and elevation or support of cast as prescribed.
10. Demonstrate compliance with prescribed therapeutic exercises and graded functional activities, with balanced rest periods.
11. Verbalize measures to reduce risk of falls and injuries in home when ambulating.
12. Demonstrate decreased level of anxiety, positive adaptation to limited mobility status.

NURSING ACTIONS/TREATMENTS

1. Assess neurovascular, musculoskeletal status of affected extremity/identify complications.
2. Assess vital signs/identify trends (e.g., elevated temperature).
3. Instruct about causative factor of fracture, safety measures with daily activities.
4. Assess/instruct to report changes in color, temperature, sensation, and movement of affected extremity, foul odor or drainage from cast, increased pain.
5. Assess nutritional status/instruct about prescribed well-balanced diet high in dietary fiber, protein, calcium, and vitamin C, adequate hydration.
6. Observe/instruct about taking medications as ordered, purpose and action, side effects/evaluate medication effectiveness.
7. Assess alteration in bowel pattern/instruct about effect of decreased activity level on bowel functioning, prescribed measures to treat or avoid constipation (e.g., increased activities, high dietary fiber, and fluids, use of stool softeners and laxatives).
8. Assess skin around cast edges for irritation or skin breakdown/instruct about good skin and cast care, areas of breakdown to report.
9. Observe/instruct in prescribed ambulatory activities with safe and correct use of assistive devices, degree of weight bearing.
10. Observe/instruct to position, elevate, or support cast as prescribed.
11. Observe/instruct about prescribed therapeutic exercises and graded functional activities with balanced rest periods.
12. Assess for increased risk of falls and injuries in home/instruct about safety measures with ambulation and daily activities with correct use of prescribed assistive devices.

13. Observe and evaluate alterations in functional skills, ambulatory activities/refer to rehabilitative services as ordered to instruct in home exercise program (e.g., strengthening exercises; gait training; use of adaptive equipment and/or assistive devices).
14. Assess level of anxiety/provide emotional support/refer to social services to assist with adaptation to limited mobility status (e.g., homemaker chore application; Meals on Wheels; transportation service).

REHABILITATION POTENTIAL

Rehabilitation potential *excellent good fair guarded poor* for *full partial* return to an independent level of functioning and increased strength and endurance as before injury.

Client's Name _____

Medical Record #_____

ONGOING/DISCHARGE EVALUATION OF TEACHING

The Client with a Fracture of Upper or Lower Extremity in a Cast

Teaching Tools:

Printed materials given: _____

Audiovisual aids used: _____

Return Information/Demonstration/Interpretation

_____ Client

_____ Caregiver

OF:	Met	Not Met	Comments
☐ Neurovascular changes, impaired mobility, drainage from cast, and increased pain of affected extremity to report to physician.	_____	_____	_____
☐ Importance of compliance with prescribed treatment regimen.	_____	_____	_____
☐ Importance of well-balanced diet high in dietary fiber, protein, calcium, and vitamin C, and adequate hydration.	_____	_____	_____

Client's Name _____

Medical Record # _____

OF:	Met	Not Met	Comments
☐ Medications and administration, purpose and action, side effects.	_____	_____	_____
☐ Effects of decreased activity level on bowel functioning, prescribed measures to manage constipation problems.	_____	_____	_____
☐ Skin and cast care; areas of skin breakdown to report.	_____	_____	_____
☐ Ambulatory activities with use of prescribed assistive devices.	_____	_____	_____
☐ Degree of weight bearing.	_____	_____	_____
☐ Positioning and elevation or support of cast.	_____	_____	_____
☐ Therapeutic exercises; graded functional activities;			

Client's Name _____

Medical Record # _____

OF:	Met	Not Met	Comments
balanced rest periods.	_____	_____	_____
☐ Risk factors for falls and injuries in home; safety measures with ambulation and daily activities.	_____	_____	_____

Signature of Home Health Nurse _____

Date _____

■ Fractured Hip with Internal Fixation or Prosthesis

The major orthopedic injury resulting in immobility and disability among the elderly is fracture of the hip and femoral neck. Osteoporosis, poor nutrition, limitation of mobility, and falls are all major contributing factors to the high incidence of this injury.

A fractured hip is a term that describes a fracture involving the proximal end of the femur, the head-neck region of the greater and lesser trochanter. Intracapsular fractures occur in the neck of the femur whereas extracapsular fractures include fractures between the base of the neck and lesser trochanter of the femur.

The location of the fracture is an important consideration in the determination of the treatment and management of the injury. Hip fractures are usually treated surgically by internal fixation of the fracture (e.g., use of pins, nails, or compression screw and side plate) or insertion of a prosthetic device to replace the femoral head (e.g., Austin-Moore or Thompson prosthesis).

POTENTIAL COMPLICATIONS

1. Infection of incisional area,
2. thrombophlebitis,
3. contractures,
4. bending or breaking of pin, crushing of bone secondary to weight bearing before ordered.

TYPES OF CLIENTS/CLINICAL CONDITIONS SEEN BY HOME HEALTH AGENCIES

1. Recent fracture with internal fixation or prosthesis: pain, prescribed weight bearing or non-weight bearing status, home-care plan of treatment rehabilitative therapy and teaching plan for management of condition.
2. Complications associated with fracture, surgical intervention: changes in prescribed home treatment and rehabilitation program, requiring instruction, supervision, and evaluation of response to therapy.

RELATED NURSING DIAGNOSIS

Activity Intolerance

related to:
1. Prolonged inactivity
2. Increased strength required for use of ambulatory assistive devices

as seen by:
Weakness and fatigue with use of walker or crutches, when attempting self-care activities; dyspnea on exertion; failure to follow graded exercise program

Anxiety

related to:
1. Pain
2. Concern for permanent disability
3. Knowledge deficit regarding prescribed rehabilitation program

as seen by:
Verbal expression of concern about returning to an independent level of functioning; apprehension regarding ability to follow through with home physical therapy program

Bowel Elimination, Alteration in: Constipation

related to:
1. Decreased mobility status
2. Inadequate intake of dietary fiber and fluids

as seen by:
Changes in frequency and pattern of bowel elimination; straining at stool; habitual use of laxatives

Comfort, Alteration in

related to:
Pain in affected extremity

as seen by:
Guarding behavior; irritability; reluctance to comply with prescribed ambulatory activities

Coping, Ineffective Individual

related to:
Disability or impaired mobility status

as seen by:
General irritability; verbalization of inability to cope

Infection, Potential for

related to:
Incisional area, breakdown of body's first line of defense

as seen by:
Increased pain; tenderness; redness; swelling; unusual drainage; tissue breakdown; fever

Injury, Potential for: Increased Risk of Falls and Injuries

related to:
1. Altered mobility status
2. Incorrect use of ambulatory assistive devices

as seen by:
Impaired balance and gait; weakness, pain, and incoordination with use of ambulatory assistive devices

Knowledge Deficit (Specify)

related to:
1. Prescribed plan of treatment, home rehabilitation program
2. Potential complications, S&S to report to home health nurse or physician

as seen by:
Verbalization of lack of information; inadequate understanding; inability to perform skills necessary to meet health-care needs at home

Mobility, Impaired Physical

related to:
1. Fracture, surgery
2. Incorrect use of ambulatory assistive devices
3. Prescribed activity restrictions

as seen by:
Pain; weakness; incoordination; inability to transfer and/or ambulate within home environment without assistance; imposed medical restrictions, limitations on weight-bearing activities

Self-Care Deficit: Feeding, Bathing/Hygiene, Dressing/Grooming, Toileting (Specify)

related to:
1. Activity intolerance
2. Impaired mobility
3. Prescribed activity restrictions

as seen by:
Inability to perform personal care activities and ADL associated with weakness and fatigue; inability to transfer and/or ambulate without assistance, to take care of physical needs; imposed medical restrictions on weight-bearing activities

Skin Integrity, Impairment of: Actual/Potential

related to:
1. Surgical incision
2. Impaired healing of incisional area secondary to infection, immobility, inadequate nutritional status

as seen by:
Increasing redness and swelling; altered circulation with prolonged unrelieved pressure; unusual drainage; pronounced tenderness

LONG-TERM GOAL

Restored continuity of the bone with return of hip joint functioning, free of complications.

SHORT-TERM GOALS

The client with a fractured hip with internal fixation or prosthesis will be able to:

1. Verbalize nature of injury and surgery.
2. Verbalize S&S of complications to report to home health nurse or physician.
3. Verbalize effect of decreased activities on bowel functioning, prescribed measures to manage constipation problems.
4. Demonstrate compliance with prescribed well-balanced diet high in protein, calcium, vitamin C, and dietary fiber and adequate hydration.
5. Demonstrate compliance with prescribed medication therapy/identify side effects.
6. Verbalize prescribed activity and positioning restrictions, alignment of affected extremity, importance of posture and body mechanics.
7. Demonstrate prescribed ambulatory activities with safe and correct use of ambulatory aids, degree of weight bearing.
8. Demonstrate compliance with prescribed therapeutic exercises, graded functional activities, transfer techniques, balanced rest periods.
9. Demonstrate compliance with prescribed wound care, S&S of infection to report to home health nurse or physician.
10. Verbalize measures to reduce risk of falls and injuries in home when ambulating.
11. Verbalize complications related to prolonged immobilization, measures to treat, activities to avoid.
12. Demonstrate effective coping mechanisms, positive adjustment to altered mobility status.

NURSING ACTIONS/TREATMENTS

1. Assess neurovascular, musculoskeletal status of lower extremities/identify complications.
2. Assess vital signs/identify trends (e.g., increased temperature).
3. Instruct as to nature of injury, surgery, importance of compliance with prescribed treatment regimen, S&S of complications to report to home health nurse or physician.
4. Assess and evaluate nutritional status/instruct about prescribed well-balanced diet, high in dietary fiber, protein, calcium, vitamin C, adequate hydration.
5. Assess alteration in bowel patterns/instruct about effect of decreased activity levels on bowel functioning, prescribed measures to treat or avoid constipation (e.g., increased activities, dietary fiber and fluids, use of stool softeners and laxatives)/evaluate effectiveness of bowel regimen.
6. Observe/instruct about taking of medications as ordered, purpose and action, side effects/evaluate medication effectiveness.

7. Observe/instruct in prescribed activity and positioning restrictions, alignment of affected extremity/importance of correct posture and body mechanics.
8. Observe/instruct in prescribed ambulatory activities, safe and correct use of prescribed ambulatory aids, degree of weight bearing.
9. Observe/instruct about prescribed therapeutic exercises and graded functional activities, transfer techniques, planned rest periods.
10. Observe and evaluate incisional area/instruct about prescribed wound care, S&S of infection to report to home health nurse or physician.
11. Assess for increased risk of falls in home/instruct about safety measures with ambulation (e.g., home environment free of hazards)/assist client with daily activities with correct use of ambulatory assistive devices.
12. Assess/instruct about complications related to prolonged immobilization, measures to treat, activities to avoid.
13. Observe and evaluate alterations in ambulatory activities/refer to physical therapy as ordered to instruct in prescribed exercises, gait training, transfer activities, use of ambulatory assistive devices with weight-bearing or non-weight-bearing activities as ordered.
14. Assess level of anxiety, expressed concerns/provide emotional support/refer to social services to assist with needed community resources to help with adjustment to limited mobility status (e.g., Meals on Wheels; transportation services, attendant care).

REHABILITATION POTENTIAL

Rehabilitation potential *excellent good fair guarded poor* for *full partial* return to an independent level of functioning and increased strength and endurance as before injury.

Client's Name _____

Medical Record # _____

ONGOING/DISCHARGE EVALUATION OF TEACHING

The Client with a Fractured Hip with Internal Fixation or Prosthesis

Teaching Tools:
Printed materials given: _____

Audiovisual aids used: _____

Return Information/Demonstration/Interpretation
_____ Client
_____ Caregiver

OF:	Met	Not Met	Comments
☐ Nature of injury, surgical procedure.	_____	_____	_____
☐ S&S of complications/ actions to take.	_____	_____	_____
☐ Importance of compliance with prescribed treatment regimen.	_____	_____	_____
☐ Importance of well-balanced diet high in dietary fiber, protein, calcium, vitamin C, and adequate hydration.	_____	_____	_____
☐ Medications and administration, purpose and action, side effects.	_____	_____	_____

Client's Name _____

Medical Record # _____

	OF:	**Met**	**Not Met**	**Comments**
☐	Activity and positioning restrictions; proper alignment of affected extremity.	_____	_____	_____
☐	Posture and body mechanics.	_____	_____	_____
☐	Effects of decreased activity level on bowel functioning; prescribed measures to manage constipation problems.	_____	_____	_____
☐	Ambulatory activities with use of prescribed ambulatory aids; degree of weight bearing.	_____	_____	_____
☐	Therapeutic exercises; graded functional activities, balanced rest periods.	_____	_____	_____
☐	Wound care management.	_____	_____	_____
☐	Risk factors for falls and injuries			

Client's Name _____

Medical Record # _____

OF:	**Met**	**Not Met**	**Comments**
in home, related safety measures.	_____	_____	_____
☐ Complications of prolonged immobilization; measures to treat; activities to avoid.	_____	_____	_____

Signature of Home Health Nurse _____

Date _____

■ Osteoarthritis

Osteoarthritis (degenerative joint disease or hypertrophic arthritis) is a chronic, slowly progressive degenerative disorder, affecting the weight-bearing joints such as the knee, hips, and spine. Osteoarthritis can be classified as primary, or idiopathic, in which an underlying factor or disease cannot be identified, or secondary, in which a cause can be identified (e.g., trauma; old fractures; other inflammatory arthritic disorders). Osteoarthritis is frequently found among the elderly as a result of the normal aging process. It is characterized by a thinning or wearing down of articular cartilage, deterioration of the joint cartilage (caused by a degeneration of chondrocytes, which are cells that make up the intercellular material of the cartilage), the formation of bony spurs at the edges of the joint, and the deposition of calcium on bone surfaces and in joint spaces.

Joint pain, the most common feature of osteoarthritis, is aggravated by weight-bearing activities and exercise and is usually relieved with rest. Other symptoms include morning joint stiffness, tenderness to touch, crepitus, bony enlargements of the distal interphalangeal joints, called Heberden's nodes, and less commonly the proximal interphalangeal joints, called Bouchard's nodes. Limitation in movement results from pain and inadequate use of the joint and/or narrowing of the joint space.

POTENTIAL COMPLICATIONS

1. Irreversible development of nodes in the hands,
2. capsular and tendon tightening,
3. flexion deformities,
4. severe pain and joint inflammation,
5. pressure sores.

TYPES OF CLIENTS/CLINICAL CONDITIONS SEEN BY HOME HEALTH AGENCIES

1. Newly diagnosed with osteoarthritis: initiation of prescribed treatment regimen and inclusive teaching plan for home management of condition, rehabilitative services to establish and instruct in home exercise program for improvement in client's functional activities.
2. Exacerbation of condition: changes in prescribed medications and treatments, instruction and supervision with evaluation of response to rehabilitation services as ordered for increased disability problems.

RELATED NURSING DIAGNOSIS

Activity Intolerance

related to:
Fatigue associated with pain and
increased strength required for use
of ambulatory assistive devices

as seen by:
Weakness; exertional dyspnea;
verbalizing lack of energy and
exhaustion with movement;
increased heart and respiratory rate
in response to activities

Anxiety

related to:
1. Limited mobility
2. Joint pain
3. Knowledge deficit regarding
prescribed treatment regimen

as seen by:
Anxious appearance; c/o increasing
helplessness; irritability; asking
numerous questions regarding
treatment regimen

Comfort, Alteration in

related to:
1. Joint pain and aching
2. Joint stiffness

as seen by:
Guarding of affected joints; moaning;
crying; fatigue

Coping, Ineffective Individual

related to:
1. Progressive loss of functional
abilities, limited mobility
2. Altered body image

as seen by:
Verbalizing inability to cope; general
irritability; inability to meet basic
needs and role expectations

Injury, Potential for: Increased Risk of Falls and Injuries

related to:
1. Loss of dexterity
2. Pain
3. Incorrect use of assistive devices
with ambulation

as seen by:
Limited mobility; impaired gait or
balance; numbness and loss of
dexterity of interphalangeal joints

Knowledge Deficit (Specify)

related to:
1. Prescribed plan of treatment for care of client with osteoarthritis
2. Potential complications, S&S to report to home health nurse or physician

as seen by:
Lack of information; inadequate understanding; inability to perform skills necessary to meet health-care needs at home

Mobility, Impaired Physical

related to:
1. Restricted joint movement
2. Pain
3. Impaired ability to transfer or ambulate without use of assistive devices
4. Prescribed activity restrictions

as seen by:
Reluctance to move; limited ROM; weakness and fatigue; inability to move purposefully within home environment; decreased muscle strength, endurance

Skin Integrity, Impairment of: Potential

related to:
1. Prolonged immobilization
2. Incorrect use of assistive devices, adaptive equipment

as seen by:
Reddened, irritated areas from pressure, immobility; tissue breakdown over bony prominences; swelling, redness, tenderness of tissues with incorrect use of splints and adaptive equipment

Self-Care Deficit: Feeding, Bathing/Hygiene, Dressing/Grooming, Toileting (Specify)

related to:
1. Activity intolerance
2. Impaired mobility
3. Prescribed activity restrictions

as seen by:
Inability to effectively manage physical needs and ADL, associated with limited joint mobility; c/o pain; weakness and fatigue; exertional dyspnea

LONG-TERM GOAL

Increase in self-care capacity with improved quality of life through efforts to restore and maintain maximal joint mobility and muscle strength.

SHORT-TERM GOALS

The client with osteoarthritis will be able to:

1. Verbalize nature of disease process, type of osteoarthritis, physical limitations, aggravating factors.
2. Verbalize S&S of complications to report to home health nurse or physician.
3. Demonstrate compliance with well-balanced diet, adequate hydration.
4. Verbalize effects of excess weight on joints.
5. Demonstrate compliance with prescribed medication therapy/identify side effects.
6. Demonstrate compliance with prescribed graded exercise program.
7. Verbalize importance of correct posture and body mechanics on joints.
8. Demonstrate joint protection techniques, measures to rest and reduce stress on joints.
9. Identify predisposing factors to skin breakdown/demonstrate good skin care measures.
10. Demonstrate compliance with prescribed measures for pain management in affected joints.
11. Demonstrate measures to reduce risk of falls and injuries with ambulation.
12. Verbalize prescribed measures to decrease level of anxiety and fear to effectively manage condition.

NURSING ACTIONS/TREATMENTS

1. Assess musculoskeletal system/identify affected joints, physical limitations, complications.
2. Assess vital signs/identify trends (e.g., increased pulse and respiratory rate).
3. Instruct as to nature of disease process, type of osteoarthritis, physical limitations, aggravating factors, importance of compliance with prescribed treatment regimen, S&S of complications to report to home health nurse or physician.
4. Assess and evaluate nutritional status/instruct about well-balanced diet, adequate hydration, effect of excess weight on joints.
5. Observe/instruct about taking medications as ordered (e.g., antispasmodics, anti-inflammatory agents, analgesics), purpose and action, side effects/evaluate medication effectiveness.
6. Observe and evaluate level of tolerance to perform physical activities/instruct about prescribed graded exercise program to preserve joint function and avoid deformities (e.g., range-of-motion exercises, extension and flexion exercises, progressive resistance exercises)/pace daily activities and balance with rest periods/avoid overexertion, emotional stress, prolonged immobility.
7. Observe/instruct about prescribed joint protection techniques, measures to rest and reduce stress on joints (e.g., correct posture, body mechanics, well-fitting

support shoes, prescribed use of splints, braces, supports, ambulatory assistive devices, adaptive equipment).

8. Assess and evaluate skin integrity/instruct about good skin care, predisposing factors to breakdown.

9. Assess and evaluate level of pain/instruct about prescribed measures of pain management to affected joints (e.g., massage, moist heat, cold therapy, paraffin dips for hands).

10. Assess for increased risk of falls and injuries/instruct about safety measures with ambulation and daily activities (e.g., home environment free of hazards, safe ambulation with use of assistive devices)/assist client with daily activities as needed.

11. Observe and evaluate alterations in functional skills, ambulatory activities/refer to rehabilitation services as ordered (e.g., ROM and strengthening exercises; progressive resistance exercises; transfer and ambulatory activities with use of assistive or protective devices; joint protection and energy conservation techniques).

12. Assess anxiety, depression regarding joint pain and limited mobility/provide emotional support/assist with establishing daily goals/refer to social services as ordered to provide counseling regarding fears of permanent disability and to provide information regarding community support systems (e.g., Meals on Wheels; transportation services; American Arthritis Foundation).

REHABILITATION POTENTIAL

Rehabilitation potential *excellent   good   fair   guarded   poor* for *full partial*   return to a maximum level of functional independence to manage self care and daily activities.

Client's Name _____

Medical Record # _____

ONGOING/DISCHARGE EVALUATION OF TEACHING

The Client with Osteoarthritis

Teaching Tools:

Printed materials given: _____

Audiovisual aids used: _____

Return Information/Demonstration/Interpretation

_____ Client

_____ Caregiver

	OF:	Met	Not Met	Comments
☐	Nature of disease process; type of osteoarthritis.	_____	_____	_____
☐	Physical limitations; aggravating factors.	_____	_____	_____
☐	S&S of complications; actions to take.	_____	_____	_____
☐	Importance of compliance with prescribed treatment regimen.	_____	_____	_____
☐	Importance of well-balanced diet, adequate hydration.	_____	_____	_____
☐	Effect of excess weight on joints.	_____	_____	_____

Client's Name _____

Medical Record # _____

OF:	**Met**	**Not Met**	**Comments**
☐ Medications and administration, purpose and action, side effects.	_____	_____	_____
☐ Graded exercise program; effect on preserving joint function and avoiding deformity.	_____	_____	_____
☐ Joint protection techniques; measures to rest and reduce stress on joints.	_____	_____	_____
☐ Predisposing factors for skin breakdown; good skin care measures.	_____	_____	_____
☐ Pain management measures for affected joints.	_____	_____	_____
☐ Risk factors for falls and injuries in home; safety measures with ambulation and daily activities.	_____	_____	_____
☐ Transfer and ambulatory activities.	_____	_____	_____

Client's Name _____

Medical Record # _____

OF:	Met	Not Met	Comments
☐ Energy conservation techniques.	_____	_____	_____

_____

Signature of Home Health Nurse _____

Date _____

■ Rheumatoid Arthritis

Rheumatoid arthritis is a chronic systemic collagen disease in which an autoimmune mechanism plays an important role. It is characterized by: recurrent inflammation of the synovial membrane (more often affecting the small joints of hands and feet in a bilateral, symmetrical manner), increased synovial effusion, and thickening of the synovium and joint capsular destruction. In active disease, the affected joints are swollen, red, enlarged, hot, tender, and painful on motion. This will result in loss of mobility of the joint, spasms, and increased wasting of muscles with eventual development of contractures, resulting in immobility. The wrists, elbows, and ankles are other commonly involved areas.

Rheumatoid or subcutaneous nodules may gradually appear over the subcutaneous tissues, usually over the hands, elbow, and forearm. The characteristic deformities of the hands include spindle-shaped proximal interphalangeal joints caused by marked swelling, hyperextension of distal phalanges, and ulnar deviation of fingers and flexion deformities of the fingers, wrists, and knees.

Because the rheumatoid process is a systemic disease, there may be an associated inflammation of connective tissue of the organ or systems of the body affected by the disease. Initially, the client with rheumatoid arthritis presents with symptoms such as fatigue, persistent low-grade fever, lymphadenopathy, anorexia, and vague joint symptoms that progress to specific joint involvement.

POTENTIAL COMPLICATIONS

1. Pain,
2. contracture deformities,
3. peripheral neuropathies,
4. infection,
5. osteoporosis,
6. pressure sores.

TYPES OF CLIENTS/CLINICAL CONDITIONS SEEN BY HOME HEALTH AGENCIES

1. Newly diagnosed with rheumatoid arthritis: initiation of prescribed treatment regimen, inclusive teaching plan for home management of arthritic condition, physical therapy for functional limitations, occupational therapy for deficits in self-care and ADL.
2. Exacerbation of condition: changes in prescribed medications and treatments, need for instruction, observation, and assessment of response to treatment changes; rehabilitative services as ordered for increased disability problems.

RELATED NURSING DIAGNOSIS

Activity Intolerance

related to:
1. Immobility secondary to inflammation and degenerative changes of joints
2. Increased strength required with use of ambulatory assistive devices

as seen by:
Weakness and fatigue; exertional dyspnea and discomfort; joint stiffness; verbalizing lack of energy and exhaustion with movement, not following prescribed energy conservation techniques

Anxiety

related to:
1. Pain
2. Limited mobility
3. Increased dependency on others for care
4. Knowledge deficit regarding prescribed treatment regimen

as seen by:
Increased helplessness; distress; verbalization of fearfulness of complete disability or dependency on others for care; irritability; uncertainty of effectiveness of new medications or treatments

Comfort, Alteration in

related to:
1. Joint pain and tenderness
2. Joint immobility
3. Degenerative changes secondary to long-term inflammatory process

as seen by:
Guarding of affected joints with movement; joint stiffness; moaning and crying from pain; decreased functional abilities

Coping, Ineffective Individual

related to:
1. Progressive loss of functional abilities
2. Altered body image
3. Life-style changes

as seen by:
General irritability; verbalization of hopelessness and inability to cope

Injury, Potential for: Increased Risk of Falls and Injuries

related to:
1. Progressive loss of dexterity
2. Joint pain and stiffness

as seen by:
Reduced joint mobility, impaired gait or balance; inability to safely carry

3. Muscle weakness
4. Incorrect use of splints or ambulatory assistive devices

out daily activities and ambulation

Knowledge Deficit (Specify)

related to:
1. Disease process and related S&S
2. Prescribed plan of treatment for management of rheumatoid arthritis
3. Potential complications, S&S to report to home health nurse or physician

as seen by:
Lack of information; inadequate understanding; inability to perform skills necessary to meet health-care needs at home

Mobility, Impaired Physical

related to:
1. Pain
2. Reduced joint mobility
3. Muscle weakness
4. Prescribed activity restrictions

as seen by:
Reluctance to move; limited range of motion; decreased muscle strength and control; inability to move purposefully within home environment without assistance; imposed medical restrictions

Powerlessness, Feelings of

related to:
Immobility or loss of functional ability secondary to rheumatic condition

as seen by:
Dependence on others to meet daily and personal needs, resulting in anger and resentment; verbal expression of lack of control over self-care or control over situations; passivity; crying

Self-Care Deficit: Feeding, Bathing/Hygiene, Dressing/Grooming, Toileting (Specify)

related to:
1. Activity intolerance
2. Impaired mobility
3. Prescribed activity restrictions

as seen by:
Inability to purposefully and independently take care of personal needs and manage daily activities without assistance, associated with weakness and fatigue, loss of joint mobility, and decreased muscle strength and control

Self-Concept, Disturbance in

related to:
1. Altered body image
2. Changes in life-style

as seen by:
Anxiety, depression, withdrawal from role responsibilities; lack of follow-through with therapy

Skin Integrity, Impairment of: Potential

related to:
1. Prolonged immobilization
2. Vascular impairments
3. Treatment with steroids
4. Pressure sores secondary to incorrect use of splints or adaptive equipment

as seen by:
Reddened areas from pressure of immobility; edema; tissue breakdown; irritation and injury to tissues from incorrect use of splints or adaptive equipment

LONG-TERM GOAL

Increased joint mobility and self-care capacity with minimization of deformities following reduction of joint pain and inflammation.

SHORT-TERM GOALS

The client with rheumatoid arthritis will be able to:

1. Verbalize nature of disease process, physical limitations, aggravating factors/S&S of complications to report to home health nurse or physician.
2. Demonstrate compliance with well-balanced diet, adequate hydration/verbalize effect of excessive weight on joints.
3. Demonstrate compliance with prescribed medication therapy/identify side effects.
4. Demonstrate compliance with prescribed ROM and therapeutic exercises, importance of daily activity schedule with frequent rest periods.
5. Verbalize importance of avoiding fatigue and emotional strain.
6. Demonstrate joint protection techniques and prescribed measures to rest and reduce stress on joints.
7. Demonstrate compliance with prescribed measures of joint pain management.
8. Identify predisposing factors in impairment of skin integrity/demonstrate good skin care.
9. Demonstrate measures to reduce risk of falls and injuries with ambulation and daily activities.

10. Verbalize complications related to prolonged immobilization, prescribed measures to treat, activities to avoid.
11. Demonstrate effective coping mechanisms to decrease level of anxiety to effectively manage arthritic condition.

NURSING ACTIONS/TREATMENTS

1. Assess musculoskeletal system/identify affected joints, contractures, deformities, immobility, paresthesias, level of functioning to manage daily activities.
2. Assess vital signs/identify trends (e.g., elevated temperature).
3. Instruct about nature of disease process, physical limitations, aggravating factors, importance of strict compliance with prescribed treatment regimen, S&S of complications to report to home health nurse or physician.
4. Assess and evaluate nutritional status, (any weight loss) instruct about well-balanced diet, adequate hydration, effect of excess weight on joints.
5. Observe/instruct about taking medications as ordered (e.g., salicylates, non-steroid anti-inflammatory agents, gold salts, corticosteroids, antimalarials, penicillamine, immunosuppressives), purpose and action, side effects.
6. Observe and evaluate level of tolerance for physical activities/instruct about prescribed ROM and therapeutic exercises, daily activity schedule with frequent rest periods, avoiding fatigue, emotional strain.
7. Observe/instruct how joint protection techniques and measures can rest and reduce stress on joints (e.g., correct body mechanics and positioning, posture, well-fitting support shoes, ambulatory assistive devices, adaptive equipment, splints).
8. Assess and evaluate level of pain/instruct about resting and supporting inflamed joints, prescribed activities to reduce stiffness, swelling, and control pain (e.g., moisture heat treatments, cold therapy, hot soaks, paraffin baths, whirlpool).
9. Assess and evaluate skin integrity/instruct about good skin care measures and predisposing factors to breakdown, S&S to report to home health nurse or physician.
10. Assess for increased risk of falls and injuries in the home associated with loss of dexterity, pain, incorrect use of splints and ambulatory assistive devices/instruct about safety measures with ambulation and ADL.
11. Assess and evaluate systems of the body for complications related to prolonged immobilization/instruct about S&S to report to home health nurse or physician, prescribed measures to treat, activities to avoid.
12. Observe and evaluate alterations in self-care activities and ADL, functional skills/refer to rehabilitation services as ordered to instruct in joint protection techniques; energy conservation; use of adaptive equipment, splints, ambulatory activities with use of assistive devices; home exercise program.

13. Assess anxiety, ineffective coping mechanisms, altered self-concept and feelings of loss of control associated with progressive loss of functional abilities and altered body image/provide emotional support and verbalization of feelings/refer to social services for counseling and to provide information regarding community support systems (e.g., Arthritis Foundation, counseling services, Meals on Wheels, transportation services, attendant care).

REHABILITATION POTENTIAL

Rehabilitation potential *excellent good fair guarded poor* for *full partial* return to a maximum level of functional independence within the limitations of arthritic condition.

Client's Name _____

Medical Record # _____

ONGOING/DISCHARGE EVALUATION OF TEACHING
The Client with Rheumatoid Arthritis

Teaching Tools:
Printed materials given: _____

Audiovisual aids used: _____

Return Information/Demonstration/Interpretation
_____ Client
_____ Caregiver

	OF:	**Met**	**Not Met**	**Comments**
☐	Nature of disease process, physical limitations, aggravating factors.	_____	_____	_____
☐	S&S of complications; actions to take.	_____	_____	_____
☐	Importance of strict compliance with prescribed treatment regimen.	_____	_____	_____
☐	Importance of well-balanced diet, adequate hydration.	_____	_____	_____
☐	Effect of excess weight on joints.	_____	_____	_____
☐	Medications and administration, purpose and			

Client's Name _____

Medical Record #_____

OF:	Met	Not Met	Comments
action, side effects.	_____	_____	_____
☐ ROM and therapeutic exercises; importance of daily activity schedule with frequent rest periods.	_____	_____	_____
☐ Energy conservation techniques.	_____	_____	_____
☐ Avoiding emotional strain.	_____	_____	_____
☐ Joint protection techniques and measures to rest and reduce stress on joints.	_____	_____	_____
☐ Measures to reduce swelling, stiffness, and pain.	_____	_____	_____
☐ Factors predisposing to skin breakdown; good skin care measures.	_____	_____	_____
☐ Risk factors for falls and injuries in home; safety measures with ambulation and daily activities.	_____	_____	_____

Client's Name _____

Medical Record # _____

OF:	**Met**	**Not Met**	**Comments**
☐ Complications of prolonged immobilization; measures to treat; activities to avoid.	_____	_____	_____

Signature of Home Health Nurse _____

Date _____

GASTROINTESTINAL DISORDERS

■ Colostomy/Ileostomy

A colostomy is a surgically created opening, in which a segment of the colon is incised and brought through the abdominal wall to the skin surface to allow the passage of feces. The colostomy may be located anywhere along the length of the colon and is referred to as an ascending, transverse, descending, or sigmoid colostomy, depending on the location of the stoma.

A double-barreled colostomy may be created in any segment of the colon. The colon is divided and has two distinct stomas. The distal opening leads to the now inactive portion of the colon, whereas the proximal stoma is the active end of the colon, through which stool is eliminated.

A loop colostomy is made by bringing the selected segment of bowel out onto the abdomen and supporting it by placing a rod (or plastic bridge) under the loop. The stoma has two openings. The proximal (or active) stoma discharges fecal material, whereas the distal (or inactive) portion of the colon has a mucus discharge. This procedure is often temporary, to allow healing of an end-to-end anastomosis after a bowel resection.

The location of the stoma, whether on the ascending, descending, transverse, or sigmoid colon, determines the consistency of the output. Management of the colostomy depends on the type of output. A colostomy located on the left transverse, descending, or sigmoid colon usually has stools that are semisoft to well-formed, with an output that is fairly predictable. A colostomy located on the ascending and right transverse colon generally has frequent, irregular discharges that are liquid to semisolid.

An ileostomy is an opening made into the distal portion of the ileum that allows elimination of fecal contents through a stoma, generally located on the right lower quadrant of the abdomen. The consistency of the fecal discharge is usually liquid to semipaste; it drains continually and is high in enzymes that are irritating and could cause damage to the skin around the stoma. A base-losing metabolic acidosis and isotonic dehydration could result as a complication of profuse discharge of ileal fluid.

In some clients a "continent" ileostomy may be created. A pouch or Kock ileostomy is a surgical procedure that creates an intra-abdominal reservoir, constructed from the terminal ileum, and an outlet valve, formed from a segment of intussuscepted ileum. The collected ileal contents are drained routinely about four times a day with a catheter that is inserted through the stoma and valve into the pouch. A pad is worn over the stoma between intubations.

Both a colostomy and an ileostomy may be temporary, depending on the indication for the surgical procedure. A temporary ostomy allows the intestine to heal or rests inflamed areas associated with diseases, injuries, or surgeries of the bowel. A permanent ostomy is generally the result of cancer of the colon or rectum or chronic inflammatory bowel disease.

POTENTIAL COMPLICATIONS

1. Suture separation,
2. wound infection,
3. stoma obstruction, constriction, prolapse, or retraction,

4. fluid and electrolyte imbalances secondary to excessive ostomy drainage,
5. peristomal skin irritation and breakdown,
6. renal calculi.

TYPES OF CLIENTS/CLINICAL CONDITIONS SEEN BY HOME HEALTH AGENCIES

1. Observation and care of surgical incision not healed.
2. Dressing changes (draining wound).
3. Wound infection.
4. Instruction and supervision of colostomy irrigations.
5. Ostomy and stomal care and instruction.
6. Postsurgical complications related to ostomy and stoma.
7. New problems or complications in long-term ostomy client: changes in prescribed plan of treatment requiring instruction, supervision, observation of response to new treatments.

RELATED NURSING DIAGNOSIS

Activity Intolerance

related to:
1. Incisional pain and discomfort
2. Inadequate nutritional status

as seen by:
Weakness and fatigue; exertional dyspnea with ambulation and daily activities

Anxiety

related to:
1. Altered body image
2. Life-style changes
3. Changes in role relationships
4. Knowledge deficit regarding prescribed treatment regimen

as seen by:
Look of anxiousness with colostomy care; verbalized fear of managing colostomy at home; expressed concern of acceptance by family and friends; numerous questions or lack of questions

Bowel Elimination, Alteration in: Constipation

related to:
1. Inadequate fluids and lack of balanced diet

as seen by:
Abdominal distension; ostomy output less than usual amount with feelings

2. Actions of certain medications and foods
3. Obstruction (e.g., food blockage, adhesions, kinking of small intestine)
4. Stenosis
5. Decreased activity levels

of fullness; nausea; vomiting; abdominal cramping

Bowel Elimination, Alteration in: Diarrhea

related to:
1. Food intolerances specific to client
2. Excessive fluid intake
3. Viral or bacterial gastroenteritis
4. Action of certain medications
5. Anxiety

as seen by:
Increased frequency of ostomy output; change in consistency of stomal effluent; abdominal pain or cramping; unusually foul-smelling stools

Breathing Pattern, Ineffective

related to:
1. Surgical incision
2. Anxiety

as seen by:
Shallow respirations; dyspnea; splinted or guarded respirations

Comfort, Alteration in: Pain

related to:
1. Surgical incision
2. Irritation or breakdown of peristomal skin
3. Stomal obstruction
4. Renal calculi

as seen by:
Verbal c/o pain; reluctance to move; splinting of incisional area with movement; increased redness and c/o burning of peristomal skin area; abdominal cramping; nausea; vomiting; flank pain; hematuria; urinary frequency or urgency

Coping, Ineffective Individual

related to:
1. Change in body apperance or functioning
2. Difficulty in managing ostomy

as seen by:
Inability to meet basic needs; increasing fatigue; fear; anxiety; verbalized inability to cope; not willing to be involved with treatment regimen

Fluid Volume Deficit

related to:
Excessive ileostomy/colostomy output

as seen by:
S&S of dehydration or electrolyte imbalance; increased pulse rate; weakness; change in mental status

Grieving

related to:
1. Changes in body appearance and usual method of bowel elimination
2. Life-style changes

as seen by:
Denial; anger; depression; crying; withdrawal from usual relationships and activities

Infection, Potential for

related to:
Incisional area or breakdown of peristomal skin secondary to breakdown of the body's first line of defense

as seen by:
Increased pain; pronounced tenderness; redness; swelling; unusual drainage; tissue breakdown

Knowledge Deficit (Specify)

related to:
1. Prescribed plan of treatment in management and adjustment to ostomy
2. Potential complications, S&S to report to home health nurse or physician

as seen by:
Verbalization of lack of information; inadequate understanding; inability to perform skills necessary to meet health-care needs at home

Mobility, Impaired Physical

related to:
1. Incisional pain and discomfort
2. Decreased strength postsurgery

as seen by:
Reluctance to attempt movement; weakness and fatigue

Nutrition, Alteration in: Less than Body Requirements

related to:
1. Inadequate oral intake
2. Diarrhea
3. Prescribed dietary restrictions

as seen by:
Anorexia; weight loss; frequent loose stools; weakness and fatigue

Self-Care Deficit: Feeding, Bathing/Hygiene, Dressing/Grooming, Toileting (Specify)

related to:
1. Activity intolerance
2. Impaired physical mobility
3. Prescribed activity restrictions

as seen by:
Dyspnea on exertion; weakness and fatigue; pain with movement when participating in self-care activities; imposed medical restrictions on ADL

Self-Concept, Disturbance in

related to:
1. Altered body image
2. Effect of ostomy on relationships and quality of life

as seen by:
Refusal to look at, touch stoma, and/or care for ostomy; increasing dependence on others for care; signs of grieving; withdrawal from relationships; verbalizes limitations or change in usual sexual behavior or activity

Skin Integrity, Impairment of: Actual/Potential

related to:
1. Surgial incision
2. Impaired healing secondary to infection
3. Improper fit of appliance with leakage of drainage
4. Improper or repeated removal of adhesives
5. Sensitivity to skin-care products
6. Inadequate nutritional status

as seen by:
Increased redness, swelling, unusual drainage, irritation, breakdown at wound site and/or peristomal skin area; burning; itching of peristomal skin with use of skin-care products

Social Isolation

related to:
Changes in body image and functioning

as seen by:
Verbalization of feelings of embarrassment and rejection with change in usual method of elimination; leakage of appliance; odor

LONG-TERM GOAL

To maintain elimination of intestinal contents through a proper functioning artificial opening of the lower alimentary canal.

SHORT-TERM GOALS

The client with a colostomy or ileostomy will be able to:

1. Verbalize understanding of indication for surgical procedure, type of ostomy, S&S of complications to report to home health nurse or physician.
2. Demonstrate compliance with prescribed diet/identify measures to avoid and relieve stomal food blockage.
3. Demonstrate compliance with prescribed medication therapy/identify complications.
4. Identify S&S of dehydration and electrolyte imbalance with excessive discharge from ostomy, prescribed measures to correct.
5. Identify predisposing factors to peristomal skin breakdown, prescribed measures to treat.
6. Verbalize importance of reporting changes in stoma to physician.
7. Demonstrate how to measure stoma, verbalize effect of decreasing stoma size on pouch size.
8. Identify measures to reduce gas formation, control odors.
9. Demonstrate prescribed technique for colostomy irrigations.
10. Demonstrate prescribed technique for draining contents and irrigation of a "continent ileostomy."
11. Demonstrate compliance with prescribed use of skin barriers, appliances and accessories and care of equipment.
12. Demonstrate compliance with prescribed wound care management, identify S&S of infection to report to home health nurse or physician.
13. Demonstrate balanced rest and activity levels.
14. Demonstrate positive adaptation to ostomy.

NURSING ACTIONS/TREATMENTS

1. Assess gastrointestinal functioning/identify complications.
2. Assess vital signs/identify trends (e.g., elevated temperature, increased pulse rate).
3. Instruct as to indication for surgical procedure, type of ostomy, importance of compliance with prescribed treatment regimen, S&S of complications to report to home health nurse or physician.
4. Assess and evaluate nutritional status, food intolerances/instruct about prescribed diet specific to ostomate, measures to avoid stomal food blockage (e.g., chewing food well, avoiding foods difficult to digest), measures to relieve stomal food blockage (e.g., actions to promote peristalsis: warm com-

presses and/or massage of abdomen), measures to shift or break up food blockage (e.g., leaning forward, knee-chest position, prescribed lavage procedure)/obtain dietary consultation as needed.

5. Observe/instruct about taking medications as ordered, purpose and action, side effects/evaluate medication effectiveness.

6. Assess and evaluate for S&S of dehydration and electrolyte imbalance caused by excessive discharge from ostomy/instruct about foods and fluids to avoid and prescribed treatment with use of antidiarrheal medications/report effects of treatment to physician.

7. Assess/instruct to inspect peristomal skin/instruct about measures to avoid irritation, breakdown, prescribed measures to treat impaired skin integrity.

8. Assess/instruct about changes in stoma (e.g., sustained color changes, increased or excess edema, bleeding)/report to physician.

9. Assess/instruct about remeasuring stoma for first two months postsurgery for changes in stomal size and need for readjustment in pouch size.

10. Assess/instruct about measures to reduce gas formation, control of odors (e.g., odor-resistant pouch, personal and appliance hygiene, avoiding gas- and odor-producing foods).

11. Observe/instruct about prescribed colostomy irrigations (type of solution, frequency, proper use of equipment)/emphasize that irrigations provide a degree of regularity and continence of bowel movements.

12. Observe/instruct about prescribed skin and stomal care procedures (e.g., proper application of skin barriers, use of appliances and accessories, cleaning and care of equipment), importance of establishing a daily time and routine for emptying and changing the appliance.

13. Observe/instruct client with a "continent" ileostomy as to prescribed technique for draining of contents and irrigation of ostomy.

14. Assess and evaluate healing of abdominal and/or perineal wound/instruct about prescribed wound care management, S&S of wound infection to report to home health nurse or physician.

15. Assess/instruct about balanced rest and activity levels.

16. Assess ineffective coping mechanisms, grieving over loss in usual method of bowel elimination/provide emotional support and encourage to verbalize feelings (e.g., concern over effect on sex life)/refer to social services to provide counseling and assistance with adaptation to condition and information regarding support groups in the community (e.g., United Ostomy Association, American Cancer Society, counseling services).

17. Refer to enterostomal therapist as needed for assistance with ostomy care.

REHABILITATION POTENTIAL

Rehabilitation potential *excellent good fair guarded poor* for *full partial* return to an independent level of functioning and improved sense of well-being to manage ostomy and ADL.

Client's Name _____

Medical Record # _____

ONGOING/DISCHARGE EVALUATION OF TEACHING
The Client with a Colostomy/Ileostomy

Teaching Tools:
Printed materials given: _____

Audiovisual aids used: _____

Return Information/Demonstration/Interpretation
_____ Client
_____ Caregiver

	OF:	Met	Not Met	Comments
☐	Indication for surgical procedure; type of ostomy.	____	____	_____
☐	S&S of complications; actions to take.	____	____	_____
☐	Importance of compliance with prescribed treatment regimen.	____	____	_____
☐	Diet specific to ostomate; measures to avoid stomal food blockage; measures to relieve stomal food blockage.	____	____	_____
☐	Medications and administration, purpose and action, side effects.	____	____	_____

Client's Name _____

Medical Record #_____

OF:	**Met**	**Not Met**	**Comments**
☐ S&S of dehydration and electrolyte imbalance with excessive ileostomy or colostomy output; prescribed measures to treat.	_____	_____	_____
☐ S&S of peristomal skin irritation, breakdown; activities to avoid; measures to treat.	_____	_____	_____
☐ Changes in stoma to report to physician.	_____	_____	_____
☐ Procedure to remeasure stoma; effect of stomal size on pouch opening.	_____	_____	_____
☐ Measures to reduce gas formation, control of odors.	_____	_____	_____
☐ Colostomy irrigations.	_____	_____	_____
☐ Draining of contents and irrigation of a "continent ileostomy."	_____	_____	_____

Client's Name _____

Medical Record # _____

	OF:	**Met**	**Not Met**	**Comments**
☐	Application of skin-care barriers.	_____	_____	_____
☐	Use of appliances and accessories.	_____	_____	_____
☐	Cleaning and care of equipment.	_____	_____	_____
☐	Wound care management.	_____	_____	_____
☐	Balanced rest and activities.	_____	_____	_____

Signature of Home Health Nurse _____

Date _____

■ Diverticulitis

Herniation of the mucosal lining through weakened muscular layers of the gastrointestinal wall, forming saclike pouches, results in a condition called diverticulosis. Predisposing factors to this muscular weakening may be associated with obesity, chronic constipation, inactivity, or aging. The most common site for the diverticula is in the sigmoid colon; generally they cause no symptoms unless they are inflamed.

Diverticula may also result from altered motility patterns of the colon and inadequate fiber in the diet. Inflammation of diverticula, a condition called diverticulitis, may produce mild symptoms of pain in the lower quadrant of the abdomen, nausea, flatulence, intermittent constipation or diarrhea. If left untreated, diverticular disease could result in abscess formation or peritonitis due to perforation, while chronic diverticulitis may cause fibrosis and adhesions, predisposing to intestinal obstruction.

POTENTIAL COMPLICATIONS

1. Hemorrhage,
2. perforation, peritonitis, abscess or fistula formation,
3. intestinal obstruction,
4. pain,
5. fluid and electrolyte imbalances with persistent diarrhea.

TYPES OF CLIENTS/CLINICAL CONDITIONS SEEN BY HOME HEALTH AGENCIES

1. Newly diagnosed with diverticulitis: initiation of prescribed treatment regimen and inclusive teaching plan for home-care management of condition.
2. Exacerbation of diverticulitis: changes in prescribed treatment regimen for management of increasing symptoms and complications (e.g., placed on antibiotic therapy for infection).
3. Recent hospitalization following an acute exacerbation and complications of diverticulitis: new medications and treatments, need for instruction, supervision and evaluation of response to treatment.

RELATED NURSING DIAGNOSIS

Anxiety

related to:
1. Pain and tenderness of abdomen
2. Diarrhea
3. Rectal bleeding
4. Knowledge deficit regarding nature of disease process and prescribed treatment regimen

as seen by:
Expression of worry and distress regarding condition; depression with intermittent exacerbation of problem

Bowel Elimination, Alteration in: Constipation

related to:
1. Incomplete bowel obstruction secondary to repeated attacks of inflammation
2. Pericolitis
3. Inadequate fluids and fiber in diet

as seen by:
Abdominal pain or cramping; distension; flatulence; decreased frequency and amount of stool; straining; hard, formed stools; ribbon-like stools; nausea

Bowel Elimination, Alteration in: Diarrhea

related to:
Irritation and inflammation of bowel

as seen by:
Increased frequency of stools; loose, liquid stools; abdominal pain or cramping; S&S of fluid and electrolyte imbalance with persistent diarrhea

Comfort, Alteration in: Pain

related to:
1. Inflammation of diverticula
2. Perianal irritation associated with diarrhea and inadequate personal hygiene

as seen by:
Pain and tenderness of the abdomen; redness, pain, discomfort of perianal area

Coping, Ineffective Individual

related to:
Pain and clinical manifestations of bowel disorder

as seen by:
General irritability; inability to meet basic needs; overeating or lack of appetite; verbalization of inability to cope.

Infection, Potential for

related to:
Abscess formation and peritonitis secondary to a perforated diverticulum

as seen by:
Pain in left lower quadrant of abdomen; tenderness; high fever and chills

Knowledge Deficit (Specify)

related to:
1. Inadequate understanding of nature of disease process, related S&S
2. Prescribed plan of treatment in management of diverticular disease

as seen by:
Verbalization of lack of information; inadequate understanding of management of diverticulitis

3. Potential complications, S&S to report to home health nurse or physician

Nutrition, Alteration in: Less than Body Requirements

related to:
1. Decreased oral intake associated with pain and GI disturbances
2. Decreased absorption of nutrients secondary to persistent diarrhea
3. Prescribed dietary restrictions

as seen by:
Pain with eating; weight loss; inadequate caloric intake; weakness and fatigue

Nutrition, Alteration in: More than Body Requirements

related to:
Excessive oral food intake

as seen by:
Weight 10 percent or more above desirable weight for height and body build; eating in response to anxiety; exacerbation of symptoms with excessive weight

Skin Integrity, Impairment of: Potential

related to:
Perianal irritation associated with diarrhea and inadequate personal hygiene

as seen by:
Redness, pain and discomfort; tissue breakdown

LONG-TERM GOAL

To reduce the inflammatory process and return to normal the motility pattern of the intestine.

SHORT-TERM GOALS

The client with diverticulitis will be able to:

1. Verbalize nature of disease process, predisposing factors, S&S of complications to report to physician.
2. Verbalize importance of adequate nutrition, good eating habits/identify difficult to digest and gastrically irritating foods.
3. Demonstrate compliance with prescribed weight control diet/verbalize effect of excessive weight in aggravating symptoms.

4. Verbalize importance of minimal- or moderate-residue diet and food and fluid restrictions during an attack of diverticulitis.
5. Demonstrate compliance with prescribed medication therapy.
6. Identify activities that increase intra-abdominal pressure, effect on diverticula.
7. Verbalize importance of good bowel habits, use of natural and bulk-forming laxatives as prescribed, avoiding use of harsh laxatives and enemas.
8. Verbalize importance of reporting problems with diarrhea to physician, good personal hygiene to perianal area to avoid irritation or breakdown.
9. Verbalize importance of exercise and planned rest periods on gastrointestinal motility.
10. Demonstrate use of effective coping mechanisms with a reduction in anxiety levels to manage ADL and prescribed treatment regimen.

NURSING ACTIONS/TREATMENTS

1. Assess gastrointestinal status, bowel elimination pattern/identify complications.
2. Assess vital signs/identify trends (e.g., elevated temperature, tachycardia, hypotension).
3. Instruct as to nature of disease process, predisposing factors, importance of compliance with prescribed treatment regimen, S&S of complications to report to physician.
4. Assess and evaluate nutritional status/instruct about prescribed increase in dietary fiber, adequate hydration, good eating habits, avoiding difficult-to-digest, irritating foods.
5. Assess and evaluate weight/instruct as to importance of prescribed weight control diet, effect of excessive weight in aggravating symptoms/weigh weekly and record.
6. Assess/instruct about minimal- or moderate-residue diet, avoiding extremely hot or cold foods and fluids, alcohol, and indigestible fiber (e.g., corn, celery) during an attack of diverticulitis.
7. Observe/instruct about taking medications as ordered (e.g., antibiotics, antispasmodics, analgesics), purpose and action, side effects/evaluate medication effectiveness.
8. Observe/instruct to avoid activities that increase intra-abdominal pressure (e.g., straining, coughing, bending, stooping), effect on diverticula.
9. Assess bowel problems with constipation and straining/instruct as to measures to establish good bowel habits, avoiding harsh laxatives and enemas, use of natural and bulk-forming laxatives as prescribed/evaluate effectiveness of bowel regimen.
10. Assess/instruct about reporting ongoing problems of diarrhea to physician, importance of good personal hygiene to perianal area to avoid irritation or breakdown.

11. Assess/instruct as to importance of exercise and planned rest periods, effect on gastrointestinal motility.
12. Assess anxiety, ineffective coping mechanisms concerning condition and treatment regimen/provide emotional support and assistance/refer to social services as needed to assist with adaptation to illness and provide information regarding needed community resources (e.g., support groups for weight loss; counseling services; Meals on Wheels).

REHABILITATION POTENTIAL

Rehabilitation potential *excellent   good   fair   guarded   poor*   for   *full partial*   return to a normal pattern of bowel elimination and symptomatic relief of diverticulitis to independently manage ADL.

Client's Name _____

Medical Record # _____

ONGOING/DISCHARGE EVALUATION OF TEACHING
The Client with Diverticulitis

Teaching Tools:
Printed mterials given: _____

Audiovisual aids used: _____

Return Information/Demonstration/Interpretation
_____ Client
_____ Caregiver

OF:	Met	Not Met	Comments
☐ Nature of disease process, predisposing factors.	_____	_____	_____
☐ S&S of complications; actions to take.	_____	_____	_____
☐ Importance of compliance with prescribed treatment regimen.	_____	_____	_____
☐ Increase in dietary fiber, adequate hydration, good eating habits.	_____	_____	_____
☐ Difficult-to-digest and irritating foods to avoid.	_____	_____	_____
☐ Weight control diet, effect on diverticula.	_____	_____	_____

Client's Name _____

Medical Record #_____

OF:	Met	Not Met	Comments
☐ Low-to-moderate residue diet, food and fluid restrictions during an attack of diverticulitis.	_____	_____	_____
☐ Medications and administration, purpose and action, side effects.	_____	_____	_____
☐ Avoiding activities that increase intra-abdominal pressure, effect on diverticula.	_____	_____	_____
☐ Good bowel habits; importance of use of natural and bulk laxatives as prescribed; avoiding harsh laxatives and enemas.	_____	_____	_____
☐ Importance of reporting to physician ongoing problems with diarrhea.	_____	_____	_____
☐ Good personal hygiene to perianal area to avoid irritation and breakdown.	_____	_____	_____

Client's Name _____

Medical Record # _____

OF:	Met	Not Met	Comments
☐ Exercise; planned rest periods.	_____	_____	_____

Signature of Home Health Nurse _____

Date _____

■ Fecal Impaction

Fecal impaction results from prolonged retention and accumulation of feces in the rectum or sigmoid colon with the inability to pass a normal stool. Rectal pain, abdominal distension, leaking of mucus and blood around the impaction (caused by irritation of the upper rectum and sigmoid), and a hardened fecal mass felt on digital exam are all characteristics that may be found with a fecal impaction.

Contributing factors to a fecal impaction are decreased activity, inadequate fluids and dietary fiber, failure to establish and maintain habituation of bowel movements, medications and systemic diseases, and conditions of the body. In the older adult, decreased colonic peristalsis, a dulling of neural impulses that sense the signal to defecate, and laxative abuse are also contributing factors to constipation or impaction.

POTENTIAL COMPLICATIONS

1. Hemorrhoids,
2. anal fissures.

TYPES OF CLIENTS/CLINICAL CONDITIONS SEEN BY HOME HEALTH AGENCIES

Clients needing assistance with restoration of bowel functioning through disimpaction and instruction in prescribed measures to achieve and maintain good bowel activity.

RELATED NURSING DIAGNOSIS

Anxiety

related to:
1. Inability to move bowels
2. Removal of impaction
3. Knowledge deficit regarding prescribed treatment regimen

as seen by:
Distress; nervousness; apprehension; numerous questions regarding treatment to resolve impaction and avoid future problems

Bowel Elimination, Alteration in: Constipation/Fecal Impaction

related to:
1. Inadequate intake of fluids and dietary fiber
2. Decreased activity levels

as seen by:
Inability to have a bowel movement; abdominal distension; cramping pain, fecal mass felt on digital exam

3. Decreased peristalsis secondary to systemic disease or condition
4. Failure to respond to defecation stimulus

Comfort, Alteration in: Pain

related to:
Abdominal cramping secondary to fecal impaction

as seen by:
Facial expression of pain or discomfort; verbalized c/o pain

Knowledge Deficit (Specify)

related to:
1. Prescribed plan of treatment in management of good bowel functioning
2. Potential complications, S&S to report to home health nurse or physician

as seen by:
Verbalization of lack of information; inadequate understanding in measures to restore good bowel functioning

LONG-TERM GOAL

To restore and maintain normal bowel motility and functioning.

SHORT-TERM GOALS

The client with a fecal impaction will be able to:

1. Verbalize predisposing factors to fecal impaction, S&S of complications to report to home health nurse or physician.
2. Demonstrate compliance with prescribed medication therapy.
3. Verbalize prescribed measures to establish and maintain good bowel habits.
4. Verbalize importance of balanced diet high in dietary fiber, adequate hydration, and effect of activities and exercise on good bowel functioning.
5. Verbalize understanding of prescribed treatments and procedures to be performed by home health nurse to restore bowel functioning.
6. Demonstrate reduction in level of anxiety regarding removal of fecal impaction and restoring of normal bowel functioning.

NURSING ACTIONS/TREATMENTS

1. Assess gastrointestinal status/identify complications.
2. Assess vital signs/identify trends (e.g., elevated temperature, rapid pulse rate, elevated BP).

3. Assess bowel elimination pattern/instruct about good bowel habits, predisposing factors to impaction.
4. Observe/instruct about taking medications (laxatives, suppositories as ordered), purpose and action, side effects/evaluate effectiveness.
5. Instruct about bowel regimen as ordered by physician for treatment of impaction (e.g., home health nurse to manually break up and remove fecal impaction, administer enema(s) as prescribed)/instruct about good bowel habits/evaluate effectiveness of bowel regimen in restoring bowel functioning.
6. Assess and evaluate dietary habits/instruct about prescribed balanced diet high in dietary fiber, adequate fluid intake, elimination of constipating foods.
7. Observe and evaluate activity levels/instruct about importance of daily activities and exercise to good bowel functioning.
8. Assess level of anxiety/give concise explanations of procedures and treatments/encourage to verbalize feelings and concerns.

REHABILITATION POTENTIAL

Rehabilitation potential   *excellent   good   fair   guarded   poor*   for   *full partial*   return to an improved level of bowel functioning.

Client's Name _____

Medical Record #_____

ONGOING/DISCHARGE EVALUATION OF TEACHING

The Client with a Fecal Impaction

Teaching Tools:

Printed materials given: _____

Audiovisual aids used: _____

Return Information/Demonstration/Interpretation

_____ Client

_____ Caregiver

	OF:	Met	Not Met	Comments
☐	Predisposing factors to fecal impaction.	_____	_____	_____
☐	S&S of complications; actions to take.	_____	_____	_____
☐	Importance of compliance with prescribed treatment regimen.	_____	_____	_____
☐	Good bowel habits.	_____	_____	_____
☐	Balanced diet, high in dietary fiber, adequate hydration.	_____	_____	_____
☐	Medications and administration, purpose and action, side effects.	_____	_____	_____

Client's Name _____

Medical Record # _____

OF:	**Met**	**Not Met**	**Comments**
☐ Importance of activities and exercise for good bowel functioning.	_____	_____	_____

Signature of Home Health Nurse _____

Date _____

■ Gastrectomy

A gastrectomy is a surgical procedure in which all or part of the stomach is resected. It is commonly performed to treat chronic peptic ulcers that continue to be symptomatic despite medical management. It is also indicated in complications of peptic ulcer disease associated with perforation, hemorrhage, pyloric obstruction, or for the removal of a malignancy. In a subtotal gastrectomy, with a gastroduodenostomy, the distal two thirds to three fourths of the stomach is resected, with anastomosis of the remaining segment of the stomach to the duodenum (Billroth I). In a subtotal gastrectomy, with a gastrojejunostomy, the distal segment of the stomach and antrum is resected, with anastomosis of the remaining stomach to the jejunum (Billroth II). Both surgical procedures reduce a large area of acid-secreting mucosa and help to restore gastric emptying. A vagotomy may be performed at the same time to further reduce the amount of gastric-acid secretion and decrease gastric motility and emptying. A total gastrectomy, with anastomosis of the esophagus to the jejunum, is a surgical procedure that may be performed to treat a gastric carcinoma.

After a gastric resection, a client may experience a condition called "dumping syndrome." This syndrome occurs when gastric contents empty too rapidly into the small intestine soon after eating, usually within the first hour. The client may complain of nausea or vomiting, dizziness, diaphoresis, abdominal distension, or diarrhea.

Alimentary or postprandial hypoglycemia is another complication that may be observed after extensive gastric surgery and is usually associated with the dumping syndrome. This dysfunction occurs when gastric contents empty into the small intestine too quickly, causing glucose to be absorbed too rapidly. This produces hyperglycemia, which stimulates excessive insulin production, with a subsequent rapid drop in blood glucose levels. Postprandial hypoglycemia usually occurs 1 to 3 hours after eating and is characterized by diaphoresis, dizziness, complaints of hunger, weakness, palpitations, and tremors.

Postgastrectomy pernicious anemia is a complication that may occur as a result of a deficiency in gastric intrinsic factor, which is essential for the absorption of vitamin B_{12}. Clinical manifestations that may occur are extreme weakness, numbness and tingling in extremities, weight loss, pallor and fever, glossitis.

POTENTIAL COMPLICATIONS

1. Hemorrhage,
2. wound infection,
3. peptic ulceration,
4. intestinal obstruction,
5. dumping syndrome,
6. postprandial hypoglycemia,
7. vitamin B_{12} deficiency.

TYPES OF CLIENTS/CLINICAL CONDITIONS SEEN BY HOME HEALTH AGENCIES

1. Postsurgical observations, initiation of prescribed treatment and teaching plan: includes wound care and/or dressing changes.

2. Development of complications related to surgery: instruction about changes in prescribed treatment regimen, observation of response to therapy.

RELATED NURSING DIAGNOSIS

Activity Intolerance

related to:
1. Incisional pain and discomfort
2. Inadequate nutritional status

as seen by:
Weakness and fatigue; exertional discomfort; dyspnea; abnormal heart rate, respiratory rate, BP, in response to activities

Anxiety

related to:
1. Incisional pain
2. Discomfort in response to activities
3. Alteration in body functioning
4. Knowledge deficit regarding prescribed treatment regimen

as seen by:
Nervousness; verbalization of uncertainty about foods allowed and prescribed measures to control dumping syndrome

Breathing Pattern, Ineffective

related to:
1. Incisional pain
2. Anxiety

as seen by:
Splinted, guarded respirations; shallow respirations

Comfort, Alteration in: Pain

related to:
Surgical incision

as seen by:
Reluctance to move; reports of pain in wound area; decreased physical activity; facial mask of pain with movement

Infection, Potential for

related to:
Incisional area and breakdown of body's first line of defense

as seen by:
Increased pain and tenderness, redness; swelling, incisional drainage; irritation and tissue breakdown

Knowledge Deficit (Specify)

related to:
1. Peptic ulcer disease
2. Prescribed plan of treatment following gastrectomy
3. Potential complications, S&S to report to home health nurse or physician

as seen by:
Verbalization of lack of information; inadequate understanding; inability to perform skills necessary to meet health-care needs at home

Nutrition, Alteration in: Less than Body Requirements

related to:
1. Decreased oral intake secondary to fear of symptoms with dumping syndrome and postprandial hypoglycemia, diet modifications, incisional pain
2. Disruption of digestion/absorption secondary to:
   a. Nutrient breakdown impeded and poor mixing of food and enzymes associated with rapid emptying of gastric contents into the jejunum (dumping syndrome)
   b. Rapid intestinal transit time with resultant diarrhea associated with loss of stomach reservoir function and vagotomy (if performed)
   c. Decreased hydrochloric acid secondary to removal of parietal cells and vagotomy (if performed)
3. Impaired absorption of vitamin B_{12} caused by gastric intrinsic factor deficiency following gastrectomy

as seen by:
Anorexia; weight loss; reluctance to eat; nausea and vomiting; abdominal distension; diarrhea; sore tongue; weakness and fatigue; peripheral neuropathy

Self-Care Deficit: Feeding, Bathing/Hygiene, Dressing/Grooming, Toileting (Specify)

related to:
1. Activity intolerance
2. Impaired mobility status

as seen by:
Decreased participation in taking care of physical needs, associated with

3. Prescribed activity restrictions

weakness and fatigue; incisional pain and reluctance to move; imposed medical restrictions

Skin Integrity, Impairment of: Actual/Potential

related to:
1. Surgical incision
2. Impaired healing secondary to infection
3. Inadequate nutritional status

as seen by:
Increased redness and swelling; unusual drainage; pain and tenderness; irritation and breakdown at wound site

LONG-TERM GOAL

To recover from surgery without evidence of complications and reduce the tendency to peptic ulcer formation through following of prescribed treatment regimen.

SHORT-TERM GOALS

The client who has had a gastrectomy will be able to:

1. Verbalize nature of peptic ulcer disease, surgical intervention, S&S of complications to report to home health nurse or physician.
2. Demonstrate compliance with prescribed diet and dietary restrictions.
3. Demonstrate compliance with prescribed medication therapy/identify complications.
4. Demonstrate prescribed wound care management.
5. Verbalize importance of exercise to tolerance with planned rest periods.
6. Describe cause of dumping syndrome, postprandial hypoglycemia, S&S, prescribed actions to take.
7. Identify stressful situations, effect on peptic ulcer disease, effective coping mechanisms, situations to avoid.

NURSING ACTIONS/TREATMENTS

1. Assess gastrointestinal status/identify S&S of complications.
2. Assess vital signs/identify trends (e.g., elevated temperature).
3. Instruct as to nature of peptic ulcer disease, surgical intervention, importance of compliance with prescribed postsurgical treatment regimen, S&S of complications to report to home health nurse or physician.
4. Assess and evaluate nutritional status/instruct about prescribed diet of small

frequent meals, avoiding difficult-to-digest and gastrically irritating foods, importance of adequate hydration.

5. Observe/instruct as to taking medications as ordered (e.g., antacids, anticholinergics, antispasmodics, analgesics, vitamin B_{12} injections)/purpose and action, side effects, avoiding ulcerogenic drugs (e.g., aspirin or aspirin-containing products, corticosteroids).

6. Assess and evaluate healing of incisional area/instruct about prescribed wound care management, S&S of infection to report to home health nurse or physician.

7. Observe/instruct about progressive, increased self-care and activities and exercise to tolerance with planned rest periods, avoiding heavy lifting or straining for 6 weeks.

8. Assess and evaluate S&S of dumping syndrome, alimentary, or postprandial, hypoglycemia/instruct about causes, prescribed measures to control (e.g., small frequent meals; eating slowly/eating foods containing more fats and protein; avoiding concentrated carbohydrates, extremely hot or cold foods, and fluids; lying down for 30 minutes to 1 hour after eating, taking medications prescribed for condition)/instruct to take a rapid-acting carbohydrate (e.g., orange juice, hard candy) with postprandial hypoglycemia.

9. Assess/instruct about measures to cope with and/or avoid stressful situations/refer to social services as needed to assist with necessary life-style changes and provide information about community services (e.g., counseling services, stress management programs).

REHABILITATION POTENTIAL

Rehabilitation potential   *excellent   good   fair   guarded   poor*   for   *full partial*   return to predisease status and stable physical condition to manage daily activities.

Client's Name _____

Medical Record # _____

ONGOING/DISCHARGE EVALUATION OF TEACHING

The Client Who Has Had a Gastrectomy

Teaching Tools:

Printed materials given: _____

Audiovisual aids used: _____

Return Information/Demonstration/Interpretation

_____ Client

_____ Caregiver

OF:	Met	Not Met	Comments
☐ Nature of disease process, surgical intervention.	_____	_____	_____
☐ S&S of complications; actions to take.	_____	_____	_____
☐ Importance of compliance with prescribed postsurgical treatment regimen.	_____	_____	_____
☐ Prescribed diet of small, frequent meals; dietary restrictions; adequate hydration.	_____	_____	_____
☐ Medications and administration, purpose and action, side effects.	_____	_____	_____

Client's Name _____

Medical Record # _____

	OF:	Met	Not Met	Comments
☐	Wound care management.	_____	_____	_____
☐	Exercise to tolerance; planned rest periods.	_____	_____	_____
☐	Cause of dumping syndrome, S&S; actions to take.	_____	_____	_____
☐	Cause of alimentary, or postprandial, hypoglycemia, S&S, actions to take.	_____	_____	_____
☐	Cause of pernicious anemia and need for vitamin B_{12} injections.	_____	_____	_____
☐	Effect of stressful situations on peptic ulcer disease.	_____	_____	_____

Signature of Home Health Nurse _____

Date _____

■ Hiatal Hernia

Hiatal hernia is a condition characterized by the herniation of a portion of the stomach into the thoracic cavity through the esophageal hiatus of the diaphragm. The incidence of hiatal hernia increases with age, with an estimation that over 50 percent of all aged persons are affected by this condition. Factors that may predispose to this condition are congenital weakness, muscle weakening associated with aging, trauma, and increased intra-abdominal pressure. The most common hiatal hernia, direct or sliding hernia, occurs when the gastroesophageal junction and a portion of the upper part of the stomach slides into the thoracic cavity above the diaphragmatic hiatus. There may be associated gastroesophageal sphincter incompetence, with subsequent gastric reflux into the esophagus. This may be characterized by heartburn, eructation, bloating, and substernal chest pain that tend to occur after meals and at bedtime (aggravated by reclining). These symptoms also tend to occur with activities that increase intra-abdominal pressure, such as coughing, bending, and lifting heavy objects. Repeated episodes of reflux may cause esophagitis and eventual ulceration, bleeding, and fibrous tissue formation.

In rolling, or paraesophageal, hernia, part of the fundus of the stomach herniates through the hiatus into the thoracic cavity beside the esophagus, while the gastroesophageal junction remains below the diaphragm. This type of hernia generally produces no symptoms and rarely any gastric reflux. There may be a feeling of fullness in the chest or angina-type pain, which can occur as a result of stretching the stomach. Compression of the herniated tissue could lead to strangulation and ischemia. This type often requires surgical intervention.

A mixed hernia includes features of both the direct hernia and the paraesophageal hernia.

POTENTIAL COMPLICATIONS

1. Weight loss,
2. bleeding,
3. esophagitis (which may be complicated by stricture or ulceration),
4. gastritis,
5. aspiration pneumonia.

TYPES OF CLIENTS/CLINICAL CONDITIONS SEEN BY HOME HEALTH AGENCIES

1. Newly diagnosed with hiatal hernia with manifestations of pain and GI disturbances: initiation of prescribed treatment regimen and inclusive teaching plan for home-care management of hiatal hernia.
2. Changes in plan of treatment for management of increasing symptoms and complications associated with gastric reflux: instruction, supervision, evaluation of response to new medications and treatments.

RELATED NURSING DIAGNOSIS

Activity Intolerance

related to:
1. Pain and sleep pattern disturbances
2. Altered nutritional status

as seen by:
Dyspnea and discomfort on exertion; c/o fatigue; abnormal heart rate; c/o heartburn on stooping or lying down

Anxiety

related to:
1. Diagnosis and related symptoms
2. Sleep disturbances
3. Knowledge deficit regarding disorder and prescribed treatment regimen

as seen by:
Distress, fearfulness of pain and related symptoms; uncertainty that treatment regimen will relieve symptoms

Comfort, Alteration in: Pain

related to:
Gastroesophageal reflux (backflow of acid contents of stomach into the esophagus)

as seen by:
Substernal chest pain; increasing changes in BP; increasing heart rate; heartburn; sleep pattern disturbances; verbalization of pain; guarding behavior

Knowledge Deficit (Specify)

related to:
1. Hiatal hernia and related S&S
2. Prescribed plan of treatment in management of hiatal hernia
3. Potential complications, S&S to report to home health nurse or physician

as seen by:
Verbalization of lack of information; inadequate understanding in management of hiatal hernia

Nutrition, Alteration in: Less than Body Requirements

related to:
1. Esophagitis caused by gastric reflux
2. Prescribed modification in diet

as seen by:
Pain; difficulty in swallowing; weight loss; decreased oral intake

Self-Care Deficit: Feeding, Bathing/Hygiene, Dressing/Grooming, Toileting (Specify)

related to:
1. Activity intolerance
2. Activities that increase gastric reflux secondary to increased intra-abdominal pressure
3. Prescribed activity restrictions

as seen by:
Heartburn on stooping or lying down; reluctance to attempt movement; imposed medical restrictions

Sleep Pattern Disturbance

related to:
1. Nighttime distress of heartburn
2. Chest pain

as seen by:
Verbal complaints of interrupted sleep due to GI distress; c/o lack of energy; irritability

LONG-TERM GOAL

To reduce or modify the amount of gastroesophageal reflux for relief of symptoms.

SHORT-TERM GOALS

The client with a hiatal hernia will be able to:

1. Verbalize nature of disorder, factors that aggravate or relieve, S&S of complications to report to home health nurse or physician.
2. Demonstrate compliance with prescribed diet, measures to decrease the amount of gastric acid secretion.
3. Verbalize importance of/demonstrate compliance with prescribed weight control diet.
4. Identify activity measures to reduce or avoid reflux.
5. Demonstrate compliance with prescribed medication therapy.
6. Demonstrate balanced rest and activity levels.
7. Identify measures to correct sleep pattern disturbances associated with gastric reflux.
8. Demonstrate reduction in level of anxiety to effectively manage daily activities and prescribed treatment regimen.

NURSING INTERVENTIONS AND TREATMENTS:

1. Assess gastrointestinal functioning, frequency and duration of S&S of distress/identify complications.

2. Assess vital signs/identify trends (e.g., increasing heart rate, declining BP).
3. Instruct on nature of disorder, factors that aggravate or relieve, S&S, importance of compliance with prescribed treatment regimen, complications to report to home health nurse or physician.
4. Assess and evaluate nutritional status, signs of weight loss/instruct about prescribed measures to decrease the amount of gastric acid secretion and increase oral food intake (e.g., eating slowly, small, frequent meals, water with meals, bland diet, stopping or decreasing smoking)/weigh weekly or more often as indicated.
5. Assess and evaluate excess weight/instruct about importance of prescribed weight control diet to decrease intra-abdominal pressure, reduce the amount of reflux/weigh and record weekly.
6. Assess/instruct about activity measures to reduce or avoid reflux (e.g., restricting activities that increase intra-abdominal pressure: coughing, straining, heavy lifting; eating sitting up and remaining in upright position for at least a half hour following meals).
7. Observe/instruct about taking prescribed medications (e.g., antacids, cholinergics, antiemetics) and other medications as ordered, purpose and action, side effects/evaluate medication effectiveness.
8. Instruct about ADL and increased self-care activities with prescribed restrictions and balanced rest periods.
9. Assess and evaluate disturbances in sleep pattern/instruct about measures to reduce gastric reflux (e.g., sleeping in semi-Fowler's position, elevating head of bed on 6-inch blocks, avoiding large meals close to bedtime).
10. Assess level of anxiety regarding unfamiliarity of disorder and related S&S/allow verbalization of feelings/explain prescribed treatment regimen and measures to relieve discomfort.

REHABILITATION POTENTIAL

Rehabilitation potential *excellent   good   fair   guarded   poor*   for   *full partial*   return to an improved state of well-being, free of symptoms associated with gastroesophageal reflux, to effectively manage daily activities.

Client's Name _____

Medical Record # _____

ONGOING/DISCHARGE EVALUATION OF TEACHING
The Client with a Hiatal Hernia

Teaching Tools:
Printed materials given: _____

Audiovisual aids used: _____

Return Information/Demonstration/Interpretation
_____ Client
_____ Caregiver

	OF:	Met	Not Met	Comments
☐	Nature of disorder, factors that aggravate or relieve.	_____	_____	_____
☐	S&S of complications, actions to take.	_____	_____	_____
☐	Importance of compliance with prescribed treatment regimen.	_____	_____	_____
☐	Effect of meal scheduling, size, and content of food in decreasing amount of gastric acid secretions.	_____	_____	_____
☐	Weight control diet; effect of excess weight on gastric acid secretions.	_____	_____	_____

Client's Name _____

Medical Record # _____

OF:	Met	Not Met	Comments
☐ Demonstrate activity measures to reduce or avoid gastric reflux.	_____	_____	_____
☐ Medications and administration, purpose and action, side effects.	_____	_____	_____
☐ Balanced rest and activities.	_____	_____	_____
☐ Measures to correct sleep disturbances associated with gastric reflux.	_____	_____	_____

Signature of Home Health Nurse _____

Date _____

■ Peptic Ulcer

Peptic ulcers are circumscribed lesions of the mucosal lining of the gastrointestinal tract that may occur in areas exposed to gastric juices containing hydrochloric acid and pepsin. Those areas that are most often exposed to gastric acid secretions are normally protected from irritation by "gastric mucosal barriers" consisting of thick, tenacious layers of gastric mucus and tight intercellular junctions of epithelial cells of the gastric mucosa. Whenever these barriers are significantly disrupted, allowing back diffusion of hydrochloric acid, underlying tissues are injured. Increased gastric secretions, decrease in vascular supply, and rapid epithelial cell renewal, alterations in normal gastric emptying time, and genetic factors are all important factors that affect the normal buffering system, predisposing to erosion of the mucosal lining.

Peptic ulcers usually occur in the duodenum (more common) or stomach and rarely in other sites such as the esophagus. Both types of ulcers are characterized by periodic attacks of epigastric pain, heartburn, and vomiting. With gastric ulcers, an associated loss of appetite and of weight may be found. This associated pain tends to occur some hours after or just before the next meal and may be relieved by food. This may be termed "hunger pains" by the client. Many times, however, food aggravates a gastric ulcer and relieves the pain of the duodenal ulcer.

Predisposing factors to the development or exacerbation of an ulceration are the use of salicylates, steroids, caffeine, or alcohol, smoking, and/or emotional stress.

POTENTIAL COMPLICATIONS

1. Hemorrhage,
2. pyloric stenosis,
3. perforation,
4. penetration (into adjacent organs),
5. intractability.

TYPES OF CLIENTS/CLINICAL CONDITIONS SEEN BY HOME HEALTH AGENCIES

1. Newly diagnosed with peptic ulcer disease: initiation of prescribed treatment regimen and inclusive teaching plan for home-care management of condition.
2. Exacerbation of peptic ulcer with complications and changes in the prescribed treatment regimen (e.g., placed on antibiotic therapy): needs instruction, supervision, and evaluation of response to therapy.
3. Recent hospitalization following an acute exacerbation and complications of peptic ulcer disease: new treatment regimen.

RELATED NURSING DIAGNOSIS

Activity Intolerance

related to:
1. Pain or GI distress
2. Inadequate nutritional status

as seen by:
Weakness and fatigue; exertional dyspnea; verbalized feelings of exhaustion

Anxiety

related to:
1. Epigastric pain
2. GI disturbances
3. Possible need for surgery
4. Knowledge deficit regarding disease process, prescribed treatment regimen

as seen by:
Appearing anxious, expressed concern about possible need for surgery; questioning new medications, treatments, their effectiveness in alleviating pain, and GI symptoms

Bowel Elimination, Alteration in: Constipation or Diarrhea

related to:
1. Dietary restrictions
2. Effects of certain medications

as seen by:
Verbalization of problem with elimination changes in frequency and amount, straining with bowel movement, urgency

Comfort, Alteration in: Epigastric Pain

related to:
Ulcerated area of the gastric mucosa exposed to secretions of gastric juices containing hydrochloric acid and pepsin

as seen by:
Tachycardia, changes in BP; restlessness; reporting of pain and rubbing or holding of area; pallor

Coping, Ineffective Individual

related to:
1. Anger or depression associated with present health status
2. Alteration in body functioning

as seen by:
Verbalization of inability to cope; fatigue; anxiety; uncontrolled internal emotions in handling of condition and daily problems of life

Knowledge Deficit (Specify)

related to:
1. Lack of understanding of disease process
2. Prescribed plan of treatment in management of peptic ulcer
3. Potential complications, S&S to report to home health nurse or physician

as seen by:
Verbalization of lack of information; inadequate understanding of prescribed treatment regimen for management of peptic ulcer disease

Nutrition, Alteration in: Less than Body Requirements

related to:
1. Decreased oral intake associated with pain
2. Prescribed dietary restrictions

as seen by:
Weight loss; weakness and fatigue; caloric intake insufficient to meet metabolic needs; c/o pain with eating

Self-Care Deficit: Feeding, Bathing/Hygiene, Dressing/Grooming, Toileting (Specify)

related to:
1. Pain and discomfort
2. Weakness and fatigue secondary to inadequate nutritional status

as seen by:
Decreased level of participation in meeting physical needs, increased dependency on others for care; dyspnea on exertion

LONG-TERM GOAL

To inhibit or buffer acid secretions of the stomach for symptomatic relief and healing of ulcer.

SHORT-TERM GOALS

The client with a peptic ulcer will be able to:

1. Verbalize nature of peptic ulcer disease, factors that aggravate or relieve pain, S&S of complications to report to home health nurse or physician.
2. Demonstrate compliance with prescribed diet (bland diet or "free choice diet")/identify difficult-to-digest or gastrically irritating foods, methods to decrease the amount of acid secretion.
3. Weigh weekly/record/report excessive weight loss to physician.
4. Demonstrate compliance with prescribed medication therapy/identify complications.

5. Verbalize effect of antacids on gastrointestinal motility.
6. Verbalize effect of prescribed medications on level of pain.
7. Verbalize importance of exercise and activities to tolerance, planned rest periods and avoiding fatigue.
8. Identify stressful situations and measures to cope/verbalize effect on peptic ulcer disease.

NURSING ACTIONS/TREATMENTS

1. Assess gastrointestinal status, S&S of distress, frequency and duration of symptoms/identify complications.
2. Assess vital signs/identify trends (e.g., hypotension, rapid pulse rate).
3. Instruct as to nature of peptic ulcer disease, factors that aggravate or relieve pain (e.g., smoking, caffeine, alcohol), importance of compliance with prescribed treatment regimen, S&S complications to report to home health nurse or physician.
4. Assess and evaluate nutritional status/instruct about prescribed diet (bland or "free choice diet," elimination of foods, fluids causing pain)/avoiding difficult-to-digest foods and gastric irritants, measures to decrease the amount of acid secretion (e.g., eating slowly; regularly scheduled, small, frequent meals; adequate hydration/obtain dietary consultation as needed.
5. Assess and evaluate for changes in weight/weigh weekly or more often as indicated/record/report excessive weight loss to physician.
6. Observe/instruct about taking medications as ordered (e.g., antacids, antispasmodics, analgesics, histamine blockers, anticholinergics), purpose and action, side effects, toxicity/avoiding ulcerogenic drugs (e.g., aspirin, corticosteroids)/evaluate medication effectiveness.
7. Assess and evaluate for alteration in bowel pattern/instruct to report problems with constipation when on aluminum-containing antacids or diarrhea when on magnesium-containing antacids, to alternate as prescribed.
8. Observe/instruct to assess level of pain before and after taking prescribed medications/report to physician.
9. Observe/instruct about activities and exercise to tolerance with planned rest periods, avoiding fatigue.
10. Assess/instruct about measures to cope with and/or avoid stressful situations, effect on ulcer.
11. Refer to social services as ordered to provide counseling in assisting with necessary life-style changes and provide information about community resources (e.g., counseling services, program to stop smoking and manage stress).

REHABILITATION POTENTIAL

Rehabilitation potential *excellent good fair guarded poor* for *full partial* return to an improved state of well-being, free of gastric symptoms and able to manage ADL.

Client's Name _____

Medical Record # _____

ONGOING/DISCHARGE EVALUATION OF TEACHING
The Client with a Peptic Ulcer

Teaching Tools:
Printed materials given: _____

Audiovisual aids used: _____

Return Information/Demonstration/Interpretation
_____ Client
_____ Caregiver

OF:	Met	Not Met	Comments
☐ Nature of peptic ulcer disease; factors that aggravate or relieve pain.	_____	_____	_____
☐ S&S of complications, actions to take.	_____	_____	_____
☐ Importance of compliance with prescribed treatment regimen.	_____	_____	_____
☐ Bland diet or "free choice" diet.	_____	_____	_____
☐ Elimination of difficult-to-digest and gastrically irritating foods.	_____	_____	_____
☐ Measures to decrease the amount of acid secretion.	_____	_____	_____

Client's Name _____

Medical Record # _____

	OF:	**Met**	**Not Met**	**Comments**
☐	Medications and administration, purpose and action, side effects.	_____	_____	_____
☐	Effects of antacids on gastrointestinal motility (laxative or constipating effect).	_____	_____	_____
☐	Report excessive weight loss to physician.	_____	_____	_____
☐	Exercise and activities to tolerance; planned rest periods.	_____	_____	_____
☐	Effect of stressful situations on peptic ulcer disease; measures to cope.	_____	_____	_____

Signature of Home Health Nurse _____

Date _____

HEPATOBILIARY DISORDERS

■ Cholecystectomy

Cholecystectomy is the surgical removal of the gallbladder performed to treat cholecystitis and cholelithiasis in those clients who have not responded to conservative treatment. It is also performed to remove a malignancy of the biliary tract.

If a choledocholithotomy is performed to remove stones from the common bile duct, the client may be discharged home with a T tube to ensure patency of the common bile duct and drainage of bile until edema of the duct subsides.

POTENTIAL COMPLICATIONS

1. Wound infection,
2. bile flow obstruction,
3. skin irritation and breakdown secondary to continual contact of skin with bile drainage,
4. abscess formation associated with accumulation of bile in the subhepatic or subdiaphragmatic space secondary to obstruction of the T-tube system with reflux of drainage or dislodgement of T tube.

TYPES OF CLIENTS/CLINICAL CONDITIONS SEEN BY HOME HEALTH AGENCIES

1. Prescribed plan of treatment and instruction-post surgery: includes observation and care of healing wound, dressing changes, T-tube management.
2. Postsurgical complications: changes in prescribed treatments, medications, need for skilled nursing observations, interventions, instructions, and evaluation of response to changes in therapy.

RELATED NURSING DIAGNOSIS

Activity Intolerance

related to:
1. Incisional pain and discomfort
2. Anxiety
3. Inadequate nutritional status

as seen by:
Exertional dyspnea; discomfort; weakness and fatigue, abnormal heart rate, BP with activity

Anxiety

related to:
1. Incisional pain
2. Knowledge deficit regarding prescribed treatment regimen

as seen by:
Restlessness, apprehension regarding T-tube management; numerous questions or lack of questions

Breathing Pattern, Ineffective

related to:
1. Surgical incision
2. Anxiety

as seen by:
Splinted or guarded respirations; shallow respirations; poor coughing efforts.

Comfort, Alteration in: Pain

related to:
Incisional pain and discomfort

as seen by:
Reluctance to move; guarding of incisional area; c/o pain

Coping, Ineffective Individual

related to:
Surgery and management of dressings and T tube

as seen by:
Anger; inability to care for self; depression; lack of follow-through with prescribed treatment regimen

Infection, Potential for

related to:
1. Dislodgement of T tube
2. Obstruction of bile flow with possible leak into peritoneum
3. Incisional area and breakdown of body's first line of defense

as seen by:
Increased pain, tenderness, redness, swelling, drainage, tissue breakdown of wound area, elevated temperature, increased pulse rate, increased WBC count

Knowledge Deficit (Specify)

related to:
1. Prescribed plan of treatment following cholecystectomy
2. Potential complications, S&S to report to home health nurse or physician

as seen by:
Verbalization of lack of information; inadequate information; inability to perform skills necessary to meet health care needs at home

Mobility, Impaired Physical

related to:
1. Activity intolerance
2. Incisional pain and discomfort
3. Prescribed activity restrictions

as seen by:
Exertional dyspnea; reluctance to attempt movement; c/o pain on movement; imposed medical restrictions

Nutrition, Alteration in: Less than Body Requirements

related to:
1. Lack of appetite
2. Prescribed dietary restrictions

as seen by:
Repeated inadequate food and fluid intake; c/o pain and not "feeling hungry"; weight loss; imposed medical restrictions regarding diet

Self-Care Deficit: Feeding, Bathing/Hygiene, Dressing/Grooming, Toileting (Specify)

related to:
1. Activity intolerance
2. Impaired physical mobility
3. Prescribed activity restrictions

as seen by:
Limited participation in meeting physical needs and ADL activities, associated with pain, weakness and fatigue; imposed medical restrictions

Skin Integrity, Impairment of: Actual/Potential

related to:
1. Surgical incision
2. Impaired healing secondary to infection
3. Continual contact of skin with bile drainage
4. Inadequate nutritional status

as seen by:
Increased redness, swelling, unusual drainage, irritation, tissue breakdown; tenderness, pain

LONG-TERM GOAL

To recover from surgery without evidence of complications and gradually resume activities of daily living.

SHORT-TERM GOALS

The client who has had a cholecystectomy will be able to:

1. Verbalize nature of biliary tract disease, purpose of surgery, S&S of complications to report to home health nurse or physician.
2. Verbalize purpose/demonstrate correct care of T tube and drainage system, skin care, dressing changes.
3. Demonstrate compliance with prescribed diet and dietary restrictions.
4. Demonstrate compliance with prescribed medication therapy/identify side effects.

5. Demonstrate compliance with prescribed wound care management, identify S&S of infection to report to home health nurse or physician.
6. Demonstrate increased participation in self-care activities with planned rest periods.
7. Demonstrate effective coping mechanisms and positive adaptation to condition postsurgery.

NURSING ACTIONS/TREATMENTS

1. Assess gastrointestinal status/identify complications.
2. Assess vital signs/identify trends (e.g., elevated temperature, rapid pulse rate, hypotension).
3. Instruct as to nature of biliary tract disease, surgical intervention, importance of compliance with prescribed postsurgical treatment regimen, S&S of complications to report to home health nurse or physician.
4. Assess and evaluate T-tube functioning/instruct as to purpose and care of tube and drainage system (e.g., how to empty T-tube drainage, frequency of emptying; color, amount, and odor to note and record; care of skin and dressings); complications to report to home health nurse or physician (e.g., T-tube dislodgement, obstruction of bile flow from kinks in tubing or blockage of T tube, flow more than 500 ml/per day, icteric skin and sclera, clay-colored stools or dark-amber urine, abdominal pain, epigastric distress).
5. Assess and evaluate nutritional status/instruct about prescribed diet (e.g., low fat, fats as tolerated, high in protein and carbohydrates), purpose of restriction for first six months, to add fats gradually, adequate fluid hydration/obtain dietary consultation as needed.
6. Observe/instruct about taking medications as ordered, purpose and action, side effects/evaluate medication effectiveness.
7. Observe and evaluate incisional area/instruct as to prescribed wound care management, S&S of infection to report to home health nurse or physician.
8. Assess and evaluate deficits in self-care/instruct about activities to tolerance with planned rest periods/instruct about avoiding heavy lifting or straining for 6 weeks.
9. Assess level of anxiety/instruct about use of ineffective coping mechanisms/provide emotional support/assist to a positive adaptation to management of condition postsurgery.

REHABILITATION POTENTIAL

Rehabilitation potential *excellent good fair guarded poor* for *full partial* return to a predisease status and improved level of functioning to manage daily activities.

Client's Name _____

Medical Record # _____

ONGOING/DISCHARGE EVALUATION OF TEACHING
The Client Who Has Had a Cholecystectomy

Teaching Tools:
Printed materials given: _____

Audiovisual aids used: _____

Return Information/Demonstration/Interpretation
_____ Client
_____ Caregiver

	OF:	Met	Not Met	Comments
☐	Nature of biliary tract disease, surgical intervention.	_____	_____	_____
☐	S&S of complications, actions to take.	_____	_____	_____
☐	Importance of compliance with postsurgical treatment regimen.	_____	_____	_____
☐	Care of T tube, drainage system, and surrounding skin.	_____	_____	_____
☐	Prescribed diet, dietary restrictions.	_____	_____	_____
☐	Medications and administration, purpose and action, side effects.	_____	_____	_____

Client's Name _____

Medical Record # _____

OF:	Met	Not Met	Comments
☐ Wound care management.	_____	_____	_____
☐ Activities to tolerance; planned rest periods.	_____	_____	_____

Signature of Home Health Nurse _____

Date _____

■ Cholelithiasis/Cholecystitis

Cholelithiasis refers to the presence of gallstones in the biliary tract, which may form from the precipitation of one or more components of bile: cholesterol, bile salts, phospholipids (mainly lecithin), bilirubin, calcium, and proteins. The etiology of gallstone formation is still not completely clear. Major predisposing factors that have been identified in the formation of gallstones include the following: (1) hepatic metabolic disturbances of biliary lipids resulting in changes in the composition of bile secreted by the liver. As a result, cholesterol secretion increases and bile salts and lecithin decrease, causing a supersaturated bile, which may precipitate in the gallbladder to form stones; (2) delayed emptying of bile from the gallbladder or failure to empty completely or to concentrate bile normally may result in biliary stasis and changes in the composition of bile (supersaturated) and precipitation of stones; or (3) foreign substances, such as bacteria, may affect the composition of bile, resulting in stone formation.

Stones may remain in the gallbladder without causing symptoms. Generally though, inflammation of the gallbladder results from the gallstones and the symptoms are often associated with a stone passing into the cystic or common bile duct (choledocholithiasis), resulting in the obstruction of the flow of bile into the duodenum. The severity of symptoms depends on the extent of bile flow obstruction.

Associated clinical manifestations may produce pain in the midepigastrium radiating to the back, nausea and vomiting, diaphoresis, fat intolerance, indigestion, and eructation and leukocytosis and elevated body temperature, secondary to inflammation.

If a stone obstructs the common bile duct, the bile, which is normally carried to the duodenum, is absorbed by the blood, resulting in jaundice of the skin and tissues and pruritus secondary to the accumulation of bile salts in the skin. As a result of the excretion of bile pigments by the kidneys, the urine turns a dark color and the feces becomes "clay-colored" from lack of bile pigments.

POTENTIAL COMPLICATIONS

1. Infectious process or abscess formation,
2. jaundice,
3. bleeding tendencies (vitamin K deficiency secondary to bile flow obstruction),
4. fluid and electrolyte imbalance (persistent nausea and vomiting).

TYPES OF CLIENTS/CLINICAL CONDITIONS SEEN BY HOME HEALTH AGENCIES

1. Newly diagnosed with gallbladder disease: initiation of prescribed treatment regimen and inclusive teaching plan for home-care management of condition.
2. Exacerbation of gallbladder disease with changes in prescribed treatment regimen: e.g., instruction and supervision of new medications, evaluation of response to treatment.
3. Recent hospitalization following an acute exacerbation associated with com-

plications of gallbladder disease: discharged home with prescribed home-treatment regimen requiring instruction, ongoing assessment of condition and response to therapy (e.g., antibiotic therapy).

RELATED NURSING DIAGNOSIS

Activity Intolerance

related to:
1. GI distress
2. Inadequate nutritional status

as seen by:
Weakness and fatigue with self-care activities; shortness of breath; exertional dyspnea

Anxiety

related to:
1. Pain and GI distress
2. Possibility of surgery
3. Knowledge deficit regarding disease process and prescribed treatment regimen

as seen by:
Nervousness; fear of surgery; asking numerous questions regarding medications and treatments

Comfort, Alteration in: Pain

related to:
1. Inflammation of gallbladder and bile ducts
2. Accumulation of bile salts in the skin as a result of obstructed bile flow

as seen by:
Facial expression of pain; c/o pain in right upper quadrant of abdomen; reluctance to move, pruritus and burning pain of skin

Infection, Potential for

related to:
1. Inflammatory process of the gallbladder
2. Debilitated condition

as seen by:
Elevated temperature; increased pulse rate; persistent pain or spasms; nausea and vomiting; weakness; elevated WBC count

Knowledge Deficit (Specify)

related to:
1. Disease process and related S&S

as seen by:
Verbalization of lack of information

2. Prescribed plan of treatment in management of gallbladder disease
3. Potential complications, S&S to report to home health nurse or physician

and inadequate understanding of prescribed treatment regimen for management of gallbladder disease

Nutrition, Alteration in: Less than Body Requirements

related to:
1. Decreased oral intake because of pain
2. GI distress
3. Nausea and vomiting secondary to intolerance of fatty foods
4. Prescribed dietary restrictions

as seen by:
Weakness and fatigue; anorexia; loss of weight; eating of high-fat foods restricted on diet; dyspepsia; nausea and vomiting

Self-Care Deficit: Feeding, Bathing/Hygiene, Dressing/Grooming, Toileting (Specify)

related to:
1. Activity intolerance
2. Pain

as seen by:
Decreased participation in self-care activities associated with weakness, fatigue; GI distress, dyspnea on exertion

Skin Integrity, Impairment of: Potential

related to:
Accumulation of bile salts in the skin

as seen by:
Itching; c/o burning pain; redness; irritation; breakdown of tissues

LONG-TERM GOAL

To relieve symptoms through resolution of infectious process and maintain nutritional status and fluid and electrolyte balance.

SHORT-TERM GOALS

The client with cholelithiasis/cholecystitis will be able to:

1. Verbalize nature of biliary tract disease, S&S, factors that aggravate or relieve, complications to report to home health nurse or physician.
2. Demonstrate compliance with prescribed diet and dietary restrictions.

3. Demonstrate compliance with prescribed medication therapy/identify side effects.
4. Verbalize S&S of bile flow obstruction to report to home health nurse or physician.
5. Demonstrate prescribed measures to relieve pruritus and burning pain.
6. Demonstrate balanced rest and activity levels.
7. Demonstrate reduction in level of anxiety to effectively manage daily activities.

NURSING ACTIONS/TREATMENTS

1. Assess gastrointestinal status, S&S of distress, frequency and duration of symptoms/identify complications.
2. Assess vital signs/identify trends (e.g., elevated temperature, increased pulse rate).
3. Instruct as to nature of biliary tract disease, S&S, factors that aggravate or relieve, importance of compliance with prescribed treatment regimen, complications to report to home health nurse or physician.
4. Assess and evaluate nutritional status/instruct about prescribed diet (e.g., low to moderate fat), effect of fat in precipitating gallbladder attack, adequate hydration/obtain dietary consultation as needed.
5. Observe/instruct about taking medications as ordered (e.g., fat-soluble vitamins, antibiotics, bile salts), purpose and action, side effects/evaluate medication effectiveness.
6. Assess/instruct about S&S of bile flow obstruction to report to home health nurse or physician (e.g., jaundice, clay-colored stools, dark urine).
7. Assess/instruct about prescribed measures to relieve pruritus and burning pain (good skin-care measures), prescribed medications (e.g., cholestyramine, antipruritic lotions), reporting any increase in symptoms to physician.
8. Observe/instruct about balanced rest and activity levels.
9. Assess level of anxiety/encourage to express concerns/provide emotional support.

REHABILITATION POTENTIAL

Rehabilitation potential   *excellent   good   fair   guarded   poor*   for   *full partial*   return to an improved level of wellness, free of symptoms, to independently manage ADL.

Client's Name _____

Medical Record # _____

ONGOING/DISCHARGE EVALUATION OF TEACHING
The Client with Cholelithiasis/Cholecystitis

Teaching Tools:
Printed materials given: _____

Audiovisual aids used: _____

Return Information/Demonstration/Interpretation
_____ Client
_____ Caregiver

	OF:	Met	Not Met	Comments
☐	Nature of biliary tract disease, S&S, factors that aggravate or relieve.	_____	_____	_____
☐	S&S of complications, actions to take.	_____	_____	_____
☐	Importance of compliance with prescribed treatment regimen.	_____	_____	_____
☐	Prescribed diet and dietary restrictions.	_____	_____	_____
☐	Medications and administration, purpose and action, side effects.	_____	_____	_____
☐	S&S of bile flow obstruction.	_____	_____	_____

Client's Name _____

Medical Record # _____

	OF:	Met	Not Met	Comments
☐	Measures to relieve pruritus and burning pain.	_____	_____	_____
☐	Balanced rest and activities.	_____	_____	_____

Signature of Home Health Nurse _____

Date _____

■ Cirrhosis

Cirrhosis is a chronic degenerative disease of the liver, characterized by necrosis of hepatic cells. This is followed in the later stages by fibrous connective scar tissue formation and nodular regenerative activity in the liver's attempt to replace damaged hepatic cells. The more common causes of cirrhosis are: (1) infections (e.g., viral hepatitis); (2) toxins (e.g., alcohol and certain drugs); (3) biliary cirrhosis (usually results from chronic biliary obstruction and infection). The main focus of this planning guide is the home-care management of the client with Laënnec's cirrhosis.

Laënnec's cirrhosis is the most common type of cirrhosis. It is the end result of toxic effects of excessive alcohol intake and nutritional deficiencies, especially dietary protein, on hepatic cells. Clinical manifestations of cirrhosis are attributed to an enlarged liver early in the disease. This is due to the accumulation of fat within the liver cells, which occurs as a result of the metabolic disturbances caused by the toxic effects of alcohol. Anorexia, fever, nausea and vomiting, weakness, changes in bowel habits, and a dull ache or heaviness in the epigastrium or right upper quadrant are found early in the disease. The liver is usually hard and palpable. Shrinkage of the liver occurs in later stages of the disease as the scar tissue contracts and the liver becomes smaller.

Clinical manifestations later in the disease are associated with portal hypertension and hepatocellular failure and their subsequent effects, culminating in major physiologic disruptions that can occur throughout the body.

These include the following: A rise in portal vein pressure, with increased resistance to blood flow through the liver and resultant passive congestion, results in signs and symptoms associated with portal hypertension: (1) ascites; (2) splenomegaly; (3) gastrointestinal disturbances (e.g., dyspepsia, bowel changes, weight loss). This predisposes to the development of points of collateral circulation and the formation of varices, which may rupture and hemorrhage (e.g., esophageal, gastric, internal hemorrhoids, caput medusae); (4) hepatic encephalopathy, occurring as a result of ammonia bypassing the liver for detoxification because of the development of an anastomotic channel of circulation.

Signs and symptoms associated with hepatocellular failure include: (1) jaundice resulting from failure to excrete bilirubin glucuronide; (2) ascites and general edema as a result of the decreased production of albumin, causing a drop in colloid osmotic pressure; (3) failure of the liver to store certain vitamins and minerals (deficiencies of fat-soluble vitamins such as A, D, E, K, especially vitamin K, resulting in bleeding tendencies; vitamin B_{12}, resulting in pernicious anemia; vitamin B_6, with associated peripheral nerve degeneration; niacin with associated sensory disturbances and paresthesias of the feet); (4) impairment in the detoxification of various metabolites (e.g., hormones of the adrenal cortex, ovaries, and testes, normally metabolized and excreted by the liver), which may result in elevated blood levels and the development of associated signs and symptoms. Excess circulating hormones of the ovaries and testes may result in spider nevi, palmar erythema, loss of axillary and pubic hair, gynecomastia, testicular atrophy, and impotence. Failure to inactivate aldosterone and antidiuretic hormone increases sodium and water retention; (5) confusion, personality and behavior changes, depression, lethargy, and finally coma occur as ammonia accumulates in the plasma as a result of the failure of hepatic detoxification mechanisms; (6) increased susceptibility and dangerous sensitivity to potential harmful drugs (e.g., barbiturates and morphine) associated with the liver's inability to detoxify drugs; (7) increased susceptibility to infections because of increased bacteria in the blood, associated with impairment of the phagocytic process of the liver (Kupffer cells).

Peripheral edema and ascites are clinical manifestations of both portal hypertension and hepatocellular failure. As portal hypertension develops, a characteristic decrease in venous return causes an increase in capillary pressure and forces fluid out of the liver's vascular compartments into the abdominal cavity.

Hepatocellular failure predisposes to ascites and peripheral edema as a result of sodium retention secondary to elevations of aldosterone and antidiuretic hormone and a drop in colloid osmotic pressure secondary to a decreased production of albumin.

POTENTIAL COMPLICATIONS

1. Jaundice,
2. pruritus,
3. ascites,
4. infection and bleeding tendencies,
5. anemia,
6. edema,
7. esophageal varices,
8. fluid and electrolyte imbalances,
9. hepatic encephalopathy,
10. hepatorenal syndrome.

TYPES OF CLIENTS/CLINICAL CONDITIONS SEEN BY HOME HEALTH AGENCIES

1. Newly diagnosed with cirrhosis: initiation of prescribed treatment regimen and inclusive teaching plan for home-care management of cirrhotic client.
2. Clients with increasingly major physiologic disruptions of the body: changes in prescribed treatment regimen and increase in frequency of skilled nurse visits for observation, evaluation, and management of deteriorating condition.
3. Recent hospitalization following increasing problems and complications associated with liver failure: new medications and treatments with instruction, supervision, and report to physician of response to treatment.

RELATED NURSING DIAGNOSIS

Activity Intolerance

related to:
1. Malnutrition

as seen by:
Verbal report of fatigue and weakness;

2. Hypoxia associated with limited lung expansion secondary to ascites
3. Anemia

exertional dyspnea; tachypnea; abnormal heart rate and BP in response to ADL; shortness of breath

Anxiety

related to:
1. Disease process, associated clinical manifestations
2. Increased dependency on others for care
3. Altered body image and life-style changes
4. Knowledge deficit regarding prescribed treatment regimen

as seen by:
Increased questioning regarding condition and treatment interventions; apprehension and distress; fear of prognosis; uncertainty about future

Bowel Elimination, Alteration in: Constipation

related to:
1. Decreased bowel activity secondary to vascular congestion of the GI tract
2. Inadequate nutritional status
3. Decreased activity levels

as seen by:
Hard, formed stools; frequency and amount less than usual pattern; decreased appetite; headache; feeling of fullness

Bowel Elimination, Alteration in: Diarrhea

related to:
Increased bowel activity secondary to vascular congestion of the GI tract

as seen by:
Urgency and frequency; loose, liquid stools; increased bowel sounds; c/o cramping and pain

Breathing Pattern, Ineffective

related to:
Limited lung expansion secondary to pressure on diaphragm from abdominal ascites

as seen by:
Increased respiratory effort; increased heart rate; hyperventilation; exertional dyspnea; report of decreased energy and fatigue

Comfort, Alteration in: Pain

related to:
1. Abdominal pain

as seen by:
C/o abdominal pain; guarding of

2. Enlargement of the liver with stretching of Glisson's capsule
3. Accumulation of bile salts in the skin
4. Bile flow obstruction with impaired fat digestion

abdomen; restlessness; pruritus with burning pain; dyspepsia

Coping, Ineffective Individual

related to:
1. Change in body appearance
2. Long-term disability with cirrhotic condition

as seen by:
Verbalizing inability to cope; inability to care for self; general irritability; withdrawn behavior; inability to abstain from alcohol

Fluid Volume, Alteration in: Excess

related to:
Pathologic changes in the cirrhotic liver

as seen by:
Peripheral edema; ascites; significant weight gain; shortness of breath; intake greater than output; increased abdominal girth; fluid wave

Grieving

related to:
1. Altered body image
2. Life-style and role relationship changes

as seen by:
Depression; anger; change in eating habits; noncompliance; withdrawal from relationships and usual activities

Infection, Potential for

related to:
1. Increased blood bacteria secondary to impaired phagocytic process of the liver
2. Anemia
3. Malnutrition

as seen by:
Elevated temperature; chills; tachycardia; S&S associated with urinary or respiratory involvement; elevated WBC count

Injury, Potential for: Increased Risk of Falls and Injuries

related to:
1. Changes in mental status secondary

as seen by:
Disorientation, forgetfulness; lethargy;

to increased blood ammonia levels
2. Fatigue and weakness or cerebral hypoxia secondary to anemia
3. Malnutrition
4. Neurologic changes associated with vitamin B_{12} and thiamin deficiencies

dizziness; lack of energy; decreased sensation in extremities; uncoordinated movements; gait disturbances and weakness in extremities; paresthesias; weakness and fatigue

Knowledge Deficit (Specify)

related to:
1. Inadequate understanding of disease process and associated clinical manifestations
2. Prescribed plan of treatment in management of liver disease
3. Potential complications, S&S to report to home health nurse or physician

as seen by:
Verbalization of lack of information; inadequate understanding; inability to perform skills necessary to meet health-care needs at home

Mobility, Impaired Physical

related to:
1. Activity intolerance
2. Neurologic changes associated with vitamin B_{12} and thiamin deficiencies
3. Prescribed activity restrictions

as seen by:
Weakness and fatigue; activity intolerance; paresthesias; weakness of extremities; ataxia; balance disturbances; imposed medical restrictions

Nutrition, Alteration in: Less than Body Requirements

related to:
1. Decreased intake of nutrients
2. Disturbances in digestion, absorption, and storage of fats and fat-soluble vitamins
3. Impaired carbohydrate and protein metabolism
4. Impaired ability to store iron, folic acid, thiamin, and vitamin B_{12} resulting in anemia

as seen by:
Weakness and fatigue; inadequate caloric intake to meet increased metabolic demands; anorexia; nausea and vomiting; stomatitis; body weight 20 percent or more under ideal weight for height, frame, and age; triceps skin fold less than normal for build

Self-Care Deficit: Feeding, Bathing/Hygiene, Dressing/Grooming, Toileting (Specify)

related to:
1. Activity intolerance
2. Impaired mobility status
3. Prescribed activity restrictions
4. Change in mental status

as seen by:
Weakness; fatigue; dyspnea on exertion; balance and gait disturbances; confusion; impaired memory

Self-Concept, Disturbance in

related to:
1. Change in body appearance and body functioning
2. Loss of self-esteem
3. Changes in life-style and role performances

as seen by:
Depression; expressed anger; withdrawal; increased dependency on others to meet daily needs; expressed fear of losing independence; noncompliance

Skin Integrity, Impairment of: Potential

related to:
1. Edema
2. Poor nutritional status
3. Accumulation of bile salts and bilirubin in the blood and body tissues secondary to hepatocellular necrosis

as seen by:
Pruritus; jaundice; tissue irritation and breakdown

Sensory-Perceptual Alteration: Mental Status, Tactile Deficit

related to:
1. Changes in mental status and lethargy associated with increase in serum ammonia levels
2. Neurologic changes associated with vitamin B_{12} and thiamin deficiencies

as seen by:
Disorientation; confusion; paresthesias, variable sensory loss; irritability

Sleep Pattern Disturbance

related to:
1. Ascites
2. Anxiety

as seen by:
Inability to assume comfortable position for sleep; restlessness; increased irritability

LONG-TERM GOAL

To maximize liver function and restore homeostasis through treatment and management of disabling symptoms.

SHORT-TERM GOALS

The client with cirrhosis of the liver will be able to:

1. Verbalize understanding of nature and progression of liver disease, cause and contributing factors, S&S of complications to report to home health nurse or physician.
2. Verbalize rationale for and demonstrate compliance with prescribed diet and fluids with dietary restrictions.
3. Demonstrate compliance with supplemental vitamin therapy.
4. Demonstrate compliance with prescribed medication therapy/identify side effects.
5. Measure and record abdominal girth according to order, intake and output, weigh and record daily or as prescribed to report to home health nurse or physician.
6. Demonstrate prescribed skin care measures to relieve itching/report to home health nurse or physician skin breakdown and failure of treatment to alleviate symptoms.
7. Verbalize cause of GI disturbances/demonstrate prescribed measures to relieve.
8. Demonstrate prescribed measures to maintain skin integrity with edematous skin/verbalize S&S of irritation or breakdown to report to home health nurse or physician.
9. Demonstrate prescribed measures to facilitate easier breathing with abdominal ascites.
10. Identify predisposing factors to activity intolerance, measures to promote rest and conserve energy.
11. Verbalize understanding of increased susceptibility to infections/identify measures to avoid exposure.
12. Identify causative factors of constipation, diarrhea, measures to correct.
13. Verbalize effect of vitamin B_{12}, thiamin deficiency on mobility, prescribed measures to treat.
14. Identify risk factors in home for falls and injuries/demonstrate safety measures with ambulatory and daily activities.
15. Verbalize cause of bleeding tendencies, signs of bleeding, measures to reduce risk.
16. Demonstrate effective coping mechanisms and adaptation to progressive changes in health and life-style associated with condition.

NURSING ACTIONS/TREATMENTS

1. Assess for clinical manifestations associated with liver disease/identify complications.
2. Assess vital signs/identify trends (e.g., elevated temperature, tachycardia, hypo- hypertension, rapid, shallow respirations).
3. Instruct as to nature and progression of liver disease, cause and contributing factors, importance of strict compliance with prescribed treatment regimen, S&S of complications to report to home health nurse or physician.
4. Assess and evaluate nutritional status (S&S of malnutrition)/instruct as to prescribed diet and fluids with restrictions based on client's metabolic condition (e.g., increase in calories, carbohydrates, proteins to promote liver cell regeneration and meet energy needs of the body; low-protein diet with elevated levels of serum ammonia; restriction of foods high in fat with impaired fat digestion; low sodium diet and fluid restrictions of 1000 to 1500 ml per day with ascites and edema; avoiding gas-producing foods; no alcohol)/obtain dietary consultation as needed.
5. Observe/instruct about purpose of prescribed supplemental vitamin therapy and minerals to treat deficiencies (e.g., vitamin B_{12}, folic acid, thiamin, iron, fat-soluble vitamins [A D E K]).
6. Observe/instruct about taking medications as ordered, purpose and action, side effects, caution associated with a cirrhotic liver.
7. Assess and evaluate degree and location of fluid retention/instruct how to measure and record abdominal girth, intake and output, weigh and record (daily or as prescribed), report weight gain of 2 pounds in a day or 5 pounds in a week.
8. Assess and evaluate jaundice and pruritus/instruct about prescribed skin measures and medications to relieve itching (e.g., cholestyramine)/report to physician skin breakdown and, failure of treatment to alleviate.
9. Assess and evaluate GI disturbances (e.g., indigestion, weight loss, nausea and vomiting, abdominal disturbances)/instruct as to cause, prescribed measures to relieve distension and gas pains (e.g., taking bile salts, eating small, frequent meals; avoiding gas-producing foods and those high in fat).
10. Assess and evaluate location, extent, severity of edema/instruct about good skin-care measures, optimal nutritional status, increased mobility, S&S of irritation or breakdown to report to home health nurse or physician.
11. Assess and evaluate abdominal pain and limited lung expansion resulting from ascites/instruct about prescribed sodium and fluid restrictions, correct positioning to facilitate easier breathing when awake or when sleeping.
12. Observe/instruct about predisposing factors to activity intolerance (e.g., paresthesias ataxic gait, weakness of extremities seen with vitamin and thiamin deficiencies), prescribed measures to treat, importance of compliance with prescribed activity restrictions with measures to promote rest and conserve energy.

13. Assess/instruct about S&S of infection, increased susceptibility with liver disease, measures to avoid exposure.
14. Assess and evaluate alterations in bowel patterns (constipation, diarrhea)/instruct about causative factors, prescribed measures to treat.
15. Assess/instruct about increased risk factors for falls and injuries in home/instruct as to safety measures with ambulation and daily activities.
16. Assess/instruct about increased tendency to bleed, measures to reduce risk (e.g., maintain a safe home environment to reduce risks of falls and injuries; use a soft toothbrush; avoid straining with bowel movement; avoid aspirin and aspirin-containing products), signs of bleeding to report to physician (e.g., blood in urine, stools; weakness; easy bruising)/educate how to apply pressure to control bleeding/report to physician.
17. Assess impaired coping mechanisms, stage of grieving, altered self-concept/provide emotional support/encourage to verbalize feelings/refer to social services as ordered to assist with modifications in life-style and adaptation to illness and needed community resources (e.g., Alcoholics Annonymous, community counseling services for client and family and rehabilitation programs).

REHABILITATION POTENTIAL

Rehabilitation potential *excellent* *good* *fair* *guarded* *poor* for *full* *partial* return to an improved level of wellness and independence to cope with ADL.

Client's Name _____

Medical Record # _____

ONGOING/DISCHARGE EVALUATION OF TEACHING
The Client with Cirrhosis

Teaching Tools:
Printed materials given: _____

Audiovisual aids used: _____

Return Information/Demonstration/Interpretation
_____ Client
_____ Caregiver

OF:	Met	Not Met	Comments
☐ Nature and progression of liver disease; cause and contributing factors.	_____	_____	_____
☐ S&S of complications; actions to take.	_____	_____	_____
☐ Importance of strict compliance with prescribed treatment regimen.	_____	_____	_____
☐ Medications and administration, purpose and action, side effects.	_____	_____	_____
☐ Purpose and indication of supplemental vitamin therapy.	_____	_____	_____

Client's Name _____

Medical Record # _____

	OF:	**Met**	**Not Met**	**Comments**
☐	Measures to assess degree of fluid retention (abdominal girth measurement, intake and output, weight).	_____	_____	_____
☐	Diet and dietary and fluid restrictions.	_____	_____	_____
☐	Measures to relieve pruritus.	_____	_____	_____
☐	Measures to relieve gastrointestinal disturbances.	_____	_____	_____
☐	Skin care of edematous areas.	_____	_____	_____
☐	Measures to facilitate adequate respiratory function with ascites.	_____	_____	_____
☐	Causative factors in constipation and diarrhea; measures to treat.	_____	_____	_____
☐	Factors predisposing to activity intolerance;			

Client's Name _____

Medical Record # _____

OF:	**Met**	**Not Met**	**Comments**
measures to treat; measures to promote rest and conserve energy.	_____	_____	_____
☐ Risk factors for infection; measures to avoid exposure.	_____	_____	_____
☐ Risk factors for bleeding; measures to avoid.	_____	_____	_____
☐ Risk factors for falls and injuries; safety measures with ambulation and daily activities.	_____	_____	_____

Signature of Home Health Nurse _____

Date _____

ENDOCRINE DISORDERS

■ Diabetes Mellitus

Diabetes mellitus is a chronic systemic disorder of heterogenous etiology, characterized by alterations in metabolism of carbohydrates, fats, and proteins. The two major classifications of diabetes are Type I, insulin-dependent diabetes (IDDM), and Type II, non-insulin-dependent diabetes (NIDDM).

In Type I diabetes, little or no endogenous insulin is secreted by the beta cells in the islets of Langerhans. Previously termed juvenile-onset or ketosis-prone diabetes, IDDM is characterized by an abrupt onset of insulin insufficiency, resulting in impaired cellular uptake and utilization of glucose. As blood glucose levels continue to increase and exceed the renal threshold, glycosuria develops. This causes an osmotic diuresis, which results in excessive urinary output, or polyuria; excessive thirst, or polydipsia (caused by excessive urinary output); and stimulation of the hypothalamus, with a resultant increase in hunger, or polyphagia (a result of glucose loss). Deprived of glucose, the body will then get most of its energy from the breakdown of fats, producing ketone bodies, which may accumulate in the blood, producing ketoacidosis if left untreated.

Type II diabetes is characterized by alterations in insulin action and secretion, in which a relative insulin deficiency exists. Previously termed adult-onset or ketosis-resistant diabetes, NIDDM accounts for approximately 80 percent of all diabetics. The individual is usually over age 40 and obese, with diabetes occurring gradually. Glycosuria is usually the first indication of NIDDM.

POTENTIAL COMPLICATIONS

Acute Metabolic Complications
1. Diabetic ketoacidosis,
2. hypoglycemia (insulin shock),
3. hyperglycemic, hyperosmolar, nonketotic coma (HHNK),
4. Somogyi phenomenon,
5. infection.

Long-Term Vascular Complications
Chronic complications of diabetes are associated with the effects of atherosclerosis and microangiopathy, resulting in vascular complications (e.g., cardiovascular disease, retinopathy). Other serious complications may be caused by an increased deposition of sorbitol (from abnormal glucose metabolism) leading to cataracts and neuropathies (e.g., peripheral neuropathy, autonomic neuropathy [e.g., orthostatic hypotension, nocturnal diarrhea]).

TYPES OF CLIENTS/CLINICAL CONDITIONS SEEN BY HOME HEALTH AGENCIES

1. Newly diagnosed diabetic,
2. newly insulin-dependent diabetic,

3. recent hospitalization following an acute exacerbation of diabetic condition,
4. long-standing diabetic with complications related to metabolic disorder and insulin therapy,
5. diabetic client with changes in prescribed treatment regimen.

RELATED NURSING DIAGNOSES

Anxiety

related to:
1. Lack of understanding of diabetes and associated symptoms
2. Unstable blood sugars with fear of complications
3. Prescribed treatment regimen of insulin therapy, caloric diet, diagnostic tests and treatments

as seen by:
Expressed concern regarding changes in health status and lack of understanding of disease process and treatment; apprehension; asking many questions or no questions; noncompliance

Bowel Elimination, Alteration in: Constipation and Diarrhea

related to:
Alternation in periods of constipation and diarrhea and nocturnal fecal incontinence related to neuropathies

as seen by:
Changes in frequency and amount of stool; loose stools or hard, formed stools; abdominal pain; cramping

Comfort, Alteration in: Pain

related to:
Diabetic neuropathies

as seen by:
Neuropathic pain: aching, dull, burning, tingling, numbness in extremities; reluctance to move; facial expression of pain; increased pulse rate

Fluid Volume: Deficit

related to:
Abnormal fluid losses secondary to osmotic diuresis from hyperglycemia

as seen by:
Poor skin turgor; excessive thirst; weak, rapid pulse; hypotension; output greater than intake

Infection, Potential for

related to:
Decreased resistance to infections with uncontrolled diabetes

as seen by:
S&S of infection (e.g., skin, urinary tract infections)

Injury, Potential for: Increased Risk of Falls and Injuries

related to:
1. Paresthesias, decreased vibratory and propriocept sensations, motor impairments secondary to neuropathies
2. Vascular insufficiency of lower extremities
3. Retinopathy
4. Hypoglycemia secondary to insulin excess

as seen by:
Decreased tactile sensations in arms and legs; loss of deep tendon reflexes; muscle weakness and atrophy; intermittent claudication; cold feet; shiny atrophic skin, decreased visual acuity; dizziness; confusion; tremors

Knowledge Deficit (Specify)

related to:
1. Lack of understanding of disease process
2. Prescribed plan of treatment
3. Potential complications, S&S to report to home health nurse or physician

as seen by:
Verbalization of lack of information; inadequate understanding; inability to perform skills necessary to meet health-care needs at home

Nutrition, Alteration in: Less than Body Requirements

related to:
1. Depletion of fat stores and breakdown of protein secondary to a lack of insulin and failure to utilize normal amounts of glucose
2. Decreased oral intake secondary to dietary restrictions

as seen by:
Weight loss; c/o fatigue and weakness; anorexia; states dislikes dietary restrictions

Nutrition, Alteration in: More than Body Requirements

related to:
1. Caloric intake in excess of energy requirements, insulin coverage
2. Obesity associated with insulin resistance

as seen by:
Weight 10 percent above that desirable for height, body build, and age; triceps skin fold greater than 15 mm in men and 25 mm in women

Self-Concept, Disturbance in:

related to:
1. Alteration in body functioning
2. Changes in life-style
3. Low self-esteem

as seen by:
Refusal to acknowledge developing problems related to condition; lack of follow-through; not taking responsibility for self-care; increased dependency on others for care

Sexual Dysfunction

related to:
Neuropathy of the autonomic pelvic nerves

as seen by:
Verbalization of limitations on usual sexual activity; depressed mood and behavior; withdrawal from spouse or significant other

Skin Integrity, Impairment of: Actual/Potential

related to:
1. Decreased tissue perfusion secondary to vascular abnormalities (e.g., athrosclerosis)
2. Alteration in nutritional state
3. Existing skin ulcerations
4. Fungal infection, pruritis secondary to hyperglycemia

as seen by:
Redness; swelling; irritation; tissue breakdown; drainage; cold feet, thickened toenails, thin and shiny atrophic skin on legs

Sensory-Perceptual Alteration: Visual and Tactile Deficits

related to:
1. Diabetic retinopathy
2. Peripheral neuropathies

as seen by:
Visual problems; tingling sensations; pain; paresthesias; loss of ability to perceive vibratory sensations.

Tissue Perfusion, Alteration in: Systemic

related to:
Vascular complications (e.g., athrosclerosis or orthostatic hypotension secondary to autonomic neuropathy

as seen by:
Skin pale; cool to touch; diminished or absent peripheral pulses; drop in blood pressure with change to sit or stand position

Urinary Elimination, Alteration in: Incontinence

related to:
Sensory or neuromuscular impairment
  associated with neuropathy

as seen by:
Frequency; hesitancy; infrequent
  voiding; nocturia; urgency

LONG-TERM GOAL

Diabetic client will understand and comply with a plan of treatment to restore glucose homeostasis and minimize long-term diabetic complications through correction of biochemical and metabolic abnormalities.

SHORT-TERM GOALS

The client with diabetes mellitus will be able to:

1. Verbalize a basic understanding of the nature and type of diabetes and effect on body systems, S&S of complications to report to home health nurse or physician.
2. Verbalize importance of compliance with prescribed treatment regimen with balance in diet, medications, and exercise.
3. Verbalize importance/demonstrate compliance with prescribed ADA diet, dietary principles, and restrictions.
4. Verbalize importance of taking meals and snacks as prescribed, effect on blood glucose levels and insulin fluctuations.
5. Verbalize importance of optimal weight in diabetic condition.
6. Demonstrate compliance with prescribed medication therapy/identify complications.
7. Demonstrate compliance with prescribed insulin therapy, correct insulin administration/identify complications.
8. Demonstrate the ability to correctly manage insulin pump as prescribed.
9. Demonstrate correct use of appropriate self-help devices for insulin administration by client with impaired vision.
10. Identify factors that precipitate hypo- and hyperglycemia, S&S to report, appropriate treatment interventions.
11. Demonstrate correct techniques in blood glucose and urine tests in assessing degree of diabetic control/identify abnormal findings to report to physician.
12. Verbalize understanding of Somogyi phenomenon, factors that precipitate, prescribed treatment interventions, S&S to report.
13. Verbalize importance of consistent exercise program with planned rest periods, effect on blood glucose levels.
14. Verbalize importance of good skin and foot care, diabetic health care and hygiene practices/identify S&S of complications to report.

15. Identify S&S of peripheral neuropathies, factors that aggravate, measures to reduce discomfort.
16. Verbalize understanding of relationship of diabetic neuropathies to alterations in bowel and bladder functioning/follow prescribed bowel and bladder program/identify S&S of complications to report.
17. Verbalize importance, purpose, and administration of prescribed glucagon.
18. Verbalize effects of physical and emotional stress on blood sugar, need for insulin adjustment.
19. Verbalize importance/wear Medic Alert bracelet.
20. Verbalize purpose of prescribed laboratory tests.
21. Demonstrate effective management and adjustment to diabetic condition.

NURSING INTERVENTIONS AND TREATMENTS

1. Assess for clinical manifestations associated with diabetes/identify complications.
2. Assess vital signs/identify trends (e.g., hypo- or hypertension, tachycardia, arrhythmias, labored respirations).
3. Instruct as to nature and type of diabetes, effect on body systems, importance of compliance with prescribed treatment regimen with balance in activities, diet, medications, and exercise.
4. Assess and evaluate nutritional status/instruct about prescribed calculated ADA diet, diabetic dietary principles and restrictions/obtain dietary consultation as needed.
5. Assess/instruct about taking meals and snacks when prescribed, effect on insulin fluctuations and blood glucose levels.
6. Assess/instruct about prescribed weight-loss diet, weighing weekly, importance of optimal weight in diabetes.
7. Observe/instruct about prescribed medications, oral hypoglycemics (e.g., Dymelor, Diabinese, Tolinase, Orinase), purpose and action, side effects, toxicity/evaluate medication effectiveness.
8. Observe/instruct about prescribed insulin therapy, preparation, purpose and action, onset, peak, duration of action, injection techniques, sites, complications, local allergic reactions/evaluate effectiveness of insulin therapy.
9. Observe/instruct client on insulin pump and prescribed management (e.g. filling syringes, changing of batteries, changing the subcutaneous needle).
10. Observe/instruct client with impaired vision in use of appropriate self-help devices (e.g., preset dosage syringe, magnifier for syringe, needle guide for insulin vial, automatic injector).
11. Observe/instruct about S&S of hypoglycemia (e.g., diaphoresis, trembling, hunger, irritability, headache, faintness, palpitations, pale, cool, moist skin) and hyperglycemia (e.g., polydipsia, polyphagia, polyuria, dry, flushed skin, lethargy, confusion, visual disturbances), factors that precipitate, appropriate treatment interventions.

12. Assess/instruct about prescribed measures to assess degree of diabetic control: urine sugar tests (e.g., Clinitest, Clinistix, Diastix, Tes-Tape), ketone level tests (e.g. Acetest, Ketostix), blood glucose level tests with use of Autolet or Autoclix with a reagent strip to test blood glucose (e.g., Visidex, Chemstrip bG) or use of a reagent strip (e.g., Dextrostix) with a blood meter, such as a glucometer, for self-testing blood glucose/record results/report values outside parameters specified by physician.
13. Assess and evaluate for S&S of Somogyi phenomenon/instruct about importance of eating 100 percent of meals and snacks as prescribed/consult physician for insulin adjustment as needed.
14. Observe and evaluate level of physical tolerance/instruct about consistent exercise program with planned rest periods, effect of exercise on blood sugar levels.
15. Assess/instruct about inspecting skin and feet daily for areas of redness or breakdown, meticulous skin and foot care, diabetic health care and hygiene practices, avoiding injury, S&S of impaired circulation and infection to report to home health nurse or physician.
16. Assess/instruct about S&S of peripheral neuropathies, factors that aggravate, and prescribed measures to reduce discomfort (e.g., to avoid temperature extremes; keep hands and feet warm in cold weather; avoid use of hot-water bottles and trauma to lower extremities).
17. Assess for bowel or bladder dysfunction/instruct about prescribed bowel and bladder program, S&S of complications to report.
18. Observe and evaluate for physical or emotional stress, methods to deal with stress/instruct about effects on blood sugar/consult with physician for insulin adjustment as needed.
19. Observe/instruct caregiver about glucagon preparation and administration, purpose and action as ordered.
20. Observe/instruct to follow safety measures related to diabetic condition (e.g., wearing Medic Alert bracelet, carrying quick-acting carbohydrates).
21. Monitor/instruct as to purpose of prescribed laboratory tests (e.g., glucose tolerance test; fasting blood sugar; two-hour postprandial).
22. Assess adjustment to diabetes and management of condition, c/o of sexual dysfunction/encourage to verbalize feelings/provide emotional support/refer to social services as ordered to assist client in adapting to diabetic condition and to provide information regarding community resources (e.g., American Diabetes Association and local affiliate; diabetic clinics; hospital support groups and community education classes, counseling services).

REHABILITATION POTENTIAL

Rehabilitation potential *excellent   good   fair   guarded   poor* for *full partial* return to a previous level of self-care and wellness with stabilized blood sugars.

Client's Name _____

Medical Record # _____

ONGOING/DISCHARGE EVALUATION OF TEACHING
The Client with Diabetes

Teaching Tools:
Printed materials given: _____

Audiovisual aids used: _____

Return Information/Demonstration/Interpretation
_____ Client
_____ Caregiver

OF:	Met	Not Met	Comments
☐ Nature and type of diabetes, effect on body systems.	_____	_____	_____
☐ S&S of complications, actions to take.	_____	_____	_____
☐ Importance of compliance with prescribed treatment regimen.	_____	_____	_____
☐ Importance of balance among activities, diet, medications, and exercise.	_____	_____	_____
☐ Calculated ADA diet; diabetic dietary principles and restrictions.	_____	_____	_____
☐ Effect of meals and snacks on			

Client's Name _____

Medical Record #_____

OF:	**Met**	**Not Met**	**Comments**
insulin fluctuations and glucose levels.	_____	_____	_____
☐ Weight-loss diet; importance of optimal weight on diabetes.	_____	_____	_____
☐ Medication administration, purpose and action, adverse reactions.	_____	_____	_____
☐ Insulin administration, purpose and action, onset, peak, duration, injection technique, sites, complications, local allergic reactions.	_____	_____	_____
☐ Purpose and management of insulin pump.	_____	_____	_____
☐ Use of self-help devices by client with impaired vision.	_____	_____	_____
☐ S&S of hypo- and hyperglycemia; factors that precipitate; appropriate treatment interventions.	_____	_____	_____

Client's Name _____

Medical Record # _____

	OF:	**Met**	**Not Met**	**Comments**
☐	Self-testing of urine sugar and/or blood glucose levels.	_____	_____	_____
☐	Somogyi phenomenon, measures to reduce risk.	_____	_____	_____
☐	Exercise program, effect on blood sugar levels.	_____	_____	_____
☐	Meticulous skin and foot care; diabetic health care and hygiene practices; S&S of complications to report.	_____	_____	_____
☐	S&S of peripheral neuropathies, factors that aggravate, measures to reduce discomfort.	_____	_____	_____
☐	Bowel and bladder program; S&S of bowel or bladder complications to report.	_____	_____	_____
☐	Effects of physical or			

Client's Name _____

Medical Record # _____

OF:	**Met**	**Not Met**	**Comments**
emotional stress on blood sugar.	_____	_____	_____
☐ Glucagon preparation and administration, purpose and action.	_____	_____	_____
☐ Safety measures related to diabetes (e.g., Medic Alert bracelet; carrying of a quick-action carbohydrate).	_____	_____	_____
☐ Purpose of prescribed laboratory tests.	_____	_____	_____

Signature of Home Health Nurse _____

Date _____

■ Hyperthyroidism

Hyperthyroidism is a metabolic imbalance characterized by an overproduction of thyroid hormone. It is more common in women than men and may take the form of Graves' disease or toxic nodular goiter, which is found to affect older individuals. Excess production of thyroid hormone accelerates metabolic processes, resulting in physiologic disturbances that affect almost all systems of the body.

The most common form of hyperthyroidism is Graves' disease, which is thought to result from an immunogenetic defect. In Graves' disease, ocular and nervous signs are the predominant findings. In toxic nodular goiter, cardiovascular findings predominate. In the elderly client presenting with an arrhythmia, angina, or heart failure, these findings may be less obvious as being clinical manifestations of hyperthyroidism.

Hyperthyroidism can appear abruptly after an emotional shock, nervous strain, or an infection, or the onset may be gradual. The most common symptoms are nervousness, tremors, diarrhea, weight loss, muscle weakness, and palpitations. In some instances a goiter or eye signs and changes such as exophthalmos may be the first signs noticed.

Thyroid crisis, or "storm," a life-threatening complication with severe manifestations of hyperthyroidism, is caused by the release into the bloodstream of increased amounts of thyroid hormones. This crisis may occur abruptly or be precipitated by factors such as stress or infection; it results from untreated or inadequately treated thyrotoxicosis.

POTENTIAL COMPLICATIONS

1. Thyroid storm,
2. cardiac dysfunction (e.g., atrial fibrillation with cardiac failure),
3. exophthalmos, which may be complicated by corneal ulcerations, visual impairments or loss and oculomotor paresis,
4. glycosuria,
5. localized pretibial myxedema,
6. osteoporosis,
7. psychosis.

TYPES OF CLIENTS/CLINICAL CONDITIONS SEEN BY HOME HEALTH AGENCIES

1. Newly diagnosed with hyperthyroidism: initiation of prescribed treatment regimen of antithyroid therapy and inclusive teaching plan for home-care management of condition.
2. Long-standing condition of hyperthroidism with complications: changes in prescribed treatment regimen requiring instruction and close monitoring of response to therapy.
3. Recent hospitalization following an acute exacerbation of hyperthyroidism:

changes in ongoing plan of treatment and additional need for skilled nursing observations and teaching.

RELATED NURSING DIAGNOSIS

Activity Intolerance

related to:
Weakness and fatigue secondary to increased metabolic rate

as seen by:
Dyspnea on exertion; tachycardia; arrhythmias; c/o weakness and fatigue

Anxiety

related to:
1. Disease process
2. Altered body image
3. Life-style changes
4. Knowledge deficit regarding prescribed treatment regimen
5. Possibility of surgery

as seen by:
Nervousness; tachycardia; tremors; increased perspiration; jittery behavior; asking numerous questions

Bowel Elimination, Alteration in: Diarrhea

related to:
Increased GI motility secondary to increased metabolic rate

as seen by:
Increased frequency of stool; loose, liquid stools; increased bowel sounds; abdominal cramping

Cardiac Output, Alteration in: Decreased

related to:
Cardiac complications that may occur with hyperthyroidism:
1. Cardiac arrhythmia with cardiac failure
2. Unrelieved rapid heart rate

as seen by:
Fatigue; dyspnea; changes in mental status; low BP; cyanosis; restlessness; edema

Communication, Impaired Verbal

related to:
1. Increased thyroxine production
2. Compression on laryngeal nerve from an enlarged thyroid

as seen by:
Rapid and excited speech; hoarseness

Coping, Ineffective Individual

related to:
1. Anxiety
2. Nervousness
3. Emotional lability associated with disease process

as seen by:
Verbalization of inablity to cope; inability to make decisions; difficulty in meeting basic needs

Injury, Potential for: Increased Risk of Falls and Injuries

related to:
1. Increased activity in the spinal cord area controlling muscle tone
2. Exophthalmos with lid retraction accompanied by paralysis of eye muscle and visual impairment

as seen by:
Weakness and fatigue; tremors; clumsiness; diplopia; impaired visual acuity; increased tearing; blurred vision

Knowledge Deficit (Specify)

related to:
1. Disease process and clinical manifestations
2. Potential complications, S&S to report to home health nurse or physician
3. Prescribed plan of treatment in management of thyroid disorder

as seen by:
Verbalization of lack of information; inadequate understanding of prescribed treatment regimen in management of thyroid disorder

Mobility, Impaired Physical

related to:
1. Activity intolerance
2. Effects of hyperthyroidism on musculoskeletal and central nervous system
3. Prescribed activity restrictions

as seen by:
Tremors; shaking; weakness and fatigue; muscle atrophy; imposed medical restrictions

Nutrition, Alteration in: Less than Body Requirements

related to:
1. Imbalance between caloric intake and increased basal metabolic rate
2. Dysphagia from compression of esophagus by thyroid enlargement

as seen by:
Loss of body weight with adequate food intake; body weight 20 percent or more under ideal weight for height, age, and frame

3. Anorexia
4. Nausea and vomiting or diarrhea
   secondary to increased GI motility

Self-Care Deficit: Feeding, Bathing/Hygiene, Dressing/Grooming, Toileting (Specify)

related to:
1. Activity intolerance
2. Impaired mobility status
3. Prescribed activity restrictions

as seen by:
Decreased ability to participate in daily activities, associated with weakness and fatigue; tremors; impaired vision

Self-Concept, Disturbance in

related to:
1. Change in appearance
2. Life-style changes

as seen by:
Withdrawal from others; denial; self-neglect; anger

Sensory-Perceptual Alteration: Visual

related to:
Visual disturbances secondary to hyperthyroidism

as seen by:
exophthalmus; diplopia; increased tearing; reports change in visual acuity; photosensitivity

Sleep Pattern Disturbance

related to:
Nervousness and excitability resulting from increased basal metabolic rate

as seen by:
C/o of not being able to sleep and/or not feeling well rested

LONG-TERM GOAL

To restore metabolic balance and diminish clinical manifestations associated with hyperthyroidism through return of client to a euthyroid state.

SHORT-TERM GOALS

The client with hyperthyroidism will be able to:

1. Verbalize nature of thyroid disorder, effect on body systems, behavior changes, S&S of complications to report to home health nurse or physician.
2. Demonstrate in taking and recording vital signs and identify alterations in rate or rhythm to report to physician.

3. Verbalize effect of increased metabolic demands on body/demonstrate compliance with prescribed diet and dietary restrictions.
4. Verbalize importance of taking vitamin and nutritional supplements as prescribed.
5. Verbalize importance of soft or semisoft foods with dysphagia, measures to avoid aspiration.
6. Weigh weekly and record/report excessive weight loss to physician.
7. Demonstrate compliance with prescribed medication therapy.
8. Verbalize measures to help counteract hypermetabolic state.
9. Verbalize importance of prescribed activity restrictions, avoiding fatigue.
10. Verbalize cause of GI disturbances, prescribed measures to decrease peristalsis.
11. Demonstrate compliance with prescribed measures to treat and protect eyes if visual disturbances or exophthalmos occur.
12. Identify risk factors for falls and injuries in home environment, safety measures with ambulation and daily activities.
13. Verbalize importance of avoiding exposure to infections, S&S to report to physician.
14. Identify S&S of hyper- or hypothyroidism to report to physician after treatment with radioactive iodine.
15. Verbalize precautions to follow after treatment with radioactive iodine.
16. Demonstrate effective coping mechanisms and positive adjustment to thyroid disorder.
17. Demonstrate compliance with prescribed speech therapy program to improve communication and swallowing.

NURSING ACTIONS/TREATMENTS

1. Assess for clinical effects of hyperthyroidism on body systems/identify complications.
2. Assess vital signs/identify trends (e.g., increased systolic BP, increased pulse rate, irregular pulse, widened pulse pressure, elevated temperature)/instruct how to take and record pulse, alterations in rate or rhythm to report to physician.
3. Instruct as to nature of thyroid disorder, effect on body systems, behavior changes, importance of strict compliance with prescribed treatment regimen, S&S of complications to report to home health nurse or physician.
4. Assess and evaluate nutritional status/instruct about effect of increased metabolic demands on body, well-balanced diet with prescribed high-caloric, protein and, carbohydrate diet, vitamins and nutritional supplements, adequate fluids, avoiding caffeine/obtain dietary consultation as needed.
5. Assess and evaluate dysphagia/instruct as to prescribed diet of semisoft and/or soft foods, measures to avoid aspiration (e.g., high Fowler's position with meals and for one half hour after eating, chewing food well).

6. Observe and evaluate for progressive weight loss/instruct to weigh and record weekly, more often as indicated/report excess weight loss to physician.
7. Observe/instruct about taking medications as ordered (e.g., thyroid hormone antagonists) purpose and action, side effects/evaluate medication effectiveness.
8. Observe and evaluate for hyperactivity, nervousness, irritability, sleep pattern disturbances/instruct about measures to help counteract hypermetabolic state (e.g., calm, nonstressful home environment, prescribed activity restrictions, avoiding fatigue).
9. Assess and evaluate GI disturbances (e.g., nausea, vomiting, diarrhea)/instruct about cause, measures to decrease peristalis (e.g., taking prescribed medications, avoiding highly seasoned and fibrous foods).
10. Assess and evaluate visual disturbances, exophthalmos/instruct about good eye care, measures to protect eyes (e.g., sunglasses, sleeping with head elevated to decrease fluid accumulation behind eyes), use of prescribed eye drops, prescribed restrictions in salt and fluid intake, complications to report to physician.
11. Assess/instruct about increased risk factors for falls and injuries, instruct about safety measures with ambulation and daily activities.
12. Observe/instruct about importance of and measures to avoid exposure to infections (may precipitate a thyroid crisis).
13. Assess/instruct about purpose of treatment with radioactive iodine, temporary increase in symptoms of hyperthyrodism that may occur on 4th or 5th day, S&S of hypothyroidism to report to physician.
14. Observe/instruct about safety precautions to follow after radioactive iodine treatment (e.g., feces, urine, saliva, and perspiration are temporarily radioactive for 48 hours after treatment: flush toilet 2–3 times after use to ensure all waste is discarded and wash hands thoroughly afterward; use disposable plates and cutlery; caregiver(s) should avoid contact with any body secretions from client; avoid close contact with infants, children, and pregnant women for one week; importance of drinking increased amounts of fluids as ordered to speed the elimination of radioactive iodine from the body; reporting to the physician of a fever accompanied by agitation, occuring within 48 hrs of treatment).
15. Assess speech and swallowing difficulties/refer to speech therapy as ordered to provide instruction in speech and swallowing training, measures to improve communication.
16. Assess emotional state and effect on family and social relationships/provide emotional support/refer to social services as ordered to provide counseling to assist with coping and adjustment to effects of disease process.

REHABILITATION POTENTIAL

Rehabilitation potential *excellent good fair guarded poor* for *full partial* return to a prehypermetabolic state and improved state of health to perform ADL independently.

Client's Name _____

Medical Record #_____

ONGOING/DISCHARGE EVALUATION OF TEACHING
The Client with Hyperthyroidism

Teaching Tools:
Printed materials given: _____

Audiovisual aids used: _____

Return Information/Demonstration/Interpretation
_____ Client
_____ Caregiver

OF:	Met	Not Met	Comments
☐ Nature of thyroid disorder; effect on body systems and behavior.	_____	_____	_____
☐ S&S of complications, actions to take.	_____	_____	_____
☐ Importance of strict compliance with prescribed treatment regimen.	_____	_____	_____
☐ How to take and record pulse rate, alterations in rate and rhythm to report to physician.	_____	_____	_____
☐ Prescribed diet for hypermetabolic state, dietary restrictions.	_____	_____	_____

Client's Name _____

Medical Record #_____

	OF:	Met	Not Met	Comments
☐	Vitamin and nutritional supplements.	_____	_____	_____
☐	Sodium and fluid restrictions with edematous condition.	_____	_____	_____
☐	Measures to improve oral intake with dysphagia, avoid aspiration.	_____	_____	_____
☐	Weighing and recording weekly, reporting excessive weight loss to physician.	_____	_____	_____
☐	Medications and administration, purpose and action, side effects.	_____	_____	_____
☐	Activity restrictions to help counteract hypermetabolic state.	_____	_____	_____
☐	Measures to decrease GI disturbances.	_____	_____	_____
☐	Measures to treat and protect eyes if visual			

Client's Name _____

Medical Record # _____

OF:	**Met**	**Not Met**	**Comments**
disturbances or exophthalmus occurs.	_____	_____	_____
☐ Risk factors for falls and injuries in the home environment; related safety measures with ambulation and daily activities.	_____	_____	_____
☐ Radioactive iodine treatment; S&S of hypo- or hyper- thyroidism; actions to take.	_____	_____	_____
☐ Safety precautions to follow after radioactive iodine treatment.	_____	_____	_____
☐ Measures to avoid infections.	_____	_____	_____

Signature of Home Health Nurse _____

Date _____

■ Hypothyroidism

Hypothyroidism is characterized by a deficiency of low serum thyroid hormone, which depresses the metabolic rate and predisposes to clinical manifestations that affect many systems of the body. Thyroid deficiency may be classified as (1) primary hypothyroidism, in which the deficiency occurs secondary to disease or deficiency of the thyroid gland itself, and which accounts for 95 percent of all cases (e.g., thyroidectomy; Hashimoto's thyroiditis, an autoimmune disorder; impaired synthesis and release of thyroid hormone; excessive iodine intake; certain antithyroid drugs); (2) secondary hypothyroidism, caused by pituitary dysfunction; and (3) tertiary hypothyroidism, which results from failure of the hypothalamus to secrete thyroid-releasing hormones.

Thyroid deficiency that occurs before or shortly after birth is called cretinism and adult hypothyroidism is called myxedema, a term used to describe a nonpitting edema associated with infiltration and accumulation of a mucinous substance in subcutaneous connective and/or muscle tissue. Clinical manifestations associated with hypothyroidism are fatigue, cold intolerance, flakey, inelastic skin, stiffness of hands and feet, decreased mental and physical abilities, constipation, hoarseness, decreased cardiac output and pulse rate, and signs of inadequate peripheral circulation.

POTENTIAL COMPLICATIONS

1. Atheromatous coronary artery disease resulting from disturbed lipid metabolism secondary to hypothyroidism,
2. decreased cardiac output secondary to thyroid hormone deficiency,
3. impaired muscle functioning associated with myxedema: (a) weakened myocardium; (b) respiratory infections; (c) urinary tract infections; (d) constipation,
4. diastolic hypertension,
5. intestinal obstruction from paralytic ileus associated with thyroid hormone deficiency,
6. myxedema coma,
7. "myxedema madness" or organic psychosis.

TYPES OF CLIENTS/CLINICAL CONDITIONS SEEN BY HOME HEALTH AGENCIES

1. Newly diagnosed with hypothroidism: initiation of prescribed treatment regimen of thyroid hormone replacement and inclusive teaching plan for home-care management of condition, close evaluation of response to initial thyroid hormone replacement, reporting client's response to physician for evaluation of need to increase or decrease medication until thyroid levels are normal.
2. Long-standing condition of hypothyroidism with complications: changes in prescribed treatment regimen with supervision, monitoring, evaluation of response to therapy changes by home health nurse.

3. Recent hospitalization following an acute exacerbation of hypothyroidism: changes in ongoing plan of treatment and additional need for skilled observations and teaching.

RELATED NURSING DIAGNOSIS

Activity Intolerance

related to:
Imbalance between oxygen supply and demand secondary to a depressed metabolic rate

as seen by:
Weakness and fatigue; exertional dyspnea; abnormal heart and respiratory rate and BP in response to activity

Anxiety

related to:
1. Disease process and associated clinical manifestations
2. Altered body image
3. Life-style changes
4. Knowledge deficit regarding prescribed treatment regimen

as seen by:
Apprehension; distress; uncertainty regarding progress and changes in treatment regimen

Bowel Elimination, Alteration in: Constipation

related to:
1. Decreased metabolism and GI motility secondary to depressed basal metabolic rate and impaired muscle functioning secondary to myxedema
2. Decreased activity levels
3. Decreased oral intake

as seen by:
Frequency and amount less than usual pattern; straining at stool; abdominal distension

Breathing Pattern, Ineffective

related to:
Decreased lung expansion secondary to mucoprotein deposits in pleural space

as seen by:
Exertional dyspnea; shortness of breath; verbal report of decreased energy and fatigue

Cardiac Output, Alteration in: Decreased

related to:
Cardiovascular involvement secondary
  to decreased thyroid hormone levels
  and depressed metabolic rate

as seen by:
Slow pulse rate; c/o fatigue;
  arrhythmias; poor peripheral
  circulation

Comfort, Alteration in: Pain

related to:
Muscular pain and stiffness in arms,
  thighs, and legs, joint stiffness and
  aching, backache secondary to
  accumulation of mucoprotein
  deposits

as seen by:
Guarded behavior; reluctance to move;
  moaning, facial mask of pain

Communication, Impaired Verbal

related to:
Infiltration of the tongue with excess
  mucoprotein substance

as seen by:
Slowed speech and hoarseness

Injury, Potential for: Increased Risk of Falls and Injuries

related to:
1. Altered mental status secondary to
   decreased cerebral blood flow
2. Ataxia
3. Intention tremors
4. Slowing of motor activity
5. Night blindness

as seen by:
Forgetfulness; confusion; weakness
  and fatigue; limited ability to
  perform ADL; reporting visual
  distortions and decrease in visual
  acuity

Knowledge Deficit (Specify)

related to:
1. Disease process and associated
   clinical manifestations
2. Prescribed treatment regimen in
   management of thyroid disorder
3. Potential complications, S&S to
   report to home health nurse or
   physician

as seen by:
Verbalization of lack of information;
  inadequate understanding of
  prescribed treatment regimen in
  management of thyroid condition

Mobility, Impaired Physical

related to:
1. Activity intolerance
2. Muscular pain and stiffness
3. Joint stiffness and aching
4. Ataxia and intention tremors secondary to clinical effects of hypothyroidism

as seen by:
Weakness and fatigue; uncoordinated movements; effects of muscle and joint discomfort

Nutrition, Alteration in: Less than Body Requirements

related to:
1. Slowed metabolic rate, with impairment in absorption of nutrients
2. Dysphagia secondary to pressure on esophagus from an enlarged thyroid
3. Pernicious anemia seen in some clients with autoimmune hypothyroidism

as seen by:
Weakness and fatigue; weight loss; difficulty swallowing; S&S of malnutrition; night blindness; stomatitis

Nutrition, Alteration in: More than Body Requirements

related to:
Imbalance between caloric intake and depressed basal metabolic rate

as seen by:
Weight 10 percent or more above that desirable for height, body build, and age; triceps skin fold greater than normal for body build

Self-Care Deficit: Feeding, Bathing/Hygiene, Dressing/Grooming, Toileting (Specify)

related to:
1. Activity intolerance
2. Impaired physical mobility
3. Prescribed activity restrictions

as seen by:
Inability to manage ADL and take care of personal needs without assistance, associated with weakness and fatigue; exertional dyspnea; joint and muscle pain, discomfort

Self-Concept, Disturbance in

related to:
1. Changes in appearance

as seen by:
Increased dependency on others;

2. Life-style changes
3. Low self-esteem

refusal to participate in care or treatment; irritability; decreased attention to grooming

Skin Integrity, Impairment of:

related to:
Dry, coarse, inelastic skin, generalized interstitial edema

as seen by:
Redness; irritation; tissue breakdown

Sensory-Perceptual Alteration: Auditory, Visual

related to:
Sensorineural hearing loss secondary to infiltration of a mucinous substance into cranial nerve VIII, night blindness related to decreased Vitamin A synthesis

as seen by:
Report of change in auditory activity; c/o auditory distortion; altered communication, behavior pattern; report in change in visual acuity; visual distortions

Sexual Dysfunction

related to:
Hypothyroidism

as seen by:
decreased libido, impotence

LONG-TERM GOAL

To restore metabolic balance and diminish clinical manifestations of hypothyroidism in the body through return of client to a euthyroid state.

SHORT-TERM GOALS

The client with hypothyroidism will be able to:

1. Verbalize nature of thyroid disorder, effect on body systems and behavior, S&S of complications to report to home health nurse or physician.
2. Demonstrate accuracy in taking and recording pulse/identify alterations in rate and rhythm to report to physician.
3. Demonstrate compliance with prescribed diet and dietary restrictions.
4. Verbalize causative factors of decreased oral intake/demonstrate compliance with prescribed diet, vitamin and nutritional supplements.
5. Verbalize importance of taking prescribed vitamins for treatment of night blindness, weakness, ataxia, and paresthesias.
6. Demonstrate compliance with prescribed weight control diet.

7. Verbalize importance of soft or semisoft foods with dysphagia, measures to avoid aspiration.
8. Demonstrate compliance with prescribed medication therapy/instruct about importance of holding thyroid hormone medications and notifying physician if pulse rate is over 100 beats per minute/verbalize need for lifelong thyroid hormone/identify side effects, toxicity.
9. Verbalize importance of reporting any cardiac problems to physician at once.
10. Verbalize importance of avoiding exposure to infection, cold temperatures, stressful situations.
11. Verbalize effect of thyroid disorder on bowel motility/identify prescribed measures to treat constipation.
12. Demonstrate prescribed skin care measures/identify S&S of skin breakdown to report to physician.
13. Verbalize causative factors to impaired activity tolerance and mobility status/demonstrate activities and exercises within physical limitations, balanced rest periods, energy conservation techniques.
14. Demonstrate prescribed measures to reduce joint and muscle pain, protection to affected extremities.
15. Demonstrate safety measures with ambulation and daily activities/identify risk factors related to disease process.
16. Verbalize purpose of prescribed diagnostic lab work.
17. Verbalize causative factors of impaired hearing and verbal communication/demonstrate prescribed measures to facilitate communication.
18. Verbalize importance/wear Medic Alert bracelet.
19. Demonstrate positive adjustment to altered body image and need for lifelong hormone therapy.

NURSING INTERVENTIONS AND TREATMENTS

1. Assess for clinical effects of hypothyroidism/identify related effects on body systems.
2. Assess vital signs/instruct how to take pulse and record alterations in rate and rhythm to report to physician/identify trends (e.g., bradycardia, hyper- or hypotension).
3. Instruct as to nature of thyroid disorder, effect on body systems, behavior changes, importance of compliance with prescribed treatment regimen, S&S of complications to report to home health nurse or physician.
4. Assess and evaluate nutritional status/instruct about prescribed diet (e.g., low caloric, high fiber, sodium restrictions, avoiding foods high in cholesterol and saturated fats) obtain dietary consultation as needed.
5. Assess/instruct about causative factors in decreased oral intake/instruct about prescribed diet, nutritional vitamins and supplements.

6. Assess and evaluate night blindness/weakness/ataxia/paresthesias/instruct about prescribed supplemental vitamins (e.g., vitamin B_{12}, vitamin A).

7. Assess/instruct about prescribed weight-control diet/weigh and record weekly.

8. Assess and evaluate problems with dysphagia/instruct about prescribed diet of semisoft or soft foods, measures to avoid aspiration (e.g., high Fowler's position with meals and for one half hour after eating, chewing foods well).

9. Observe/instruct to take medications as ordered, purpose and action, side effects, toxicity, importance of taking same time each day to maintain constant hormone level, lifelong need for thyroid hormone replacement therapy; educate about not taking any medications unless ordered by physician (since metabolism is decreased, any medication taken will be prolonged with a risk of drug toxicity).

10. Assess and evaluate response to thyroid hormone medication (e.g., cardiac problems may develop if replacement of thyroid hormone too rapid)/assess BP, pulse rate, volume, regularity/instruct about taking pulse prior to taking medications, holding and reporting to physician pulse rate over 100 beats per minute; importance of reporting cardiac problems to physician at once (e.g., angina, dyspnea, pulse irregularities, or tachycardia).

11. Observe and evaluate for progressive weight loss with initiation of thyroid hormone replacement therapy/instruct to weigh and record weekly, more often as indicated/report significant weight change so that physician can determine if thyroid hormone dosage adequate or too high.

12. Observe/instruct about importance of avoiding exposure to infections, cold temperatures, stressful situations.

13. Assess effect of hypothyroidism on slowing bowel motility/instruct about measures to increase peristalsis (e.g., prescribed increase in dietary fiber, use of prescribed laxatives or stool softeners, increased activities, avoiding straining), educate as to effect on a compromised cardiovascular system/evaluate effectiveness of bowel regimen.

14. Observe and evaluate skin for dryness, nonpitting edema, instruct about prescribed skin-care measures, fluid restrictions, S&S of breakdown and bleeding to report to physician.

15. Observe and evaluate activity tolerance, mobility status/instruct about causative factors of decreased energy and impaired muscle function/instruct about prescribed activities and exercises within physical limitations, balanced rest periods, energy conservation techniques.

16. Assess/instruct about prescribed measures to reduce discomfort of back, stiff aching joints and muscles (e.g., application of heat, splints)/protection against injury to affected extremities.

17. Assess for forgetfulness, confusion, paresthesias, ataxia, night blindness, bleeding tendencies/instruct about safety measures to decrease risk of falls and injuries in the home.

18. Assess and evaluate impairment in verbal communication (e.g., slowed speech

and hoarseness), hearing/instruct as to cause, measures to improve communication (e.g., hearing-impaired device installed on phone, allow client time to communicate, answer questions)/refer to speech therapy as ordered to provide instruction in speech and swallowing training, measures to improve communication.

19. Observe/instruct about importance of wearing Medic Alert bracelet with information on thyroid hormone replacement.

20. Monitor/instruct about purpose of prescribed diagnostic lab work (e.g., measuring thyroxine levels in blood until correct maintenance dose has been reached).

21. Assess adjustment to alterations in body image and behavior changes/provide emotional support/refer to social services as ordered to provide counseling and information regarding community services (e.g., attendant services; Meals on Wheels).

REHABILITATION POTENTIAL

Rehabilitation potential   *excellent*   *good*   *fair*   *guarded*   *poor*   for   *full*
partial   return to an improved metabolic state and state of well-being to independently manage ADL.

Client's Name _____

Medical Record # _____

ONGOING/DISCHARGE EVALUATION OF TEACHING
The Client with Hypothyroidism

Teaching Tools:
Printed materials given: _____

Audiovisual aids used: _____

Return Information/Demonstration/Interpretation
_____ Client
_____ Caregiver

OF:	Met	Not Met	Comments
☐ Nature of thyroid disorder, effect on body systems and behavior.	_____	_____	_____
☐ S&S of complications, actions to take.	_____	_____	_____
☐ Importance of compliance with prescribed treatment regimen.	_____	_____	_____
☐ How to take pulse and record; alterations in rate and rhythm to report to physician.	_____	_____	_____
☐ Prescribed diet, dietary restrictions.	_____	_____	_____
☐ Causative factors of			

Client's Name _____

Medical Record #_____

OF:	Met	Not Met	Comments
decreased oral intake; prescribed diet; vitamins and nutritional supplements.	_____	_____	_____
☐ Weight control diet.	_____	_____	_____
☐ Measures to improve oral intake with dysphagia, avoid aspiration.	_____	_____	_____
☐ Medications and administration, purpose and action, side effects, toxicity.	_____	_____	_____
☐ Weighing and recording weekly when starting on thyroid hormone replacement therapy; reporting significant weight changes to physician.	_____	_____	_____
☐ Taking pulse before taking thyroid hormone; holding and reporting to physician pulse rate over 100 beats per minute.	_____	_____	_____

Client's Name _____

Medical Record #_____

OF:	**Met**	**Not Met**	**Comments**
☐ Importance of avoiding exposure to infections, cold temperatures, stressful situations.	_____	_____	_____
☐ Effect of hypothyroidism on bowel motility; measures to treat constipation.	_____	_____	_____
☐ Skin-care measures; S&S of breakdown to report to physician.	_____	_____	_____
☐ Balanced rest and activities.	_____	_____	_____
☐ Energy conservation techniques.	_____	_____	_____
☐ Measures to reduce discomfort in aching joints and muscles; protection of affected extremities.	_____	_____	_____
☐ Risk factors for falls and injuries in the home environment; related safety measures.	_____	_____	_____

Client's Name _____

Medical Record # _____

OF:	Met	Not Met	Comments
☐ Measures to improve communication.	_____	_____	_____
☐ Medic Alert bracelet.	_____	_____	_____
☐ Purpose of prescribed diagnostic lab work.	_____	_____	_____

Signature of Home Health Nurse _____

Date _____

URINARY TRACT/RENAL DISORDERS

■ End-Stage Renal Disease/Hemodialysis

Chronic renal failure (CRF) is characterized by progressive and irreversible destruction of the total number of functioning nephrons in the kidneys. This progressive destruction ultimately results in physiologic disruptions of cellular homeostasis throughout the body. Some examples of factors responsible for CRF are chronic glomerulonephritis, chronic renal and bladder infections, and systemic diseases such as diabetes and hypertension.

CRF may be divided into three stages based upon the ability of the total number of functioning nephrons to regulate fluid and electrolyte and acid-base balance to maintain homeostasis. In stage one (decreased renal reserve), there is some degree of impaired renal functioning but the serum creatinine and blood urea nitrogen (BUN) levels are normal and the client is usually asymptomatic, except at times of illness and stress. In the second stage (renal insufficiency), 75 percent of functional renal tissue has been destroyed. The BUN and creatinine levels are becoming elevated and symptoms of decreased mental acuity, polyuria, nocturia, and increased blood pressure are beginning to appear as the kidneys are unable to concentrate urine. There may be more severe signs if the client is stressed physically as renal function becomes further impaired. In the third stage (end-stage renal failure) 90 percent of functional renal tissue has been destroyed and there is a marked increase in the BUN and creatinine levels and fluid and electrolyte imbalances, with resultant biochemical changes, called uremic syndrome, that affect all systems of the body. Oliguria is characteristic of this stage.

Clinical manifestations of CRF are related to the severity and duration of renal dysfunction in relation to the kidneys' ability to excrete acids, regulate fluid and electrolyte balance, synthesize ammonia, and remove excess hydrogen ions. Some primary manifestations and complications of CRF are weakness and fatigue, arrhythmias, gastrointestinal bleeding, anemia, malnutrition, neuropathies, congestive heart failure, and hypertension. As the glomerular filtration rate is significantly reduced, end-stage renal failure results, with subsequent systemic dysfunction. Hemodialysis, peritoneal dialysis, or kidney transplantation will be necessary if the client with renal failure does not respond to treatment. The client in end-stage renal failure who is undergoing hemodialysis is the main focus of this home health-nursing care plan.

The purpose of hemodialysis is to shunt blood from the body to a dialyzer to remove excess water and toxic wastes from the blood and to correct and restore acid–base and fluid and electrolyte imbalances. These activities of renal function are accomplished by bringing blood into contact with the semipermeable material of the dialyzer for purification. The dialysate solution, an aqueous solution that diffuses across the semipermeable material into the blood, contains essential electrolytes (sodium, potassium, calcium, magnesium, and chlorides) and acetate and glucose. This dialysate solution is modified slightly from normal blood composition, to correct the fluid and electrolyte disorders of renal failure.

Long-term intermittent hemodialysis requires access to the client's bloodstream. Access is achieved by the placement of two small catheters necessary for hemodialysis, one in the vein, the other in the artery. Examples of hemodialysis access sites are the arteriovenous shunt, arteriovenous fistula, and the arteriovenous vein graft. The most commonly used access for long-term treatment is the arteriovenous fistula. From these catheters, blood leaves the body to circulate through the dialyzer and return to the body after the purification process.

POTENTIAL COMPLICATIONS

Chronic Renal Failure:
1. Fluid and electrolyte imbalances,
2. anuria,
3. gastrointestinal bleeding,
4. congestive heart failure,
5. hypertension,
6. pericarditis,
7. anemia,
8. renal osteodystrophy/pathologic fractures,
9. peripheral neuropathies,
10. uremia,
11. uremic encethalopathy,
12. malnutrition,
13. bleeding tendencies,
14. infection,
15. metabolic acidosis.

Hemodialysis/Vascular Access:
1. Spontaneous bleeding associated with anticoagulant therapy,
2. thrombosis,
3. infection,
4. hemorrhage secondary to disconnection of shunt cannula,
5. shunt clotting.

TYPES OF CLIENTS/CLINICAL CONDITIONS SEEN BY HOME HEALTH AGENCIES

1. Newly diagnosed in renal failure: initiation of prescribed treatment regimen and inclusive teaching plan for home-care management of client in renal failure.
2. Progression of disease process associated with renal impairment with worsening of symptoms related to fluid and electrolyte and acid–base imbalances: changes in therapy; home health nurse to provide instruction and supervision in new medications and/or treatments; assessment of physical status and response to changes in therapy.
3. Recent hospitalization for renal failure: new plan of treatment.
4. Initiation of hemodialysis treatments.

RELATED NURSING DIAGNOSIS

Activity Intolerance

related to:
1. Imbalance between oxygen supply and demand secondary to anemia
2. Inadequate nutritional status
3. Acid–base imbalance

as seen by:
Weakness and fatigue; exertional dyspnea; abnormal heart rate and BP in response to activities; decreased tolerance of self-care activities

Anxiety

related to:
1. Psychological and physiologic stress of disease process
2. Need for hemodialysis to live
3. Altered body image
4. Unpredictable medical status
5. Life-style and role changes
6. Knowledge deficit regarding prescribed treatment regimen

as seen by:
Verbal report of fearfulness; apprehension; anger; hostility; restlessness; asking numerous questions or lack of questions regarding medical condition and home plan of care

Bowel Elimination, Alteration in: Constipation

related to:
1. Side effects of aluminum- or calcium-containing antacids
2. Decreased activity levels
3. Dietary and fluid restrictions
4. Electrolyte imbalance

as seen by:
Frequency and amount less than usual pattern; hard, formed stools; c/o constipation, feeling of pressure

Bowel Elimination, Alteration in: Diarrhea

related to:
1. Irritation of intestinal mucosa secondary to increased levels of nitrogenous wastes
2. Fluid and electrolyte imbalances
3. Unrelieved stress levels
4. Side effect of magnesium-containing antacids

as seen by:
Frequent, loose stools; hyperactive bowel sounds, abdominal pain and discomfort

Cardiac Output, Alteration in: Decreased

related to:
Arrhythmias secondary to fluid and

as seen by:
Dyspnea; changes in BP and heart

electrolyte and acid–base imbalances

rate; cold, clammy skin; abnormal heart sounds; restlessness; changes in mental state

Comfort, Alteration in: Pain

related to:
Physiologic changes in body systems with inability to maintain homeostasis secondary to fluid and electrolyte, acid–base imbalances, and high serum levels of nitrogenous wastes

as seen by:
Pruritus or burning pain; paresthesias; muscle and joint pain

Coping, Ineffective Individual

related to:
Depression in response to chronic renal failure and need for hemodialysis

as seen by:
Feelings of helplessness; verbalization of inability to cope and feelings of rejection; inability to meet basic needs

Fluid Volume, Alteration in: Excess

related to:
1. Decreased excretion of sodium secondary to a decrease in the number of functioning nephrons
2. Compromised regulatory mechanisms
3. Excess fluid and sodium intake

as seen by:
Peripheral edema; elevated BP prior to dialysis; weight gain; intake greater than output; dyspnea

Gas Exchange, Impaired

related to:
1. Altered oxygen supply secondary to anemia as a result of decreased production of erythropoietin by the failing kidneys
2. Early breakdown of red blood cells as a result of toxic fluid environment

as seen by:
Pallor; increased cardiac and respiratory rate; shortness of breath; irritability; lack of energy

Grieving

related to:
1. Anger, depression, or denial associated with loss of normal kidney function
2. Changes in quality of life and role relationships
3. Fear of death
4. Dietary and fluid restrictions

as seen by:
Withdrawal from friends and usual activities; sorrow; distress over health status; expression of feelings of desperation

Infection, Potential for

related to:
Venous access site

as seen by:
Redness; swelling and warmth around access site; pain over access site; drainage; elevated temperature; elevated WBC count

Infection, Potential for

related to:
1. Debilitated condition, lowered resistance to infection
2. Anemia secondary to bone marrow depression as a result of decreased or absent production of erythropoietin by failing kidneys

as seen by:
Elevated temperature; increased pulse rate; adventitious breath sounds; cloudy or foul-smelling urine

Injury, Potential for: Increased Risk of Falls and Injuries

related to:
1. Paresthesias associated with peripheral neuropathies (secondary to anemia and fluid and electrolyte imbalances)
2. Pathologic fractures associated with renal osteodystrophy
3. Impairment in thought processes secondary to increased serum levels of nitrogenous wastes
4. Cerebral hypoxia secondary to decreased tissue oxygenation

as seen by:
Weakness and fatigue; pain; burning; decreased sensation in legs and feet; pain in spine; decreased endurance; shortened memory; confusion; poor judgment

Knowledge Deficit (Specify)

related to:
1. Prescribed plan of treatment in management of renal condition and shunt care
2. Potential complications, S&S to report to home health nurse or physician

as seen by:
Verbalization of lack of information, inadequate understanding; inability to perform skills necessary to meet health-care needs at home

Mobility, Impaired Physical

related to:
1. Activity intolerance
2. Motor and sensory deficits
3. Prescribed activity restrictions

as seen by:
Weakness and fatigue; pain; burning and decreased sensation in legs and feet; muscle and joint pain; imposed medical restrictions

Nutrition, Alteration in: Less than Body Requirements

related to:
Decreased oral intake secondary to:
1. Anorexia
2. Nausea and vomiting
3. Fatigue
4. Stomatitis
5. Prescribed dietary restrictions

as seen by:
Body weight 20 percent ore more under ideal weight for height, frame, and age; triceps skin-fold measurement less than normal for build; weakness (inability to prepare food on diet); mouth discomfort; lack of interest in foods prescribed

Oral Mucous Membrane, Alteration in

related to:
1. Dry mouth secondary to restricted fluids
2. Stomatitis associated with decomposing urea

as seen by:
Oral pain; discomfort; inflammation or ulceration of oral mucous membrane; leukoplakia

Powerlessness, Feelings of

related to:
Chronic renal failure, hemodialysis

as seen by:
Verbalization of no control over situation; c/o inability to perform previous tasks, activities; depression over condition; dependency on others

Self-Care Deficit: Feeding, Bathing/Hygiene, Dressing/Grooming, Toileting (Specify)

related to:
1. Activity intolerance
2. Impaired mobility
3. Prescribed activity restrictions

as seen by
Decreased participation in personal care and ADL associated with weakness and fatigue; motor and sensory deficits and altered musculoskeletal functioning; imposed medical restrictions

Self-Concept, Disturbance in

related to:
1. Altered body image, effect on relationships and quality of life
2. Lowered self-esteem

as seen by:
Depression; increased dependency on others to meet physical needs; withdrawal; self-destructive behavior

Sexual Dysfunction

related to:
Altered body structure or function associated with chronic renal failure, hemodialysis

as seen by:
Verbalization of alteration in relationship with spouse or significant other; limitation imposed by disease process; expressed concern about problem

Skin Integrity, Impairment of: Actual/Potential

related to:
1. Scratching, secondary to pruritus
2. Decreased mobility
3. Inadequate nutritional status
4. Edema
5. Tissue hypoxia secondary to anemia
6. Vascular access site, hemodialysis

as seen by:
Dry, scaly skin; redness; warmth; irritation; pitting edema; tissue breakdown; drainage; pain

Social Isolation

related to:
1. Altered body image
2. Changes in life-style and role function

as seen by:
Withdrawn behavior; verbalized feelings of aloneness and rejection; expressed anger; hostility caused by

3. Decreased mobility   not being able to tolerate activities and/or having previous functional skills necessary for independence

LONG-TERM GOAL

To maintain an optimal physiologic state with an improved quality of life through measures to correct and maintain fluid and electrolyte and acid–base balances in the body.

SHORT-TERM GOALS

The client with end-stage renal disease and on hemodialysis will be able to:

1. Verbalize nature and progression of disease process, stage of CRF, predisposing factors, S&S of complications to report to home health nurse or physician.
2. Demonstrate how to accurately take pulse rate and blood pressure and record/identify alterations outside parameters set by physician.
3. Demonstrate compliance with prescribed diet and dietary restrictions.
4. Identify predisposing factors to decreased oral intake, measures to improve nutritional status.
5. Demonstrate compliance with prescribed vitamin and mineral supplements.
6. Demonstrate compliance with prescribed medication therapy/identify side effects.
7. Demonstrate compliance with daily fluid requirements.
8. Verbalize importance of reporting to physician daily weight gain of more than one pound a day or a continued weight loss.
9. Demonstrate how to measure and record daily intake and output.
10. Verbalize increased susceptibility to infection, measures to reduce risk of exposure.
11. Demonstrate good oral hygiene with stomatitis.
12. Demonstrate progressive activities within physiologic limits, balanced rest and exercise periods, avoiding fatigue.
13. Identify contributing factors to constipation, measures to avoid, prescribed treatment measures.
14. Identify contributing factors to diarrhea, measures to avoid, prescribed treatment measures.
15. Identify S&S of impaired skin integrity, contributing factors, prescribed treatment regimen, S&S of complications to report to home health nurse or physician.
16. Verbalize complications of prolonged immobility, S&S to report to home health nurse or physician, prescribed measures to treat, activities to avoid.
17. Verbalize increased risks for falls and injuries/identify self-protection mea-

sures, environmental hazards in the home to avoid with ambulatory and daily activities.

18. Identify S&S of bleeding, cause, measures to reduce risk.
19. Verbalize purpose of hemodialysis and access site/demonstrate how to check blood flow/verbalize physical restrictions to avoid.
20. Demonstrate prescribed measures to protect and care for access site.
21. Identify complications, emergency situations with access site, actions to take.
22. Demonstrate compliance with prescribed anticoagulant therapy, safety factors with use, adverse reactions to report to physician.
23. Verbalize purpose of prescribed blood studies for coagulation times and other diagnostic lab work.
24. Verbalize importance of wearing Medic Alert bracelet.
25. Demonstrate effective coping mechanism for altered body image and changes in life-style with positive adaptation to chronic progression of disease process.
26. Demonstrate compliance with specific energy-conservation techniques and exercise and activity program.
27. Identify measures to avoid and treat pathologic fractures.
28. Demonstrate compliance with keeping emergency phone numbers by phone.

NURSING INTERVENTIONS AND TREATMENTS

1. Assess systems of the body for S&S of renal and urologic dysfunction/identify complications.
2. Assess vital signs/identify trends (e.g., rapid pulse rate, irregular pulse, hypertension, elevated temperature)/instruct how to take pulse rate and BP, record, report alterations outside parameters set by physician.
3. Instruct as to nature and progression of disease process, present stage of CRF, importance of strict compliance with prescribed treatment regimen, S&S of major changes in body systems to report to physician.
4. Assess and evaluate nutritional status/instruct about prescribed diet (e.g., low-protein, high-calorie diet with sodium, potassium, phosphorus restrictions)/obtain dietary consultation as needed.
5. Assess and evaluate predisposing factors to decreased oral intake/instruct about prescribed measures to improve nutritional status (e.g., small, frequent meals, good oral hygiene).
6. Observe/instruct about importance of taking prescribed vitamin and mineral supplements.
7. Observe/instruct about taking medications as ordered, purpose and action, side effects, dangers of toxic serum levels in the uremic client when taking any medication not prescribed.
8. Assess and evaluate hydration status/instruct about daily fluid restrictions or to increase fluids as prescribed.
9. Assess/instruct to weigh and record at the same time every day, on same scale

with same clothing/report daily weight gain of more than one pound a day or continued weight loss to physician.

10. Observe/instruct how to measure and record daily intake and output as ordered.

11. Assess/instruct about increased susceptibility to infections, measures to reduce risk of exposure, S&S to report to home health nurse or physician.

12. Assess and evaluate stomatitis/instruct as to cause, good oral hygiene, avoiding spicy foods, ingesting maximal fluids as allowed.

13. Observe and evaluate for activity intolerance, skeletal disorders, motor and sensory deficits/instruct to perform progressive activities within physiologic limits as ordered, balanced with rest periods, avoid fatigue.

14. Assess problems with constipation/instruct about contributing factors, measures to treat (e.g., increase in activities, in dietary fiber/use of prescribed medications based on metabolic condition)/evaluate effectiveness of bowel regimen.

15. Assess and evaluate problems with diarrhea/instruct about contributing factors, measures to treat (e.g., use of prescribed medications depending on metabolic status), prescribed measures to decrease accumulation of nitrogenous wastes (e.g., decreased intake of proteins, treatment of underlying disease, avoiding gas-producing and spicy foods, caffeine).

16. Assess/instruct about S&S of impaired skin integrity, contributing factors/instruct about good skin care measures, prescribed medications, S&S of irritation and breakdown to report to home health nurse or physician.

17. Assess and evaluate systems of the body for complications related to prolonged immobility/instruct about S&S to report to home health nurse or physician, prescribed measures to treat, activities to avoid.

18. Assess/instruct about increased risk of falls and injuries/instruct about self-protection measures (e.g., use of ambulatory assistive devices, nonskid soles on shoes, avoiding temperature extremes on areas with decreased sensation, avoiding environmental hazards in home with ambulation and daily activities).

19. Assess/instruct as to S&S of bleeding, cause of increased susceptibility (because o. platelet deficiencies), measures to reduce risks (e.g., reducing risks of falls and injuries in home, using soft toothbrush, shaving only with electric razor, avoiding straining, avoiding use of aspirin and aspirin-containing products), use of pressure to control any bleeding, reporting to physician.

20. Assess/instruct as to purpose of hemodialysis, access site (e.g., atriovenous shunt, atriovenous graft, or atriovenous fistula), how to check blood flow (e.g., palpating for thrills and auscultating for bruits), physical restrictions (e.g., avoiding pressure or constriction, bending/blood drawing from access site).

21. Observe/instruct about prescribed measures to protect and care for vascular access site (e.g., cleaning, bandaging, avoiding showering or bathing for several hours after dialysis, prescribed exercises for affected arm to promote venous dilation and blood flow), S&S of infection to report to physician.

22. Assess/instruct about S&S of complications of arteriovenous shunt, arteriovenous fistula, arteriovenous graft (e.g., bleeding, clotting, hematoma,

infection)/instruct about emergency situations (e.g., separation of shunt at connection site, dislodging of shunt tubing from exit site, actions to take, report to physician).

23. Observe/instruct about prescribed anticoagulant therapy, safety factors with use, adverse reactions to report to physician.
24. Monitor/instruct about purpose of prescribed blood studies for coagulation times and other diagnostic lab work.
25. Observe/instruct about importance of wearing Medic Alert bracelet with information on medical condition, hemodialysis.
26. Refer to rehabilitative services as ordered to instruct in specific energy conservation techniques, exercise, activity program, measures to avoid and treat pathologic fractures.
27. Assess ability to cope with chronic renal failure/provide emotional support/encourage to express feelings/refer to social services as ordered to assist with grieving process, assist to set realistic goals for life, to provide counseling and information regarding community support groups (e.g., National Kidney Foundation; National Association of Patients on Hemodialysis and Transplantation, Inc.)
28. Observe/instruct to keep emergency phone numbers by phone, including the dialysis center.

REHABILITATION POTENTIAL

Rehabilitation potential   *excellent   good   fair   guarded   poor*   for   *full partial*   achievement of an improved physiologic state and well-being, able to manage personal and daily activities.

■ Incontinence and Retention/Care of the Client with an Indwelling Urethral Catheter

Insertion of an indwelling catheter (also known as a Foley or retention catheter) into the bladder through the urethra for continuous urinary drainage may be indicated for a variety of reasons (e.g., unable to void; after certain genitourinary operations; neurogenic bladder secondary to trauma or spinal cord lesion). Instructions to the client and caregiver to ensure that a properly functioning urinary drainage system will be established and maintained without the development of complications is the primary objective of this home health-nursing care plan.

POTENTIAL COMPLICATIONS

1. Urinary tract infection,
2. urinary retention secondary to obstruction of drainage tube (e.g., sediment buildup and calculi deposits; inadvertent removal of catheter; reflux of urine associated with drainage bag above bladder level),
3. injury to urethral lumen or bladder wall secondary to undue tension on catheter,
4. skin irritation and breakdown associated with tape or antiseptic cleansing solution.

TYPES OF CLIENTS/CLINICAL CONDITIONS SEEN BY HOME HEALTH AGENCIES

1. Insertion of Foley catheter: no prior knowledge or training in care of catheter, tubing, drainage bag, irrigations.
2. Catheter maintenance: changing every four weeks or more often as ordered, PRN for emergency care.

RELATED NURSING DIAGNOSIS

Anxiety

related to:
1. Loss of urinary control
2. Catheter insertion and maintenance
3. Knowledge deficit regarding prescribed treatment regimen for management of urethral catheter

as seen by:
Feelings of helplessness; fearfulness of inadequacy; uncertainty about ability to understand and perform skills needed to manage urinary catheter

Comfort, Alteration in: Pain

related to:
1. Tissue trauma associated with use of catheter with larger diameter size than urinary meatus
2. Tenderness and swelling of tissue around urinary meatus
3. Bladder spasms associated with obstruction to urinary outflow
4. Frank pain or tenderness over bladder secondary to urinary infection

as seen by:
Verbal c/o pain or discomfort; crying or moaning; changes in pulse and BP; restlessness and increased anxiety

Infection, Potential for

related to:
1. Introduction of bacteria into bladder during catheter insertion
2. Migration of bacteria into bladder with poor catheter care or improper catheter irrigations
3. Inadequate nutritional status or fluid intake

as seen by:
Cloudy urine; increased sediment; elevated temperature; bladder pain and discomfort; hematuria; fever and chills; foul-smelling urine.

Knowledge Deficit (Specify)

related to:
1. Prescribed plan of treatment in management of indwelling urethral catheter
2. Potential complications, S&S to report to home health nurse or physician

as seen by:
Verbalization of lack of information; inadequate understanding or inability to perform skills necessary to meet health-care needs at home

Self-Concept, Disturbance in

related to:
Loss of self-esteem secondary to loss in usual method of urinary elimination

as seen by:
Withdrawn behavior; refusal to participate in own care; fear of rejection; verbalized displeasure at altered body functioning

Skin Integrity, Impairment of: Potential

related to:
1. Repeated or improper removal of taped area of catheter to skin

as seen by:
Irritation and hypersensitivity of skin; tissue breakdown; tenderness and

2. Inadequate catheter care   swelling of tissue around urinary
                                               meatus

Urinary Elimination Pattern, Alteration in: Retention

related to: **as seen by:**
Obstruction of drainage tube secondary   Bladder distension; sensation of
to: bladder fullness; no urinary output
1. Urinary sediment and calculi
   deposits or kinks and twists in
   tubing
2. Inadvertent removal of catheter
3. Reflux of urine associated with
   drainage bag above bladder level

LONG-TERM GOAL

To maintain a continuous drainage of urine, free of complications, through use of an indwelling urethral catheter.

SHORT-TERM GOALS

The client with an indwelling urethral catheter will be able to:

1. Verbalize nature of renal or urologic disorder/indication for catheter, S&S of complications to report to home health nurse or physician.
2. Verbalize importance of prescribed diet, increased fluids as prescribed.
3. Demonstrate compliance with prescribed medication therapy/identify side effects.
4. Identify effect of various foods and medications on color of urine.
5. Verbalize procedure and purpose of urinary catheterization, frequency of change, size and type of catheter used, changes in color, amount, and consistency of the urine to report to home health nurse or physician.
6. Demonstrate prescribed management of urinary catheter, tubing, drainage collection bag/verbalize measures to maintain patency and avoid urinary retention.
7. Verbalize importance of good personal hygiene/demonstrate correct procedure in cleaning of perineal and rectal area.
8. Demonstrate correct procedure for urinary irrigations.
9. Demonstrate daily recording of output/report minimal or no urinary drainage to physician.
10. Demonstrate a positive adjustment to need for an indwelling urethral catheter.

NURSING ACTIONS/TREATMENTS

1. Assess urinary functioning, character of urine, patency of catheter and drainage system/identify complications.
2. Assess vital signs/identify trends (e.g., elevated temperature).
3. Instruct as to nature of renal or urologic disorder, indication for an indwelling urethral catheter, importance of compliance with prescribed treatment regimen, S&S of complications to report to home health nurse or physician.
4. Assess and evaluate nutritional status/instruct to eat well-balanced diet, increased fluids of 2000 to 3000 ml per day, acid–ash foods and fluids as prescribed.
5. Observe/instruct about taking medications as ordered, purpose and action, side effects/evaluate medication effectiveness.
6. Observe color of urine/instruct about the effect various foods and medications have on color of urine.
7. Instruct about procedure and purpose of urinary catheterization, frequency of change, size and type of catheter used, changes in color, amount, and consistency of urine to report to home health nurse or physician.
8. Observe and evaluate functioning of urinary catheter/instruct in care of catheter, tubing, drainage bag, use of leg bag, measures to maintain patency and avoid urinary retention (e.g., how to secure tubing and leg bag, drainage tube free of kinks and twists, keeping drainage bag below bladder level to avoid reflux of urine and chance of infection, emptying drainage bag at least every eight hours and leg bag when half full/changing drainage tube and bag monthly or PRN as needed, periurethral care and cleaning of catheter junction twice a day or more often as needed).
9. Assess/instruct as importance of good personal hygiene (e.g., good hand-washing technique before and after handling catheter and drainage system, cleaning of perineal and rectal area twice a day and after each bowel movement).
10. Assess and evaluate bladder spasms/instruct about prescribed urinary irrigations (solution, amount, frequency).
11. Observe/instruct to daily record output, report to physician minimal or no urinary drainage.
12. Assess level of anxiety/provide reassurance and positive reinforcement when instructing in catheter care and maintenance.

REHABILITATION POTENTIAL

Rehabilitation potential *excellent good fair guarded poor* for *full partial* return to a secure and satisfying life-style, able to manage urinary catheter and ADL.

Client's Name _____

Medical Record #_____

ONGOING/DISCHARGE EVALUATION OF TEACHING

The Client with an Indwelling Urethral Catheter

Teaching Tools:

Printed materials given: _____

Audiovisual aids used: _____

Return Information/Demonstration/Interpretation

_____ Client

_____ Caregiver

OF:	Met	Not Met	Comments
☐ Nature of renal or urologic disorder; indication for indwelling urethral catheter.	____	____	_____
☐ S&S of complications; actions to take.	____	____	_____
☐ Importance of compliance with prescribed treatment regimen.	____	____	_____
☐ Importance of well-balanced diet, increased fluids.	____	____	_____
☐ Prescribed acid–ash foods and fluids.	____	____	_____
☐ Medications and administration,			

Client's Name _____

Medical Record # _____

OF:	**Met**	**Not Met**	**Comments**
purpose and action, side effects.	_____	_____	_____
☐ Effect of various foods and medications on color of urine.	_____	_____	_____
☐ Procedure and purpose of urinary catheterization; frequency of change; size and type of catheter used.	_____	_____	_____
☐ Changes in color, amount, and consistency of urine to report to physician.	_____	_____	_____
☐ Care of urinary catheter, tubing, drainage bag.	_____	_____	_____
☐ Use of Leg Bag.	_____	_____	_____
☐ Periurethral care and cleaning of catheter junction twice a day or more often as needed. Measures to maintain patency and avoid urinary retention.	_____	_____	_____

Client's Name _____

Medical Record # _____

OF:	**Met**	**Not Met**	**Comments**
☐ Good hand-washing technique.	_____	_____	_____
☐ Cleaning of perineal and rectal area.	_____	_____	_____
☐ Urinary irrigations.	_____	_____	_____
☐ Recording of urinary output.	_____	_____	_____

Signature of Home Health Nurse _____

Date _____

Client's Name _____

Medical Record # _____

ONGOING/DISCHARGE EVALUATION OF TEACHING

The Client in End-Stage Renal Failure on Hemodialysis

Teaching Tools:

Printed materials given: _____

Audiovisual aids used: _____

Return Information/Demonstration/Interpretation

_____ Client

_____ Caregiver

	OF:	Met	Not Met	Comments
☐	Nature and progression of disease process; stage of CRF.	_____	_____	_____
☐	How to take pulse rate and blood pressure, record; reporting of alterations outside parameters set by physician.	_____	_____	_____
☐	S&S of complications of CRF, actions to take.	_____	_____	_____
☐	Importance of compliance with prescribed treatment regimen.	_____	_____	_____
☐	Diet and dietary restrictions.	_____	_____	_____

Client's Name _____

Medical Record #_____

OF:	Met	Not Met	Comments
☐ Predisposing factors in decreased oral intake, measures to improve nutritional status.	_____	_____	_____
☐ Vitamin and mineral supplements.	_____	_____	_____
☐ Daily fluid restrictions or increased fluids.	_____	_____	_____
☐ Medications and administration, purpose and action, side effects.	_____	_____	_____
☐ Daily recording of weight; reporting a daily weight gain of more than one pound a day or continued weight loss to physician.	_____	_____	_____
☐ Daily intake and output.	_____	_____	_____
☐ Increased susceptibility to infections; measures to reduce risk of exposure.	_____	_____	_____

Client's Name _____

Medical Record #_____

OF:	**Met**	**Not Met**	**Comments**
☐ Oral hygiene.	_____	_____	_____
☐ Progressive activities within physiologic limits, balanced rest periods.	_____	_____	_____
☐ Contributing factors in constipation, measures to treat.	_____	_____	_____
☐ Contributing factors in diarrhea, measures to treat.	_____	_____	_____
☐ S&S of impaired skin integrity, contributing factors, measures to treat.	_____	_____	_____
☐ Complications of prolonged immobility, treatment measures, activities to avoid.	_____	_____	_____
☐ Increased risk of falls and injuries; self-protection measures.	_____	_____	_____
☐ Environmental hazards in home			

Client's Name _____

Medical Record #_____

OF:	**Met**	**Not Met**	**Comments**
environment with ambulatory and daily activities to avoid.	_____	_____	_____
☐ Increased risk of bleeding, measures to reduce and control any bleeding.	_____	_____	_____
☐ Purpose of hemodialysis.	_____	_____	_____
☐ Access site and how to check blood flow.	_____	_____	_____
☐ Access site and physical restrictions.	_____	_____	_____
☐ Complications, emergency situations with access site, actions to take.	_____	_____	_____
☐ Measures to protect and care for access site.	_____	_____	_____
☐ Emergency situations with shunt, actions to take.	_____	_____	_____
☐ Anticoagulant therapy.	_____	_____	_____

Client's Name _____

Medical Record # _____

OF:	Met	Not Met	Comments
☐ Prescribed blood studies for coagulation time and other diagnostic lab work.	_____	_____	_____
☐ Energy-conservation techniques.	_____	_____	_____
☐ Exercise and activity program.	_____	_____	_____
☐ Measures to avoid and treat pathologic fractures.	_____	_____	_____
☐ Medic Alert bracelet.	_____	_____	_____
☐ Emergency numbers listed by phone.	_____	_____	_____

Signature of Home Health Nurse _____

Date _____

■ Lower Urinary Tract Infection

Lower urinary tract infections (UTIs) are associated with infections of the bladder and the urethra. The condition is more commonly found in women than men, possibly as a result of the shortness of the urethra and greater chance of infection from the bacteria found in the vagina and rectum. Most of these UTIs generally result from an ascending infection caused by a single gram-negative bacteria, most commonly *Escherichia coli*. UTIs are frequently found in clients with a neurogenic bladder or a Foley catheter. In these situations, bacteria enter the bladder mucosa and multiply, resulting in an infection that occurs following a local breakdown in the bladder's defense mechanisms. Clinical manifestations associated with UTIs are urinary frequency, urgency, burning, and dysuria, spasms of the bladder, elevated temperature, and chills.

POTENTIAL COMPLICATIONS

1. Hematuria,
2. pyuria,
3. dysuria,
4. pyelonephritis.

TYPES OF CLIENTS/CLINICAL CONDITIONS SEEN BY HOME HEALTH AGENCIES

1. Newly diagnosed with lower urinary tract infection: prescribed treatment with antimicrobial therapy, urinary analgesics, or urinary antiseptics.
2. Exacerbation of lower urinary tract infection: continuance or change in medication therapy.

RELATED NURSING DIAGNOSIS

Anxiety

related to:
1. Dysuria
2. Urgency and frequency
3. Recurrence of urinary tract infections, new medication therapy

as seen by:
Expressed concern over recurrence of urinary tract infections and effectiveness of prescribed medications; distress associated with symptoms of urinary infection and effectiveness of prescribed medications

Comfort, Alteration in: Pain

related to:
Urinary tract infection

as seen by:
Dysuria; bladder spasms; low back pain; elevated temperature; chills; malaise; tenderness over the bladder area; flank pain

Knowledge Deficit (Specify)

related to:
1. Prescribed plan of treatment
2. Potential complications, S&S to report to home health nurse or physician

as seen by:
Verbalization of lack of information; inadequate understanding of prescribed therapy for treatment of urinary tract infection

Nutrition, Alteration in: Less than Body Requirements

related to:
Anorexia, secondary to nausea and bladder spasms

as seen by:
Repeated inadequate dietary and fluid intake: weight loss

Urinary Elimination Pattern Alteration in: Obstruction

related to:
Urinary tract infection

as seen by:
Dysuria; frequency; nocturia; hematuria

LONG-TERM GOAL

To maintain fluid and electrolyte balance and normal pattern of urinary elimination through resolution of the inflammatory process within the urinary tract.

SHORT-TERM GOALS

The client with a lower urinary tract infection will be able to:

1. Verbalize nature of disease process, predisposing factors, S&S of recurrence to report to home health nurse or physician.
2. Verbalize importance of prescribed diet, increased fluids to 2000 to 3000 ml per day, food and fluids to avoid.
3. Demonstrate compliance with prescribed medication therapy.
4. Verbalize importance of activities as tolerated, with planned rest periods.

5. Demonstrate measures to relieve perineal discomfort.
6. Verbalize measures to avoid urinary tract infections.

NURSING ACTIONS/TREATMENTS

1. Assess systems of the body for S&S of renal or urologic dysfunction as well as alterations in character of urine or urinary patterns/identify complications.
2. Assess vital signs/identify trends (e.g., elevated temperature).
3. Instruct as to nature of disease process, predisposing factors/instruct as to importance of compliance with prescribed treatment regimen, S&S to report to home health nurse or physician.
4. Assess and evaluate nutritional status/instruct about well-balanced diet, prescribed increased fluids 2000 to 3000 ml per day, prescribed acid–ash foods and fluids (e.g., cranberry juice, prune juice, grapes, whole grains, meat, eggs, poultry, fish), avoiding caffeine beverages, alcohol, pepper.
5. Observe/instruct about taking medications as ordered (antimicrobial therapy, urinary analgesics, or urinary antiseptics), purpose and action, side effects/evaluate medication effectiveness.
6. Assess/instruct about daily activities as tolerated, with planned rest periods.
7. Assess/instruct about specific measures to relieve perineal discomfort (e.g., sitz baths, warmth to lower abdomen)/evaluate effectiveness of measures to relieve discomfort.
8. Assess/instruct about measures to avoid urinary tract infections (e.g., completely empty bladder every 4 to 6 hours, practice good personal hygiene, increase fluids).

REHABILITATION POTENTIAL

Rehabilitation potential   *excellent   good   fair   guarded   poor*   for   *full partial*   return to a level of wellness to manage daily activities as prior to urinary tract infection.

Client's Name _____

Medical Record # _____

ONGOING/DISCHARGE EVALUATION OF TEACHING

The Client with a Lower Urinary Tract Infection

Teaching Tools:

Printed materials given: _____

Audiovisual aids used: _____

Return Information/Demonstration/Interpretation

_____ Client

_____ Caregiver

OF:	Met	Not Met	Comments
☐ Nature of disease process, predisposing factors.	_____	_____	_____
☐ S&S of complications, actions to take.	_____	_____	_____
☐ Importance of compliance with prescribed treatment regimen.	_____	_____	_____
☐ Well-balanced diet, increased fluids, and foods to avoid.	_____	_____	_____
☐ Prescribed acid–ash foods and fluids.	_____	_____	_____
☐ Medications and administration, purpose and action, side effects.	_____	_____	_____

Client's Name _____

Medical Record #_____

OF:	Met	Not Met	Comments
☐ Activities as tolerated, planned rest periods.	_____	_____	_____
☐ Measures to relieve perineal discomfort.	_____	_____	_____
☐ Measures to avoid urinary tract infections.	_____	_____	_____

Signature of Home Health Nurse _____

Date _____

■ Urinary Diversion/Ileal Conduit

Urinary diversion is a surgical procedure that provides an alternative avenue for the excretion of urine when the bladder is no longer functional or has been removed. Permanent urinary diversion surgery may be done for a number of reasons, some of which are: malignancies of the bladder or ureters; chronic urinary infections; neurogenic bladder; ureteral or urethral stricture; trauma; or prostatic carcinoma. A temporary urinary diversion may be done in cases of urinary obstruction secondary to ureteral edema or calculi. Some of the more common types of urinary diversions are the ileal conduit, ileal conduit reservoir, cutaneous ureterostomy, nephrostomy, and cystostomy.

The ileal conduit, or ileal loop, is a surgically created opening in which a segment of ileum is excised and one end brought through the lower abdominal wall to form a stoma. The other end is closed and the two ureters are stitched into a created pouch. Since there is urinary output from the time the stoma is created, the client must always wear a collecting appliance. Home care of the client with an ileal conduit is the primary focus of this care plan.

POTENTIAL COMPLICATIONS

1. Ureteral obstruction,
2. urinary or wound infection,
3. skin irritation or breakdown,
4. hematuria,
5. ileal stoma prolapse, edema, or stenosis,
6. unusual pain.

TYPES OF CLIENTS/CLINICAL CONDITIONS SEEN BY HOME HEALTH AGENCIES

1. Newly created ileal conduit: initiation of prescribed treatment regimen and inclusive treatment plan in management of ostomy.
2. Complications associated with physical condition and with ileal conduit requiring changes in prescribed treatment regimen: home health nurse needed for skilled observations, instruction, and supervision of new medications and treatments, evaluation of response to changes in therapy.
3. Recent hospitalization for exacerbation of physical condition and complications related to ileal conduit.

RELATED NURSING DIAGNOSIS

Activity Intolerance

related to:
1. Incisional pain and discomfort

as seen by:
Exertional dyspnea; weakness and

2. Anxiety
3. Inadequate nutritional status

fatigue; abnormal heart rate, respiratory rate, and BP in response to activity

Anxiety

related to:
1. Altered body image
2. Effect on life-style and relationships
3. Increased dependency on others
4. Knowledge deficit regarding treatment regimen

as seen by:
Verbalization of feelings of inadequacy and lack of understanding in management of ostomy; increased helplessness; expressed concern and uncertainty about future acceptance by significant others

Breathing Pattern, Ineffective

related to:
1. Incisional pain
2. Anxiety

as seen by:
Altered depth of respirations; reluctance to attempt movement; shortness of breath

Comfort, Alteration in: Pain

related to:
1. Surgical incision
2. Irritation or breakdown of peristomal skin

as seen by:
Guarding of incisional area; moaning with movement; verbalization of pain or burning discomfort; reluctance to move

Coping, Ineffective Individual

related to:
1. Loss in usual method of urinary elimination
2. Management of ostomy

as seen by:
Depression; anxiety; verbalization of inability to cope; anger and hostility; withdrawal and isolation; inability to care for self

Grieving

related to:
1. Change in body image
2. Effects on life-style

as seen by:
Depression; anger; denial; crying; changes in eating habits; noncompliance with teaching

Infection, Potential for

related to:
Impaired healing of incisional area

as seen by:
Increased redness and warmth; swelling; pain; tissue breakdown; unusual drainage; elevated temperature; elevated WBC count

Knowledge Deficit (Specify)

related to:
1. Prescribed plan of treatment after urinary diversion
2. Potential complications, S&S to report to home health nurse or physician

as seen by:
Verbalization of lack of information; inadequate understanding; inability to perform skills necessary to meet health-care needs at home

Self-Care Deficit: Feeding, Bathing/Hygiene, Dressing/Grooming, Toileting (Specify)

related to:
1. Activity intolerance
2. Ineffective coping and depression
3. Prescribed activity restrictions

as seen by:
Impaired ability to perform self-care activities in response to pain; weakness and fatigue; lack of interest in taking care of self; imposed medical restrictions

Self-Concept, Disturbance in

related to:
Effect of altered body image on lifestyle and relationships

as seen by:
Increasing dependence on others for care; signs of grieving; lack of follow-through on teaching; not wanting to care for ostomy

Sexual Dysfunction

related to:
Alteration in body image and self-concept

as seen by:
Withdrawn behavior; alteration in relationship with spouse or significant other; verbalization of the problem

Skin Integrity, Impairment of: Actual/Potential

related to:
1. Surgical incision
2. Impaired healing secondary to infection
3. Improper fit of appliance, with continual contact of skin with urine
4. Improper or repeated removal of adhesives
5. Sensitivity to skin-care products

as seen by:
Increased redness, warmth; swelling; unusual drainage; irritation and breakdown; pronounced tenderness or pain

Social Isolation

related to:
Altered body image

as seen by:
Isolation, verbalized feelings of embarrassment and rejection; seeking to be alone

LONG-TERM GOAL

To restore and maintain optimal urinary functioning and achieve a positive adaptation to an altered body image.

SHORT-TERM GOALS

The client with a urinary diversion/ileal conduit will be able to:

1. Verbalize indication for urinary diversion, type of ostomy, S&S of complications to report to home health nurse or physician.
2. Verbalize importance of well-balanced diet, maximal daily fluids/identify food and substances affecting urinary output.
3. Identify measures to control urine odor.
4. Demonstrate compliance with prescribed medication therapy/identify side effects.
5. Verbalize purpose of remeasuring stoma periodically for readjustment in pouch size.
6. Demonstrate prescribed stoma and skin care, use of skin barriers, appliances, accessories, cleaning and care of equipment.
7. Verbalize unusual changes in stoma to report to physician.
8. Verbalize prescribed care of peristomal skin, measures to avoid irritation and breakdown.

9. Demonstrate prescribed wound care management.
10. Demonstrate compliance with progressive activities, balanced rest periods, prescribed restrictions.
11. Demonstrate effective strategies in coping with alteration in body image.

NURSING ACTIONS/TREATMENTS

1. Assess systems of the body for S&S of renal and urologic dysfunction/identify complications.
2. Assess vital signs/identify trends (e.g., elevated temperature).
3. Instruct about indication for a urinary diversion, type of ostomy, importance of compliance with prescribed treatment regimen, S&S of complications to report to home health nurse or physician.
4. Assess and evaluate nutritional status/instruct about well-balanced diet, maximal daily fluid intake allowed, food and substances that affect output (e.g., diuretic effects of caffeine and alcohol).
5. Assess/instruct about prescribed measures to control urine odor (e.g., drink cranberry juice, use deodorizing tablets, avoid foods with strong odor).
6. Observe/instruct about taking medications as ordered, purpose and action, side effects/evaluate medication effectiveness.
7. Assess/instruct about remeasuring stoma for the first 2 to 4 months postsurgery for changes in stomal size and need for readjustment in pouch size.
8. Observe/instruct about prescribed stoma and skin care, proper application of skin barriers, use of appliances and accessories, cleaning and care of equipment.
9. Observe/instruct about unusual changes in stoma (e.g., color changes, increased edema, bleeding)/report to physician.
10. Observe/instruct about inspecting peristomal skin, measures to avoid irritation and breakdown, prescribed measures to treat.
11. Assess and evaluate healing of incisional area/instruct about prescribed wound care management, S&S of infection to report to home health nurse or physician.
12. Observe and evaluate level of tolerance to manage ADL/instruct about progressive activities balanced with rest periods, prescribed restrictions (e.g., avoiding heavy lifting 4 to 6 weeks postsurgery).
13. Refer to enterostomal therapist as ordered for assistance and instruction in ostomy care.
14. Assess grieving over loss in usual method of urinary elimination/provide emotional support and encourage to verbalize feelings/refer to social services to provide counseling in assisting with adaptation to condition, information regarding community resources (e.g., American Cancer Society, support groups, transportation assistance, Meals on Wheels).

REHABILITATION POTENTIAL

Rehabilitation potential *excellent   good   fair   guarded   poor* for *full partial* return to an independent level of functioning and sense of well-being, able to manage the physical aspects of stomal care and psychological adjustment to alteration in body image.

Client's Name _____

Medical Record # _____

ONGOING/DISCHARGE EVALUATION OF TEACHING

The Client with a Urinary Diversion/Ileal Conduit

Teaching Tools:

Printed materials given: _____

Audiovisual aids used: _____

Return Information/Demonstration/Interpretation

_____ Client

_____ Caregiver

OF:	Met	Not Met	Comments
☐ Indication for urinary diversion; type of ostomy.	_____	_____	_____
☐ S&S of complications, actions to take.	_____	_____	_____
☐ Importance of compliance with prescribed treatment regimen.	_____	_____	_____
☐ Well-balanced diet, maximal daily fluids.	_____	_____	_____
☐ Food and substances affecting urinary output.	_____	_____	_____
☐ Medications and administration, purpose and action, side effects.	_____	_____	_____

Client's Name _____

Medical Record #_____

	OF:	Met	Not Met	Comments
☐	Unusual stomal changes to report to physician.	_____	_____	_____
☐	Measures to control urine odor.	_____	_____	_____
☐	Stomal and peristomal skin care.	_____	_____	_____
☐	Application of skin barriers, use of appliances and accessories, cleaning and care of equipment.	_____	_____	_____
☐	Periodic remeasuring of stoma, readjustment in pouch size.	_____	_____	_____
☐	Wound care management.	_____	_____	_____
☐	Progressive activities with planned rest periods, prescribed activity restrictions.	_____	_____	_____

Signature of Home Health Nurse _____

Date _____

DISORDERS OF THE REPRODUCTIVE SYSTEM

■ Anterior and Posterior Colporrhaphy/Vaginal Hysterectomy

Downward displacement of the uterus with subsequent relaxation of the pelvic musculature and ligaments may result in herniation of the bladder (cystocele) and rectum (rectocele) into the vagina. The relaxation of the muscles of the pelvic floor is most often attributed to injuries sustained during childbirth. However, relaxation may also be caused by a congenital weakness or occur as a result of aging.

Colporrhaphy is the term given to the surgical repair of the vaginal walls and ligaments of the pelvic floor. An anterior colporrhaphy is the term for repair of a cystocele and posterior colporrhaphy for repair of a rectocele. Uterine prolapse with severe downward displacement may also occur in conjunction with a cystocle and rectocele. Surgery is indicated when conservative measures (e.g., use of a pessary or perineal exercises) have been ineffective in controlling urinary symptoms of urgency, frequency, and incontinence, bowel problems of constipation or fecal incontinence, or pelvic pressure and pain.

Uterine prolapse with severe downward displacement may be treated surgically, either by suturing the uterus back in place or by removal through the vagina (vaginal hysterectomy). This procedure may be the treatment of choice if the client is postmenopausal. The fallopian tubes and the ovaries may also be removed during this surgery, depending on the age and condition of the client.

POTENTIAL COMPLICATIONS

1. Wound infection,
2. vaginal hemorrhage,
3. thrombophlebitis,
4. reherniation of bladder or rectum.

TYPES OF CLIENTS/CLINICAL CONDITIONS SEEN BY HOME HEALTH AGENCIES

1. Postsurgical observations: initiation of prescribed treatment and teaching plan.
2. Development of complications associated with surgery: instruction about changes in prescribed treatment regimen, evaluation of responses to therapy (e.g., antibiotic therapy).

RELATED NURSING DIAGNOSIS

Anxiety

related to:
1. Alteration in body image

as seen by:
Regretfulness; insomnia, uncertainty

2. Effect of surgery on femininity and sexuality
3. Knowledge deficit regarding prescribed treatment regimen

about relationships and sexuality; asking nummerous questions after surgery

Bowel Elimination, Alteration in: Constipation

related to:
1. Decreased activities
2. Inadequate fluids and dietary fiber

as seen by:
Straining at stool; decrease in frequency and amount from usual pattern

Comfort, Alteration in: Pain/Discomfort

related to:
Pelvic edema following surgical procedure

as seen by:
Verbal c/o pelvic pressure and low back pain

Grieving

related to:
1. Depression associated with loss of body part and function
2. Implications of loss of femininity
3. Threat to sexuality

as seen by:
Depression; sadness; anger; alteration in eating habits and activity levels

Infection, Potential for

related to:
Surgical incision, breakdown in the body's first line of defense

as seen by:
Excessive, unusual or odorous vaginal discharge; c/o increased pelvic pressure; elevated temperature

Knowledge Deficit (Specify)

related to:
1. Prescribed plan of treatment
2. Potential complications, S&S to report to home health nurse or physician

as seen by:
Verbalization of lack of information, inadequate understanding of prescribed home-care treatment regimen after surgery

Mobility, Impaired Physical

related to:
1. Pain and discomfort

as seen by:
Weakness and fatigue; decreased

2. Prescribed activity restrictions

strength and endurance; imposed medical restrictions

Self-Concept, Disturbance in

related to:
Altered body image

as seen by:
Signs of grieving; withdrawn behavior; verbal response to changes in body structure and function

Sexual Dysfunction

related to:
Altered body image

as seen by:
Verbalization of problem; change of interest in self and spouse or significant other; expressed concern about effect of hysterectomy on sexual performance

LONG-TERM GOAL

To attain maximal comfort and emotional well-being following vaginal hysterectomy.

SHORT-TERM GOALS

The client who has had an anterior and posterior colporrhaphy and vaginal hysterectomy will be able to:

1. Verbalize indication for surgical procedure, S&S of complications to report to home health nurse or physician.
2. Verbalize importance of well-balanced diet, adequate hydration.
3. Demonstrate compliance with prescribed medication therapy/identify side effects.
4. Verbalize importance of reporting excessive or unusual, odorous vaginal discharge to physician.
5. Verbalize purpose/Demonstrate compliance with prescribed activity restrictions, report heavy bleeding and cramping to physician.
6. Verbalize importance of not straining at stool, prescribed measures to avoid constipation.
7. Verbalize importance of not douching or having sexual relations for six weeks or as prescribed.
8. Verbalize importance of good personal hygiene, avoiding tub baths for six weeks or as prescribed.

9. Verbalize importance of Kegel exercises.
10. Demonstrate effective coping mechanisms, positive adjustment to hysterectomy.

NURSING ACTIONS/TREATMENTS

1. Assess cardiovascular status, alterations in urologic functioning/identify complications.
2. Assess vital signs/identify trends (e.g., elevated temperature).
3. Instruct about indication for surgical procedure, importance of compliance with prescribed postsurgical treatment regimen, S&S of complications to report to home health nurse or physician.
4. Assess and evaluate nutritional status/instruct about well-balanced diet, adequate hydration.
5. Observe/instruct about taking medications as ordered, purpose and action, side effects/evaluate medication effectiveness.
6. Assess and evaluate vaginal discharge/instruct to report excessive or unusually odorous vaginal discharge.
7. Observe/instruct about prescribed activity restrictions to lessen pressure in suture line and chance of reherniation of bladder and rectum (e.g., avoiding prolonged sitting, heavy lifting, strenous exercise, bladder distension, voiding at least every 3 hours)/report heavy bleeding and cramping to physician.
8. Assess bowel elimination pattern/instruct about increased dietary fiber and fluids and activities as prescribed, use of stool softeners and laxatives as ordered, avoiding straining/evaluate effectiveness of bowel regimen.
9. Instruct to avoid sexual relations or douching for six weeks or as prescribed.
10. Assess/instruct about importance of cleanliness, perineal hygiene, avoiding tub baths for six weeks or as prescribed.
11. Assess/instruct about prescribed perineum-tightening exercises (Kegel exercises) to improve vaginal tone.
12. Assess psychological and emotional status, sexual dysfunction related to alteration in self-concept/provide emotional support/encourage to verbalize feelings/refer to social services as ordered to provide counseling to assist with adjustment to hysterectomy.

REHABILITATION POTENTIAL

Rehabilitation potential *excellent   good   fair   guarded   poor* for *full partial* return to an independent level of functioning to effectively manage daily activities.

Client's Name _____

Medical Record # _____

ONGOING/DISCHARGE EVALUATION OF TEACHING

The Client who Has Had an Anterior and Posterior Colporrhaphy/Vaginal Hysterectomy

Teaching Tools:
Printed materials given: _____

Audiovisual aids used: _____

Return Information/Demonstration/Interpretation
_____ Client
_____ Caregiver

OF:	Met	Not Met	Comments
☐ Indication for surgical intervention.	_____	_____	_____
☐ S&S of complications/ actions to take.	_____	_____	_____
☐ Importance of compliance with prescribed treatment regimen.	_____	_____	_____
☐ Importance of well-balanced diet, adequate hydration.	_____	_____	_____
☐ Medications and administration, purpose and action, side effects.	_____	_____	_____
☐ Changes in vaginal			

Client's Name _____

Medical Record # _____

OF:	**Met**	**Not Met**	**Comments**
discharge to report to physician.	_____	_____	_____
☐ Activity restrictions.	_____	_____	_____
☐ Measures to avoid constipation.	_____	_____	_____
☐ Importance of no sexual relations or douching for six weeks or as prescribed.	_____	_____	_____
☐ Importance of cleanliness and good personal hygiene, avoiding tub baths for six weeks or as prescribed.	_____	_____	_____
☐ Kegel exercises.	_____	_____	_____

Signature of Home Health Nurse _____

Date _____

■ Benign Prostatic Hypertrophy or Prostatic Cancer/Prostatectomy

A prostatectomy is the surgical removal of part or all of the prostate gland for the treatment of benign hypertrophy or prostatic carcinoma.

Benign prostatic hypertrophy (BPH) is a condition that is frequently seen in men after the age of 50. This condition is usually progressive and eventually the adenomatous growth partially obstructs the urethra, predisposing to alterations in urinary functioning (e.g., decreased force of urinary stream, difficulty starting stream, and nocturia). When conservative treatment for BPH is no longer effective, the adenomatous tissue is removed by one of four surgical approaches: the transurethral, transabdominal-retropubic, suprapubic or perineal. A transurethral resection is the surgery most frequently performed. A special surgical instrument is inserted into the urethra and the excess prostatic tissue that blocks urinary flow is removed. In a suprapubic prostatectomy, an incision is made in the lower abdomen and bladder neck for removal of the excess prostatic tissue. In a retropubic prostatectomy an incision is made in the lower abdomen, directly over the prostate, without entering the bladder. In the fourth type of prostatectomy surgery, the prostate gland is approached from behind and removed through an incision that is made above the rectum. Factors considered in the surgical approach are age of the client, health status, and diagnosis.

In prostatic carcinoma, the entire prostatic gland is removed, including the capsule and adjacent tissues and possibly the pelvic lymph nodes, using the perineal or retropubic approach.

POTENTIAL COMPLICATIONS

1. Urinary or wound infection,
2. alterations in patterns of urinary elimination (retention or incontinence),
3. hematuria or blood clots,
4. increased bladder spasms,
5. occlusion of urinary catheter or drainage system (if discharged home with catheter),
6. impotence.

TYPES OF CLIENTS/CLINICAL CONDITIONS SEEN BY HOME HEALTH AGENCIES

1. New surgery: postsurgical observations, instructions in prescribed treatment regimen for home-care management of client who has had a prostatectomy.
2. Postsurgical complications with changes in prescribed plan of treatment: instruction and supervision of new medications, treatments, evaluation of response to therapy.

3. Client discharged home with urinary catheter: knowledge deficit regarding catheter care and maintenance.

RELATED NURSING DIAGNOSIS

Anxiety

related to:
1. Altered body image
2. Effect of surgery on sexual functioning
3. Pain and discomfort
4. Knowledge deficit regarding prescribed treatment regimen

as seen by:
Apprehension; increased questioning regarding progress and home-care treatment regimen; expressed concern about potential sexual dysfunction

Bowel Elimination, Alteration in: Constipation

related to:
1. Inadequate fluids and dietary fiber
2. Decreased mobility postsurgery

as seen by:
Straining; changes in amount and frequency from usual pattern; c/o constipation

Bowel Elimination, Alteration in: Incontinence

related to:
1. Relaxation of perineal musculature
2. Damage to rectum and external sphincter with radical perineal prostatectomy

as seen by:
Involuntary passage of stool

Comfort, Alteration in: Pain

related to:
Bladder spasms, blood clots secondary to resection

as seen by:
Verbal report of sharp, intermittent suprapubic pain; restlessness; guarded behavior over bladder region

Grieving

related to:
1. Depression associated with changes in body functioning

as seen by:
Anger; sadness; difficulty in expressing feelings about altered

2. Implications of loss of masculinity
3. Threat to sexual functioning

body functioning; lack of interest in participating in daily activities

Infection, Potential for

related to:
Incisional area, breakdown in body's first line of defense

as seen by:
Swelling; c/o increased pain; increased redness; warmth; irritation and tissue breakdown; unusual drainage; elevated temperature; cloudy urine

Knowledge Deficit (Specify)

related to:
1. Prescribed plan of treatment following a prostatectomy
2. Potential complications, S&S to report to home health nurse or physician

as seen by:
Verbalization of lack of information; inadequate understanding; inability to perform skills necessary to meet health-care needs at home

Mobility, Impaired Physical

related to:
1. Pain
2. Prescribed activity restrictions

as seen by:
Weakness and fatigue; reluctance to attempt movement; inability to move purposefully within home environment

Self-Concept, Disturbance in

related to:
1. Changes in body functioning
2. Lowered self-esteem

as seen by:
Expressed concern regarding masculinity; verbalization of negative feelings of self-worth; unwillingness to adapt to changes and accept positive reinforcement; withdrawn behavior

Skin Integrity, Impairment of: Actual/Potential

related to:
1. Surgical incision
2. Impaired healing secondary to infection

as seen by:
Increased redness, swelling, and drainage of incisional area; irritation and tissue breakdown

Sexual Dysfunction

related to:
1. Disturbance in self-concept
2. Depression associated with altered body functioning
3. Impotence related to parasympathetic nerve damage which may occur with perineal approach or a radical prostatectomy

as seen by:
Expressed concern regarding masculinity and sexual functioning; inability to maintain relationship with spouse or significant other

LONG-TERM GOAL

To restore optimal urinary functioning following removal of obstructing prostatic tissue.

SHORT-TERM GOALS

The client who has had a prostatectomy will be able to:

1. Verbalize understanding of nature of disease process, surgical intervention, S&S of complications to report to home health nurse or physician.
2. Verbalize importance of well-balanced diet, prescribed increase in fluids of 3000 ml per day, avoiding alcohol, caffeine.
3. Demonstrate compliance with prescribed medication therapy/identify side effects.
4. Verbalize purpose/identify prescribed areas of activity restrictions.
5. Identify measures to gain and maintain urinary control.
6. Demonstrate prescribed wound care management.
7. Verbalize purpose and procedure of sitz baths.
8. Demonstrate good skin care with suprapubic drain.
9. Demonstrate prescribed measures to manage alterations in bowel functioning.
10. Demonstrate correct techniques in management of urinary catheter, tubing, and collection bag.
11. Demonstrate effective coping mechanisms in adaptation to altered body image.

NURSING ACTIONS/TREATMENTS

1. Assess systems of the body for S&S of renal and urologic dysfunction/identify complications.
2. Assess vital signs/identify trends (e.g., elevated temperature, hypotension).

3. Instruct as to nature of disease process, surgical intervention, importance of compliance with prescribed postsurgical treatment regimen, S&S of complications be report to home health nurse or physician.
4. Assess and evaluate nutritional status/instruct about well-balanced diet, prescribed increase in fluids of 3000/ml per day, avoiding alcohol, caffeine.
5. Observe/instruct about taking medications as ordered, purpose and action, side effects/evaluate medication effectiveness.
6. Assess/instruct about S&S of bleeding (slightly blood-tinged urine normal for first few weeks after surgery), prescribed activity restrictions (e.g., avoiding heavy lifting, prolonged sitting, strenuous exercise, sexual activity for 4 to 6 weeks or as prescribed).
7. Assess and evaluate for incontinence, retention/instruct about S&S of infection and measures to regain or maintain urinary control (e.g., prescribed perineum-tightening exercises (Kegel exercises) 10 to 20 times per hour when awake until urinary control regained, avoiding caffeine and alcohol, urinating when urge is felt and/or at least every 2 to 3 hours).
8. Assess and evaluate incisional area/instruct about prescribed wound care management, S&S of infection to report to home health nurse or physician.
9. Observe/instruct about purpose and procedure of sitz baths as prescribed.
10. Assess skin for drainage or urine around suprapubic drain/instruct about good skin care.
11. Assess problems with constipation/instruct to increase dietary fiber, fluids, and activities, use stool softeners and laxatives as prescribed/avoid straining, evaluate effectiveness of bowel regimen.
12. Assess and evaluate problems with fecal incontinence/instruct about cause with radical perineal approach, prescribed bowel program.
13. Assess and evaluate functioning of urinary catheter/instruct in care of catheter, tubing, and drainage collection bag, measures to maintain patency and avoid urinary retention, S&S of complications to report to home health nurse or physician.
14. Assess emotional status, coping mechanisms/encourage to verbalize feelings/refer to social services as ordered to provide counseling and assist in positive adaptation to changes in body functioning/provide information about community support groups (e.g., American Cancer Society; sexual counseling).

REHABILITATION POTENTIAL

Rehabilitation potential *excellent good fair guarded poor* for *full partial* return to a previous level of urinary functioning and satisfying life-style.

Client's Name _____

Medical Record # _____

ONGOING/DISCHARGE EVALUATION OF TEACHING

The Client Who Has Had a Prostatectomy

Teaching Tools:

Printed materials given: _____

Audiovisual aids used: _____

Return Information/Demonstration/Interpretation

_____ Client

_____ Caregiver

OF:	Met	Not Met	Comments
☐ Nature of disease process, surgical intervention.	_____	_____	_____
☐ S&S of complications, actions to take.	_____	_____	_____
☐ Importance of compliance with prescribed treatment regimen.	_____	_____	_____
☐ Importance of well-balanced diet, increased fluids.	_____	_____	_____
☐ Medications and administration, purpose and action, side effects.	_____	_____	_____
☐ Activity restrictions to reduce risk of bleeding.	_____	_____	_____

Client's Name _____

Medical Record # _____

OF:	Met	Not Met	Comments
☐ Measures to regain urinary control.	_____	_____	_____
☐ Wound care management.	_____	_____	_____
☐ Sitz baths.	_____	_____	_____
☐ Skin care with suprapubic drain.	_____	_____	_____
☐ Measures to avoid constipation.	_____	_____	_____
☐ Bowel program (fecal incontinence).	_____	_____	_____
☐ Management of urinary catheter.	_____	_____	_____

Signature of Home Health Nurse _____

Date _____

DISORDERS OF THE
HEMATOLOGIC SYSTEM

■ Iron Deficiency Anemia

Iron deficiency anemia is a microcytic, hypochromic anemia resulting from an inadequate supply of iron. It is the most common form of anemia in all age groups. Two thirds of total body iron is found in the hemoglobin and the other one third is found mostly in the liver, spleen, and bone marrow. When dietary intake of iron and iron from disintegrating red blood cells are inadequate to maintain the body's iron supplies, iron stores of the body become depleted, causing a decrease in hemoglobin and the eventual development of associated symptoms.

Causative factors in the development of an iron deficiency anemia are: (1) inadequate dietary intake of iron; (2) chronic blood loss, which is the most important cause and may be seen with conditions such as peptic ulcers, malignant diseases of the stomach or large bowel, or gastric bleeding induced by drugs (e.g., anticoagulant therapy, steroids, aspirin); (3) impaired iron absorption (e.g., seen with a partial or total gastrectomy, celiac disease, chronic diarrhea, and malignant disease of the stomach or large bowel); (4) increased iron requirements.

Clinical manifestations are symptoms associated with oxygen deficiency such as fatigue, pallor, dyspnea on exertion, headache, tachycardia, stomatitis, glossitis, irritability, changes in epithelial tissues (seen in prolonged iron deficiency) such as brittle, spoon-shaped nails, split hair that breaks off, and cracked areas of the corner of mouth. Associated neurologic involvement includes neuralgic pain, numbness and tingling of the extremities, and vasomotor disturbances.

POTENTIAL COMPLICATIONS

1. Infections,
2. cardiovascular disturbances,
3. associated neurologic effects with severe anemia.

TYPES OF CLIENTS/CLINICAL CONDITIONS SEEN BY HOME HEALTH AGENCIES

1. Newly diagnosed with iron deficiency anemia: initiation of iron supplement therapy, teaching plan for home-care management of anemic condition.
2. Development of complications associated with iron deficiency: new orders or changes in ongoing plan of treatment; home health nurse to observe, instruct, evaluate response to prescribed therapy.
3. Acute exacerbation of anemic condition: requiring an increase or change in iron replacement therapy.

RELATED NURSING DIAGNOSIS

Activity Intolerance

related to:
1. Hypoxia associated with iron deficiency anemia
2. Inadequate nutritional status

as seen by:
Dyspnea on exertion; weakness; easily fatigued; decreased endurance; abnormal cardiac, respiratory, and/or BP in response to activity; shortness of breath

Anxiety

related to:
1. Anemic condition and associated clinical manifestations
2. Knowledge deficit regarding prescribed treatment regimen

as seen by:
Expressed concern regarding clinical manifestations and effectiveness of treatment; anxious appearance; asking numerous questions regarding iron therapy

Comfort, Alteration in: Pain

related to:
1. Headache
2. Neuralgic pain
3. Glossitis
4. Stomatitis

as seen by:
Holding of head, c/o head hurting; severe stabbing pain with neuralgia; beefy red, sore tongue; sore mouth; cracked corners of mouth

Gas Exchange, Impaired

related to:
Altered oxygen-carrying capacity of the blood associated with low hemoglobin content of the red blood cells

as seen by:
Confusion; restlessness; irritability; labored respirations; dyspnea; tachycardia; pallor

Infection, Potential for

related to:
Increased susceptibility to infection secondary to weakened condition

as seen by:
Signs and symptoms of an infection (e.g., fever and chills; weakness and fatigue; adventitious breath sounds; cloudy urine; burning on urination; elevated WBC count)

Injury, Potential for: Increased Risk of Falls and Injuries

related to:
1. Cerebral hypoxia
2. Associated neuromuscular effects of iron deficiency

as seen by:
Inability to concentrate; dizziness; tendency to fainting; changes in alertness; vasomotor disturbances; neuralgic pain; numbness and tingling of extremities

Knowledge Deficit (Specify)

related to:
1. Nature of anemia, clinical manifestations
2. Prescribed plan of treatment for management of anemic condition
3. Potential complications, S&S to report to home health nurse or physician

as seen by:
Verbalization of lack of information; inadequate understanding; inability to perform skills necessary to meet health-care needs at home

Mobility, Impaired Physical

related to:
1. Activity intolerance
2. Neuralgic pain
3. Neuromuscular effects of anemia
4. Prescribed activity restrictions

as seen by:
Weakness and fatigue; decreased muscle strength; vasomotor disturbances; numbness and tingling of extremities; pain and discomfort; imposed medical restrictions

Nutrition, Alteration in: Less than Body Requirements

related to:
1. Insufficient oral intake of iron
2. Dysphagia
3. GI disturbances

as seen by:
Inadequate intake of foods high in iron; weight loss; anorexia; painful eating with glossitis or stomatitis; difficulty swallowing

Oral Mucous Membrane, Alteration in

related to:
1. Glossitis
2. Stomatitis

as seen by:
Sore mouth and tongue; c/o oral pain

Self-Care Deficit: Feeding, Bathing/Hygiene, Dressing/Grooming, Toileting (Specify)

related to:
1. Intolerance of activities
2. Impaired mobility
3. Prescribed activity restrictions

as seen by:
Decreased participation in self-care activities, associated with weakness and fatigue; decreased endurance; dyspnea on exertion; abnormal changes in cardiac, respiratory rate and/or BP in response to activity

Sensory–Perceptual Alteration: Mental Status

related to:
Cerebral hypoxia with changes in mental status

as seen by:
Impaired concentration; irritability; anxiety

LONG-TERM GOAL

To arrest course and progress of anemic disease and alleviate symptoms through correction of iron deficiency.

SHORT-TERM GOALS

The client with an iron deficiency anemia will be able to:

1. Verbalize nature of anemia, underlying cause, S&S of complications to report to home health nurse or physician.
2. Verbalize importance of well-balanced diet, iron-rich foods, adequate hydration.
3. Demonstrate compliance with prescribed medication therapy/identify side effects and toxicity.
4. Verbalize side effects of iron therapy in GI functioning/report to physician for adjustment in dosage.
5. Verbalize therapeutic importance of prescribed iron injections.
6. Verbalize change in color of stool while on iron therapy.
7. Identify signs of bleeding and associate with anemic condition/demonstrate correct procedure to check stool for occult blood/record/report abnormal finding to physician.
8. Verbalize cause of tongue and mouth ulcerations, iron deposits on teeth and gums/demonstrate good oral hygiene, avoiding irritating foods.

9. Demonstrate balanced rest and activities, energy conservation techniques.
10. Verbalize importance of/identify measures to avoid exposure to infections.
11. Identify increase risk factors for falls and injuries/demonstrate safety measures with ambulation and daily activities.
12. Verbalize purpose of prescribed lab work for serum iron determinations and other diagnostic lab tests.

NURSING ACTIONS/TREATMENTS

1. Assess for clinical manifestations of iron deficiency anemia/identify complications.
2. Assess vital signs/identify trends (e.g., tachycardia, palpitations, increased respiratory rate, orthostatic hypotension).
3. Instruct as to nature of anemia, underlying cause, importance of compliance with prescribed treatment regimen, S&S of recurrence or complications to report to home health nurse or physician.
4. Assess and evaluate nutritional status/instruct about well-balanced diet of iron-rich foods and fluids, adequate hydration.
5. Observe/instruct about taking medications as ordered (e.g., reducing gastric distress with iron supplements by taking with or shortly after meals, though iron is best absorbed on an empty stomach; not taking dairy products, eggs, whole-grain breads, coffee, tea or antacids within 2 hours of taking iron therapy because interferes with absorption; encouraging foods high in vitamin C because enhance iron absorption), purpose and action, side effects, toxicity (e.g., alterations in GI functioning: constipation, diarrhea, nausea, vomiting)/report to physician for adjustment in dosage.
6. Administer prescribed iron injections using Z-track method/instruct about therapeutic importance.
7. Observe stool/instruct about color change in stool while on iron supplements (e.g., black or green).
8. Assess/instruct about signs of bleeding associated with anemic condition, procedure to check stools for occult blood/record/report abnormal findings to physician.
9. Assess/instruct about cause of tongue and mouth ulcerations, iron deposits on teeth and gums/instruct about good oral hygiene, avoiding irritating foods, fluids, drinking liquid form of iron through straw to avoid staining teeth.
10. Observe and evaluate fatigue and weakness/instruct about activities as tolerated with planned rest periods, energy conservation techniques.
11. Assess/instruct about measures and importance of avoiding exposure to infections.
12. Assess/instruct about changes in mental status, numbness and tingling of extremities associated with anemia/instruct about increased risk of falls and inju-

ries in home environment, safety measures with ambulatory and daily activities (e.g., avoiding use of heating pads or hot water, changing positions slowly).
13. Monitor/instruct as to purpose of prescribed lab work for serum-iron-level determinations and other diagnostic lab tests.

REHABILITATION POTENTIAL

Rehabilitation potential   *excellent   good   fair   guarded   poor*   for   *full partial*   return to a level of wellness and activity tolerance to effectively manage daily activities.

Client's Name _____

Medical Record # _____

ONGOING/DISCHARGE EVALUATION OF TEACHING
The Client with Iron Deficiency Anemia

Teaching Tools:
Printed materials given: _____

Audiovisual aids used: _____

Return Information/Demonstration/Interpretation
_____ Client
_____ Caregiver

OF:	Met	Not Met	Comments
☐ Nature of iron deficiency anemia, underlying cause.	_____	_____	_____
☐ S&S of complications, actions to take.	_____	_____	_____
☐ Importance of compliance with prescribed treatment regimen.	_____	_____	_____
☐ Well-balanced diet, foods and fluids high in iron; adequate hydration.	_____	_____	_____
☐ Medications and administration, purpose and action, side effects, toxicity.	_____	_____	_____
☐ Alterations in GI functioning;			

Client's Name _____

Medical Record # _____

OF:	Met	Not Met	Comments
need for adjustment in iron supplements.	_____	_____	_____
☐ Iron injections.	_____	_____	_____
☐ Color of stool while on iron therapy.	_____	_____	_____
☐ Procedure to check for occult blood, signs of bleeding to report to physician.	_____	_____	_____
☐ Good oral hygiene; irritating foods, fluids to avoid.	_____	_____	_____
☐ Balanced rest and activities.	_____	_____	_____
☐ Energy conservation techniques.	_____	_____	_____
☐ Importance of avoiding exposure to infections.	_____	_____	_____
☐ Increased risk of falls and injuries; safety measures with ambulation and daily activities in home environment.	_____	_____	_____

Client's Name _____

Medical Record # _____

OF:	Met	Not Met	Comments
☐ Purpose of prescribed lab work.	_____	_____	_____

Signature of Home Health Nurse _____

Date _____

■ Pernicious Anemia

Pernicious anemia is a megaloblastic, macrocytic hyperchromic anemia. It is thought to result from an inherited autoimmune mechanism, causing atrophy of the mucous membrane in the fundus of the stomach and subsequent decreased production of hydrochloric acid and intrinsic factor (IF). IF combines with vitamin B_{12}, making it more soluble for the absorption of the vitamin from the lower ileum. Vitamin B_{12} is essential for growth by all cells of the body, and a deficiency in this vitamin results in depressed growth of tissues. This is especially true of those cells that grow rapidly and proliferate, like the cells found in the bone marrow and gastrointestinal tract. A deficiency not only inhibits the rate of red blood cell (RBC) production, but causes failure of maturation in the process of erythropoiesis, with the resultant formation of RBCs with poor oxygen-carrying capacity. Pernicious anemia may also occur when most of the stomach has been removed for treatment of peptic ulcer or gastric carcinoma.

Some of the symptoms of pernicious anemia include a sore tongue, digestive disturbances, loss of appetite and weight, weakness and bowel changes, symptoms associated with peripheral nerve degeneration (which may gradually extend to the spinal cord), numbness and paresthesias, lack of coordination, ataxia, loss of position and vibratory sense in the distal extremities, loss of touch sense, loss of bowel and bladder control, and cerebral changes such as loss of memory, headache, and depression. Cardiovascular symptoms are due to impaired oxygen-carrying capacity of the blood secondary to overall lowered hemoglobin and result in symptoms of fatigue, weakness, dyspnea, tachycardia, light-headedness; if left untreated they may progress to congestive heart failure.

POTENTIAL COMPLICATIONS

1. Infection,
2. gastrointestinal disturbances,
3. sensory and motor deficits,
4. cardiovascular disturbances,
5. bowel and bladder incontinence.

TYPES OF CLIENTS/CLINICAL CONDITIONS SEEN BY HOME HEALTH AGENCIES

1. Newly diagnosed with pernicious anemia: initiation of prescribed vitamin B_{12} injections; injections once a month as ordered when blood values normal; teaching plan based on management of symptoms associated with vitamin B_{12} deficiency.
2. Exacerbation of anemic condition: requiring additional injections based on lab work and/or treatment of complications related to vitamin B_{12} deficiency.

RELATED NURSING DIAGNOSIS

Activity Intolerance

related to:
1. Hypoxia secondary to decreased oxygen supply to cells
2. Inadequate nutritional status

as seen by:
Weakness and fatigue; dyspnea on exertion; abnormal cardiac, respiratory and/or BP rate in response to activity

Anxiety

related to:
1. Anemic condition and associated clinical manifestations
2. Knowledge deficit regarding prescribed treatment regimen

as seen by:
Anxiousness regarding need for injections; apprehension; numerous questions regarding treatment and potential complications related to anemia

Bowel Elimination, Alteration in: Diarrhea or Constipation

related to:
Impaired digestion secondary to gastric mucosal atrophy and decreased hydrochloric acid production or removal of parietal cells (gastrectomy) with decreased hydrochloric acid production

as seen by:
Increased frequency of stool; loose liquid stools or hard, formed stools; amount and frequency less than usual pattern

Comfort, Alteration in: Pain

related to:
1. Sore, inflamed tongue and mouth
2. Headache
3. Neuritis

as seen by:
C/o sore tongue and mouth; painful eating; holding of head; c/o pain; neuralgia

Gas Exchange, Impaired

related to:
Altered oxygen-carrying capacity of the blood associated with insufficient and deformed red blood cells

as seen by:
Dyspnea; restlessness; confusion; irritability; labored respirations or tachycardia; cyanotic skin; postural hypotension

Infection, Potential for

related to:
Increased susceptibility secondary to
   weakened condition (especially
   urinary and respiratory infections)

as seen by:
S&S of an infection (e.g., chills and
   fever; fatigue; cloudy urine; urinary
   frequency and urgency; adventitious
   breath sounds; elevated WBC count)

Injury, Potential for: Increased Risk of Falls and Injuries

related to:
1. Cerebral hypoxia
2. Neurologic changes associated with
   pernicious anemia

as seen by:
Changes in alertness; memory
   impairment; impaired judgment;
   light-headedness; weakness and
   fatigue; lack of coordination; ataxia;
   paresthesias of hands and feet;
   disturbed position and vibratory
   sense; loss of touch sensation;
   diplopia; blurred vision

Knowledge Deficit (Specify)

related to:
1. Nature of anemia, clinical
   manifestations
2. Prescribed plan of treatment for
   management of anemic condition
3. Potential complications, S&S to
   report to home health nurse or
   physician

as seen by:
Verbalization of lack of information;
   inadequate understanding; inability
   to perform skills necessary to meet
   health-care needs at home

Mobility, Impaired Physical

related to:
1. Weakness in extremities
2. Prescribed activity restrictions
3. Loss of vibratory and position
   sense
4. Peripheral numbness and
   paresthesias

as seen by:
Balance and gait disturbances; ataxia;
   fatigue; imposed medical restrictions

Nutrition, Alteration in: Less than Body Requirements

related to:
1. Decreased oral intake secondary to

as seen by:
Inadequate oral intake of foods high in

glossitis, stomatitis, GI
disturbances
2. Pathologic condition of the small
intestine that inhibits absorption of
vitamin B_{12}
3. Insufficient oral intake of vitamin
B_{12}

vitamin B_{12}; anorexia; loss of
weight; weakness and fatigue;
nausea and vomiting, painful eating
with glossitis or stomatitis

Oral Mucous Membrane, Alteration in

related to:
Stomatitis, glossitis associated with
vitamin B_{12} deficiency

as seen by:
A sore mouth and tongue; c/o oral
pain; gingival bleeding

Self-Care Deficit: Feeding, Bathing/Hygiene, Dressing/Grooming, Toileting (Specify)

related to:
1. Intolerance of activities
2. Impaired mobility
3. Prescribed activity restrictions

as seen by:
Decreased participation in self-care
activities, associated with dyspnea
on exertion; abnormal changes in
cardiac and respiratory rate;
weakness and fatigue; motor and
sensory deficits; imposed medical
restrictions

Sensory–Perceptual Alteration: Visual/Tactile/ Mental Status

related to:
1. Cerebral hypoxia with changes in
mental status
2. Visual disturbances
3. Sensory changes

as seen by:
Impaired memory; irritability; slowed
verbal responses; confusion;
depression; dyspnea; blurred vision;
loss of touch sense

LONG-TERM GOAL

To alleviate manifestations and arrest the course and progress of pernicious anemia
through correction of the vitamin B_{12} deficiency.

SHORT-TERM GOALS

The client with pernicious anemia will be able to:

1. Verbalize nature of anemia, underlying cause, S&S of recurrence or complications to report to home health nurse or physician.

2. Verbalize importance of a well-balanced diet with foods high in vitamin B_{12}.
3. Weigh weekly/record/report continued weight loss to physician.
4. Demonstrate compliance with prescribed medication therapy/identify side effects.
5. Verbalize need for life-long treatment/demonstrate correct technique in self-administration of vitamin B_{12} injections as ordered.
6. Verbalize cause of stomatitis, glossitis, or gingival bleeding/demonstrate good oral hygiene.
7. Verbalize importance of avoiding exposure to infections, S&S to report to home health nurse or physician.
8. Demonstrate compliance with prescribed bowel and bladder program.
9. Verbalize importance of balanced rest and activities.
10. Identify energy conservation techniques.
11. Identify increased risk factors for falls and injuries/demonstrate safety factors with ambulation and daily activities in the home environment.
12. Verbalize purpose of prescribed lab work for vitamin B_{12} deficiency and other diagnostic lab tests.

NURSING ACTIONS/TREATMENTS

1. Assess for clinical manifestations of pernicious anemia/identify complications.
2. Assess vital signs/identify trends (e.g., palpitations, tachycardia, changes in rhythm, increased respiratory rate, postural hypotension).
3. Instruct as to nature of anemia, underlying cause, importance of compliance with prescribed treatment regimen, S&S of recurrence or complications to report to home health nurse or physician.
4. Assess and evaluate nutritional status (e.g., effects of anorexia, nausea and vomiting, dysphagia)/instruct about well-balanced diet with foods high in vitamin B_{12}.
5. Observe and evaluate for weight loss/instruct to weigh and record weekly/report continued weight loss to physician.
6. Observe/instruct about taking medications as ordered, purpose and action, side effects.
7. Administer vitamin B_{12} injections as prescribed/instruct about therapeutic importance, need for life-long treatment, self-administration as ordered.
8. Observe and evaluate stomatitis or glossitis, gingival bleeding/instruct about good oral hygiene, avoiding irritating foods.
9. Assess/instruct about measures to avoid exposure to infections, S&S of infection to report to home health nurse or physician.
10. Assess and evaluate for alteration in bowel elimination (diarrhea or constipation)/instruct about prescribed bowel program.
11. Observe and evaluate fatigue and weakness/instruct to plan activities balanced with rest periods/teach measures to conserve energy.
12. Observe and evaluate for motor and sensory deficits/instruct about increased

risk factors for falls and injuries (e.g., light-headedness, blurred vision, diplopia, ataxia, paresthesias of hands and feet)/safety measures with ambulatory and daily activities in the home environment, changing position slowly.
13. Monitor/instruct as to purpose of prescribed lab work for pernicious anemia and other diagnostic lab tests.

REHABILITATION POTENTIAL

Rehabilitation potential *excellent good fair guarded poor* for *full partial* return to an independent level of functioning with alleviation of symptoms and improved activity tolerance, management of self-care needs and ADL.

Client's Name _____

Medical Record # _____

ONGOING/DISCHARGE EVALUATION OF TEACHING
The Client with Pernicious Anemia

Teaching Tools:
Printed materials given: _____

Audiovisual aids used: _____

Return Information/Demonstration/Interpretation
_____ Client
_____ Caregiver

OF:	Met	Not Met	Comments
☐ Nature of anemia, underlying cause.	_____	_____	_____
☐ S&S of recurrence or complications, actions to take.	_____	_____	_____
☐ Importance of compliance with prescribed treatment regimen.	_____	_____	_____
☐ Importance of life-long compliance with prescribed treatment regimen.	_____	_____	_____
☐ Well-balanced diet with foods high in vitamin B_{12}.	_____	_____	_____
☐ Medications and administration,			

Client's Name _____

Medical Record # _____

OF:	**Met**	**Not Met**	**Comments**
purpose and action, side effects.	___	___	_____
☐ Vitamin B$_{12}$ injections.	___	___	_____
☐ Good oral hygiene.	___	___	_____
☐ Importance of avoiding exposure to infection.	___	___	_____
☐ Bowel and bladder program.	___	___	_____
☐ Balanced rest and activities.	___	___	_____
☐ Energy conservation techniques.	___	___	_____
☐ Increased risk factors for falls and injuries; safety measures with ambulation and daily activities in home environment.	___	___	_____
☐ Purpose of diagnostic lab test.	___	___	_____

Signature of Home Health Nurse _____

Date _____

DISORDERS OF THE
INTEGUMENTARY SYSTEM

■ Burns

Burns are a major cause of accidental death in the nation. Thermal burns are the most common type of burn injury and may result from factors such as flame, steam, scalding water or foods, and hot surfaces. Other causes of burn injuries are excessive exposure to electricity, chemicals such as strong acids and alkalies, poisonous gases, and radiation. The extent of the burn injury is dependent upon the causative agent, duration of exposure, and thickness of the skin.

Burns are classified as partial-thickness or full-thickness depending on the depth of damage to the integument.

Partial-thickness burn injuries to the skin involve the entire epidermis, including the germinal layer and part of the dermis. Since part of the hair follicles and sweat and sebaceous glands that are found deeper in the dermis layer are not destroyed, epithelial cells are available for regeneration of the epidermis. A partial-thickness burn is equivalent to a first or second degree burn, in the traditional classification of burns. Sensations of pain and temperature are normal or increased.

In a full-thickness burn injury, both the dermis and epidermis are destroyed and no sensations of pain or temperature are felt. A full-thickness burn is equivalent to a third or fourth degree burn.

POTENTIAL COMPLICATIONS

1. Infection,
2. bleeding,
3. contractures,
4. falls and injuries associated with musculoskeletal impairments,
5. opening of a healed wound,
6. separation of grafted areas.

TYPES OF CLIENTS/CLINICAL CONDITIONS SEEN BY HOME HEALTH AGENCIES

1. Recent burn injuries with prescribed management of healing wounds: includes dressing changes; instruction in aseptic technique; use of pressure garments, elastic wraps; physical therapy, occupational therapy to establish home program for management of impaired musculoskeletal status, contractures; instruction in prescribed exercises and use of braces, splints, self-help devices or ambulatory aids.
2. Discharged home from hospital following grafting of burn areas: wound care management, antibiotic therapy.
3. Postburn complications: prescribed treatments requiring skilled observation by home health nurse; instruction in new treatments; evaluation of response to therapy and resolution of complications.

RELATED NURSING DIAGNOSIS

Anxiety

related to:
1. Pain
2. Altered body image
3. Knowledge deficit regarding prescribed treatment regimen

as seen by:
Fearfulness of response by others to appearance of burn areas; expressed concern and nervousness in home management of burn or graft areas

Comfort, Alteration in: Pain

related to:
Burn injury areas and donor sites

as seen by:
Verbalization of pain; guarded behavior of injury areas; grimaces

Coping, Ineffective

related to:
1. Change in body appearance
2. Pain
3. Increased dependency on others for care

as seen by:
Depression; anxiety; inability to care for self; withdrawn behavior; anger

Infection, Potential for

related to:
Burn areas, graft or donor sites

as seen by:
S&S of infection (e.g., increased warmth; redness; swelling; pain); graft site separation; unusual drainage; opening of healing burn area

Injury, Potential for: Increased Risk of Falls and Injuries

related to:
1. Sensory deficits
2. Decreased range of motion secondary to contractures
3. Musculoskeletal involvement secondary to burns

as seen by:
Limited ability to perform ADL; weakness and fatigue; reduced tactile sensation; lack of muscle coordination

Knowledge Deficit (Specify)

related to:
1. Prescribed plan of treatment in management of burns
2. Potential complications, S&S to report to home health nurse or physician

as seen by:
Verbalization of lack of information; inadequate understanding; inability to perform skills necessary to meet health-care needs at home

Mobility, Impaired Physical

related to:
Extensive burn areas, contractures, musculoskeletal involvement

as seen by:
Inability to move purposefully within the home environment without assistance; reluctance to move; limited ROM; impaired coordination

Nutrition, Alteration in: Less than Body Requirements

related to:
Oral intake inadequate to meet increased metabolic demands of the body for healing of burn injury or graft areas

as seen by:
Generalized weakness; poor wound healing; repeated inadequate food intake; weight loss

Self-Care Deficit: Feeding, Bathing/Hygiene, Dressing/Grooming, Toileting (Specify)

related to:
1. Activity intolerance
2. Impaired physical mobility
3. Prescribed activity restrictions

as seen by:
Inability to perform self-care activities, associated with weakness and fatigue; sensory deficits; musculoskeletal involvement; imposed medical restrictions

Self-Concept, Disturbance in

related to:
1. Altered body image
2. Life-style changes
3. Loss of self-esteem

as seen by:
Depression; anxiety; decreased attention to grooming; lack of follow-through in assisting with burn care

Skin Integrity, Impairment of: Actual/Potential

related to:
1. Burn injury areas
2. Skin grafts
3. Impaired healing related to infection
4. Inadequate nutritional status
5. Decreased mobility

as seen by:
S&S of impaired wound healing or infection (e.g., increased redness; warmth; swelling; pain; irritation; breakdown; necrosis in burn areas; separation of grafted areas)

LONG-TERM GOAL

To promote healing and restore skin integrity.

SHORT-TERM GOALS

The client with a burn injury will be able to:

1. Verbalize burn safety behavior and practices.
2. Verbalize S&S of complications to report to home health nurse or physician.
3. Verbalize importance of adequate hydration, prescribed well-balanced diet for healed burn areas, graft and donor sites, diet high in proteins and calories for healing burn areas, graft and donor sites.
4. Demonstrate compliance with prescribed medication therapy/identify side effects.
5. Identify prescribed pain management measures.
6. Demonstrate principles of asepsis, proper hand-washing techniques before wound care.
7. Demonstrate prescribed wound care management.
8. Verbalize importance of avoiding trauma and excessive exposure of grafted areas to sunlight.
9. Demonstrate correct use of prescribed stretch fabric garments and elastic wraps/verbalize purpose in controlling scarring.
10. Demonstrate compliance with prescribed exercise program with correct use of supports, self-help devices, splints, braces, or ambulatory aids as ordered.
11. Verbalize importance of personal hygiene and good skin care of unburned areas.
12. Verbalize importance of proper turning, positioning, and therapeutic exercises to correct and avoid contractures.
13. Identify complications related to prolonged immobilization, prescribed measures to treat, activities to avoid.
14. Demonstrate positive adjustment to alterations in body image and life-style changes.

NURSING ACTIONS/TREATMENTS

1. Assess burn area, graft and donor sites/identify complications.
2. Assess vital signs/identify trends (e.g., elevated temperature).
3. Assess cause of burn/instruct as to safety behavior and practices in the home, importance of compliance with prescribed treatment regimen, S&S of complications to report to home health nurse or physician.
4. Assess and evaluate nutritional status/instruct about prescribed well-balanced regular diet for healed burn areas, graft and donor sites, high-protein, high-calorie diet for healing burn areas, graft and donor sites, adequate fluid intake.
5. Observe/instruct about taking medications as ordered, purpose and action, side effects.
6. Assess and evaluate level of skin sensitivity/instruct about prescribed pain management measures.
7. Observe/instruct as to principles of asepsis and proper hand-washing techniques before wound care.
8. Observe/instruct about prescribed care of wound, graft and donor sites with use of topical medications, dressings, elastic bandages, or stockings/evaluate healing of wound areas.
9. Assess/instruct about S&S of infection, opening of a healed wound, separation of grafted burn areas to report to home health nurse or physician.
10. Observe/instruct to avoid trauma and excessive exposure of graft areas to sunlight.
11. Observe/instruct as to purpose and use of prescribed stretch fabric garments and elastic wraps for control of scarring.
12. Observe and evaluate mobility status, activity levels/instruct about prescribed exercise program, use of ambulatory aids or self-help devices as ordered; proper fit and use of splints, braces.
13. Assess/instruct about importance of personal hygiene of unburned areas, good skin care.
14. Observe/instruct about importance of proper turning, positioning, prescribed therapeutic exercises to correct and avoid contractures.
15. Assess and evaluate for complications related to prolonged immobilization/instruct about prescribed measures to treat, activities to avoid.
16. Observe and evaluate alterations in functional skills, ambulatory activities/refer to rehabilitative services as ordered for establishment of home exercise program for impaired musculoskeletal status with contractures caused by burn areas; instruction in use of self-help aids, ambulatory assistive devices, braces, splints.
17. Assess psychological and emotional responses to burns/provide emotional support/refer to social services as ordered for counseling to assist with adjustment to body and life-style changes and to provide information regarding needed community resources (e.g., attendant services, Meals on Wheels, transportation services, counseling services).

REHABILITATION POTENTIAL

Rehabilitation potential   *excellent   good   fair   guarded   poor*   for   *full   partial*   achievement of an improved level of independence and functioning consistent with physical limitations to manage daily activities.

Client's Name _____

Medical Record #_____

ONGOING/DISCHARGE EVALUATION OF TEACHING
The Client with Burn Injury

Teaching Tools:
Printed materials given: _____

Audiovisual aids used: _____

Return Information/Demonstration/Interpretation
_____ Client
_____ Caregiver

OF:	Met	Not Met	Comments
☐ Burn safety behavior and practices.	_____	_____	_____
☐ S&S of complications, actions to take.	_____	_____	_____
☐ Importance of compliance with prescribed treatment regimen.	_____	_____	_____
☐ Prescribed diet and fluid requirements.	_____	_____	_____
☐ Medications and administration, purpose and action, side effects.	_____	_____	_____
☐ Pain management measures.	_____	_____	_____

Client's Name _____

Medical Record # _____

OF:	**Met**	**Not Met**	**Comments**
☐ Principles of asepsis and proper hand-washing techniques.	_____	_____	_____
☐ Wound care management.	_____	_____	_____
☐ Stretch fabric garments, elastic wraps for control of scarring.	_____	_____	_____
☐ Graft areas: avoid trauma and excessive exposure to sun.	_____	_____	_____
☐ Exercise program with prescribed use of splints, braces, self-help devices, ambulatory aids.	_____	_____	_____
☐ Personal hygiene, good skin care of unburned areas.	_____	_____	_____
☐ Proper turning and positioning; therapeutic exercises.	_____	_____	_____
☐ Complications related to prolonged			

Client's Name _____

Medical Record # _____

OF: **Met**   **Not Met**   **Comments**

immobilization;
activities to
avoid; measures
to treat.   _____   _____   _____

Signature of Home Health Nurse _____

Date _____

■ Decubitus Ulcers

Decubitus ulcers are areas of cellular necrosis that occur as a result of any condition that impairs or interferes with the exchange of nutrients and metabolic wastes between the cells and the blood. There are various factors that predispose to ulcer formation, but generally any client whose condition is debilitated or deteriorating is at high risk. Two major groups of high-risk clients are those with decreased sensory input who are unable to recognize warning signs of ulcer formation (e.g., clients with neurologic conditions such as spinal cord injuries and cerebral vascular accidents) and those clients who are able to receive and recognize sensory input but are unable to react to the warning signs (e.g., those with paralysis, motor deficits, weakness). Predisposing factors for ulcer formation are nutritional deficiencies, age, preexisting conditions, decreased mobility, radiation, chemotherapy, sensory and motor deficits. The sacrum, ischial tuberosities, trochanter area of the leg, heel, and malleolus of the ankle are the most frequent locations of pressure ulcer development.

Treatment modalities for decubitus ulcers are numerous, but whatever the prescribed treatment, it is imperative that the following factors be considered to eliminate any that could compromise the healing of the ulcer: (1) Impaired tissue oxygenation resulting from sustained pressure on the decubitus ulcer; (2) necrotic tissue that interferes with the formation of granulation tissue; (3) infection of the ulcer area; (4) ineffectiveness of decubitus ulcer treatment; (5) debilitated or preexisting conditions in the client.

POTENTIAL COMPLICATIONS

1. Infection,
2. development of new ulcers,
3. extension of necrotic areas.

TYPES OF CLIENTS/CLINICAL CONDITIONS SEEN BY HOME HEALTH AGENCIES

1. Ulcers that are open and draining: daily treatments and dressings.
2. Discharged home from hospital following debridement and grafting of ulcer area: prescribed ulcer care and/or dressings; close observation of healing process and the development of any complications; reporting to physician effectiveness of prescribed treatments.

RELATED NURSING DIAGNOSIS

Anxiety

related to:
1. Healing of ulcer

as seen by:
Verbalized concern regarding ulcer not

2. Altered body image
3. Impaired functional status
4. Prescribed treatment regimen

healing; expressed concern regarding effectiveness of new medications and treatments

Comfort, Alteration in: Pain

related to:
Inflammation, edema, and ulceration of skin and subcutaneous tissue

as seen by:
Protection of involved area; c/o pain; moaning; increased pulse rate

Fluid Volume, Alteration in: Excess

related to:
Increased tissue fragility associated with edema (specify causal and contributing factors specific to medical condition (e.g., congestive heart failure; peripheral edema secondary to cirrhosis)

as seen by:
Edematous areas; weight gain

Infection, Potential for

related to:
Decubitus ulcer, breakdown of the body's first line of defense

as seen by:
Increased redness; swelling; necrotic tissue; unusual drainage; foul odor; fever; elevated WBC count

Injury, Potential for: Increased Risk of Accidental Tissue Injury

related to:
Decreased tactile sensitivity

as seen by:
Decreased sensation in superficial tissue of body parts and disregard for teaching to avoid use of heating pad and hot-water bottle to feet and legs

Knowledge Deficit (Specify)

related to:
1. Causative factors
2. Prescribed plan of treatment for care and management of decubitus ulcers

as seen by:
Verbalization of lack of information; inadequate understanding; inability to perform skills necessary to meet health-care needs at home

3. Potential complications, S&S to report to home health nurse or physician

Mobility, Impaired Physical

related to:
Specify causal and contributing factors specific to medical condition, (e.g., stroke; spinal cord trauma; arthritis; multiple sclerosis)

as seen by:
Inability to move independently

Nutrition, Alteration in: Less than Body Requirements

related to:
Specify causal and contributing factors specific to medical condition (e.g., peptic ulcer; diverticulitis; renal failure; depression)

as seen by:
S&S of malnutrition

Self-Care Deficit: Feeding, Bathing/Hygiene, Dressing/Grooming, Toileting (Specify)

related to:
Specify causal and contributing factors specific to medical condition (e.g., stroke, rheumatoid arthritis)

as seen by:
Inability to wash body or body parts; inability to get to toilet or carry out proper toilet hygiene

Self-Concept, Disturbance in

related to:
1. Altered body image
2. Effect of ulcers on life-style
3. Low self-esteem

as seen by:
Depression; not looking at or touching area of ulcer; expressed anger; withdrawal; increased dependency on others to meet physical and daily needs; lack of follow-through

Skin Integrity, Impairment of: Actual/Potential

related to:
Irritation and breakdown (specify causal and contributing factors specific to medical condition [e.g., tissue ischemia secondary to prolonged pressure and immobility;

as seen by:
Erythema; destruction of skin layers

nutritional deficiencies; radiation or chemotheraphy; sensory and motor deficits; edema; anemia; chronic illness; incontinence)

Sensory–Perceptual Alteration: Tactile

related to:
Impairment in ability to feel or perceive pressure (specify causal and contributing factors specific to medical condition e.g., neurologically impaired client)

as seen by:
Inability to feel pain or pressure

LONG-TERM GOAL

To promote healing and restore skin integrity without the development of complications.

SHORT-TERM GOALS

The client with a decubitus ulcer will be able to:

1. Verbalize nature of decubitus ulcers, predisposing factors to formation, S&S of complications to report to home health nurse or physician.
2. Verbalize importance of prescribed high-calorie, high-protein diet, vitamin and mineral supplements, adequate fluid intake.
3. Verbalize importance of taking prescribed nutritional supplements.
4. Demonstrate compliance with prescribed medication therapy/identify side effects.
5. Demonstrate compliance with prescribed skin care program.
6. Verbalize importance/identify measures to relieve pressure and shearing force on skin.
7. Demonstrate prescribed wound care management.
8. Verbalize S&S of complications related to prolonged immobility, prescribed measures to treat, activities to avoid.
9. Verbalize knowledge of measures to decrease risk of tissue damage with sensory loss.
10. Demonstrate prescribed exercises and activities to increase circulation and muscle tone.
11. Demonstrate follow-through with prescribed treatment regimen.

NURSING ACTIONS/TREATMENTS

1. Assess location and character of skin changes/grade existing ulcers (e.g., depth, length, and width; color and amount of any exudate; presence or absence of pain or odor; the color of exposed tissue; increased warmth)/identify complications.
2. Assess vital signs/identify trends (e.g., elevated temperature).
3. Instruct about nature and predisposing factors in decubitus ulcer formation, importance of compliance with prescribed treatment regimen, S&S of complications to report to home health nurse or physician.
4. Assess nutritional status/evaluate nutritional condition that predisposes to pressure sore formation (e.g., obesity, underweight, anorexia)/instruct about high-calorie, high-protein diet with vitamin and mineral supplements (e.g., vitamin C for collagen formation), adequate fluid intake as prescribed.
5. Observe/instruct as to purpose of taking nutritional supplements as prescribed.
6. Observe/instruct about taking medications as ordered, purpose and action, side effects/evaluate medication effectiveness.
7. Inspect skin for breakdown (e.g., potential breakdown from continual contact with urine and feces)/instruct about daily skin care program (e.g., reddened skin areas are indicative of skin damage and should not be massaged/evaluate skin integrity).
8. Observe/instruct about purpose of measures to relieve pressure and shearing force on skin (e.g., pressure relief aids, turning, repositioning, moving client carefully from a bed or chair to avoid injury to skin).
9. Assess/instruct about good hand-washing technique; consistent approach to treatment; to clean wound and apply topical preparations to debride and treat ulcers, pack wounds, apply dressings as prescribed (e.g., slightly moist surface of wound enhances epithelial cell migration); to use sterile technique and sterile equipment when ulcer is infected/explain that infectious diseases can be transmitted in exudate; how to dispose of contaminated dressings.
10. Assess and instruct about S&S of complications related to prolonged immobility, prescribed measures to treat, activities to avoid.
11. Assess for S&S of sensory loss/instruct about safety measures to decrease risk of tissue damage (e.g., inability to feel pain or pressure, importance of not using heating pads or hot-water bottles).
12. Observe and evaluate alterations in mobility status, functional skills/instruct about prescribed exercises (e.g., ROM and isometric exercises) and activities to increase circulation and muscle tone.
13. Assess feelings of low self-esteem and lack of follow-through with prescribed treatment regimen/encourage verbalization of feelings/provide emotional support/refer to social services to assist with needed community resources (e.g., Meals on Wheels, attendant services).

REHABILITATION POTENTIAL

Rehabilitation potential   *excellent   good   fair   guarded   poor*   for   *full partial*   return to an improved level of wellness and restoration of skin integrity for maximal independence in ADL.

Client's Name _____

Medical Record # _____

ONGOING/DISCHARGE EVALUATION OF TEACHING
The Client with a Decubitus Ulcer

Teaching Tools:
Printed materials given: _____

Audiovisual aids used: _____

Return Information/Demonstration/Interpretation
_____ Client
_____ Caregiver

	OF:	Met	Not Met	Comments
☐	Nature of decubitus ulcers; predisposing factors to formation.	_____	_____	_____
☐	S&S of complications; actions to take.	_____	_____	_____
☐	Importance of compliance with prescribed treatment regimen.	_____	_____	_____
☐	High-calorie, high-protein diet, vitamin and mineral supplements, adequate fluid intake.	_____	_____	_____
☐	Nutritional supplements.	_____	_____	_____
☐	Medications and administration,			

Client's Name _____

Medical Record # _____

OF:	**Met**	**Not Met**	**Comments**
purpose and action, side effects.	_____	_____	_____
☐ Skin care program.	_____	_____	_____
☐ Measures to relieve pressure and shearing force on skin.	_____	_____	_____
☐ Application of topical preparations.	_____	_____	_____
☐ Packing of wounds.	_____	_____	_____
☐ Application of dressings.	_____	_____	_____
☐ Complications related to prolonged immobility, measures to treat, activities to avoid.	_____	_____	_____
☐ Exercises and activities to increase circulation and muscle tone.	_____	_____	_____
☐ S&S of sensory loss; measures to decrease risk of tissue injury.	_____	_____	_____

Signature of Home Health Nurse _____

Date _____

DISORDERS OF THE EYE

■ Cataract Extraction

With or Without an Intraocular Lens Implant

A cataract is a progressive clouding or opacity of the crystalline lens or capsule of the eye, occurring primarily as a complication of aging. This is called a senile cataract and is the focus of this planning guide. Predisposition to cataracts is hereditary but they may result from other causes such as trauma, congenital (usually hereditary but may be due to maternal rubella during first trimester), and toxic causes or may be secondary to other eye conditions.

Senile cataracts are progressive, degenerative changes that occur in the crystalline lens and usually occur bilaterally, each progressing independently of the other. These degenerative changes most often occur after 50 years of age. Cataract symptoms may include blurred or dim vision, sensitivity to glare and bright lights, and impaired visual acuity.

Cataracts may develop within the cortex or the nucleus of the lens. Cortical cataracts are characterized by various stages of development, with opacities starting in the periphery of the lens, then progressing to the pupillary area with eventual decreased visual acuity, and progressing until the entire lens becomes opaque. The nuclear cataract does not go through stages of development but is characterized by a slowly progressive central opacity, which may have a yellow discoloration and result in interference with certain colors reaching the retina.

Cataract surgery becomes necessary when the client is no longer able to carry out certain activities as a result of impaired visual acuity. The intracapsular cataract extraction removes the entire lens and surrounding capsule. The extracapsular cataract extraction is used to remove the nucleus, the cortex, and the anterior portion of the lens capsule. During surgery, after the cataractous lens is removed, useful vision may be restored through an intraocular lens implant (IOL) that is surgically placed behind the cornea and in the iris. The client's visual deficit may also be corrected with glasses and contact lenses.

POTENTIAL COMPLICATIONS

1. Hyphema,
2. iris prolapse,
3. infection,
4. wound rupture secondary to loosening of sutures,
5. loss of vitreous,
6. increased intraocular pressure.

TYPES OF CLIENTS/CLINICAL CONDITIONS SEEN BY HOME HEALTH AGENCIES

1. Cataract surgery: inclusive teaching plan about prescribed eye medications, dressings, activities and observations for complications.
2. Discharged home following treatment for postoperative complications secondary

to cataract surgery: home health nurse to closely observe operative eye, provide treatments, report response to therapy.

RELATED NURSING DIAGNOSIS

Anxiety

related to:
1. Pain and discomfort and limited vision postsurgery
2. Knowledge deficit regarding prescribed treatment regimen

as seen by:
Verbalized fear of complications or surgery not improving vision; fear and apprehension of being unable to put in eye drops, manage prescribed eye care, and take care of ADL

Comfort, Alteration in: Pain

related to:
1. Slight pain
2. Discomfort with cataract extraction
3. Severe pain secondary to postoperative complication of hemorrhage or infection

as seen by:
Verbalization of pain and discomfort; facial mask of pain; protective behavior with affected eye; crying

Infection, Potential for

related to:
Cataract removal

as seen by:
Increased redness; sharp pain; edema; unusual drainage; fever

Knowledge Deficit (Specify)

related to:
1. Prescribed plan of treatment in postoperative cataract care
2. Potential complications, S&S to report to home health nurse or physician

as seen by:
Lack of information; inadequate understanding; inability to perform skills necessary to meet health-care needs at home

Injury, Potential for: Increased Risk of Falls and Injuries

related to:
Loss of depth perception secondary to prescribed covering of operative eye or if IOL has not been implanted

as seen by:
Bumping into furniture with ambulation; bruised areas on extremities; missing a step on stairs

Mobility, Impaired Physical

related to:
1. Limited vision
2. Prescribed restrictions
3. Loss of depth perception

as seen by:
Unsteady gait; bumping into furniture with one eye covered; medical restrictions regarding bending and lifting; progressive decrease in activities.

Self-Care Deficit: Feeding, Bathing/Hygiene, Dressing/Grooming, Toileting (Specify)

related to:
1. Visual impairment
2. Prescribed activity restrictions after cataract surgery

as seen by:
Limited ability to perform self-care activities as a result of decreased vision, imposed medical restrictions

Sensory–Perceptual Alteration: Visual

related to:
Postoperative cataract surgery: hand-motion vision only in the involved eye and limited depth perception if an IOL has not been implanted or loss of depth perception if involved eye is patched

as seen by:
Bumping into furniture; clumsy behavior; report of changes in visual acuity; missing a step on the stairs.

LONG-TERM GOALS

To restore useful vision without evidence of complications through strict compliance with postoperative care and restrictions.

SHORT-TERM GOALS

The client who has had cataract surgery will be able to:

1. Verbalize nature of cataract disorder, surgical procedure, S&S of complications to report to home health nurse or physician.
2. Verbalize importance of well-balanced diet, adequate hydration.
3. Demonstrate compliance with prescribed medication therapy/identify side effects.
4. Demonstrate compliance with prescribed postoperative eye care and eye protection measures.

5. Verbalize importance/identify measures to avoid increased intraocular pressure/identify S&S to report promptly to home health nurse or physician.
6. Verbalize importance of a gradual increase in activities with balanced rest periods as prescribed.
7. Demonstrate safety precautions with daily activities and ambulation to reduce risk of falls and injuries in home environment.
8. Demonstrate compliance in use of prescribed glasses or cataracts.

NURSING ACTIONS/TREATMENTS

1. Examine both eyes/identify pathologic changes in affected eye/report to physician.
2. Assess vital signs/identify trends (e.g., elevated temperature).
3. Instruct as to nature of cataract disorder, surgical removal of lens, intraocular lens implant, importance of compliance with prescribed treatment regimen, S&S of complications to report to home health nurse or physician.
4. Assess and evaluate nutritional status/instruct as to importance of well-balanced diet, adequate hydration.
5. Observe/instruct about correct instillation of prescribed eye drops or ointments (e.g., mydriatic drops, antibiotic drops or ointments, steroid drops), purpose and action, side effects.
6. Observe/instruct about taking medications as ordered, purpose and action, side effects/evaluate medication effectiveness.
7. Inspect and evaluate the lids, conjunctiva, and sclera for edema, discharge, or redness/instruct to wash hands before cleaning eye, clean eye twice a day or more often as ordered (e.g., clean discharge and crusts from eyelids with warm compresses)/apply prescribed eye shield or eye patch.
8. Assess eye for increased intraocular pressure (IOP) (e.g., complaints of inordinate amount of pain in operated eye, pupil semidilated, cornea hazy)/instruct about measures to avoid increased IOP (e.g., heavy lifting, bending, coughing, straining, lying flat, rubbing or hitting eye)/report any problems promptly to physician.
9. Observe and evaluate ambulatory activities/instruct to gradually increase activities as ordered with balanced rest periods as prescribed.
10. Assess and evaluate limited vision/instruct safety factors with ambulation and daily activities to reduce risk of fall and injuries in the home environment.
11. Observe/instruct about prescribed use of glasses or contacts.

REHABILITATION POTENTIAL

Rehabilitation potential   *excellent   good   fair   guarded   poor*   for   *full partial*   return to a previous level of independence and productive life-style through restoration of useful vision.

Client's Name _____

Medical Record # _____

ONGOING/DISCHARGE EVALUATION OF TEACHING

The Client with a Cataract Extraction with or without an Intraocular Lens Implant

Teaching Tools:
Printed materials given: _____

Audiovisual aids used: _____

Return Information/Demonstration/Interpretation
_____ Client
_____ Caregiver

OF:	Met	Not Met	Comments
☐ Nature of disease process, surgical procedure.	_____	_____	_____
☐ S&S of complications, actions to take.	_____	_____	_____
☐ Importance of compliance with prescribed treatment regimen.	_____	_____	_____
☐ Well-balanced diet, adequate hydration.	_____	_____	_____
☐ Eye drops and eye ointments and their administration.	_____	_____	_____
☐ Medications and administration, purpose and action, side effects.	_____	_____	_____

Client's Name _____

Medical Record # _____

OF:	Met	Not Met	Comments
☐ Cleaning of eye as prescribed.	———	———	———————————
☐ Eye shield application.	———	———	———————————
☐ Eye patch application.	———	———	———————————
☐ Measures to avoid increased intraocular pressure.	———	———	———————————
☐ Progressive activities with balanced rest periods.	———	———	———————————
☐ Safety factors with ambulation and daily activities.	———	———	———————————
☐ Demonstrate prescribed use of glasses or contacts.	———	———	———————————

Signature of Home Health Nurse _____

Date _____

NEOPLASTIC DISORDERS/ANTINEOPLASTIC TREATMENT

■ Breast Cancer/Mastectomy

A mastectomy is the surgical removal of one or both breasts, usually performed for the treatment of breast carcinoma. The surgical options considered by the surgeon take into account the stage of the disease process, prevention of the spread of the carcinoma, and minimization of disfigurement.

The Halsted radical procedure involves removing the entire breast with underlying muscles, axillary lymph nodes, fat and fascia. This was once the surgery of choice for local as well as regional breast carcinoma. More widely used today is a modified radical procedure that involves leaving the large muscles of the chest and removing the entire breast, some axillary nodes, and fat. A simple mastectomy may be performed when there is no carcinoma involvement of muscle or lymph nodes. In this procedure the entire breast and some fat tissue is removed.

In those surgeries involving lymph node dissection, severe edema secondary to removal of lymph nodes and restricted shoulder mobility continue to be a complication.

POTENTIAL COMPLICATIONS

1. Wound infection,
2. lymphedema of arm on operated side,
3. motor or sensory impairment of arm and/or shoulder on operated side.

TYPES OF CLIENTS/CLINICAL CONDITIONS SEEN BY HOME HEALTH AGENCIES

1. New surgery: postsurgical observations; instruction in prescribed treatment regimen for home-care management of mastectomy client (e.g., care of incisional area, dressing changes).
2. Postsurgical complications: changes in prescribed plan of treatment; instruction in new therapy; evaluation of response to treatment.
3. Mastectomy performed within last six months: complications of restricted mobility of arm and/or shoulder on operated side, associated with motor impairment.

RELATED NURSING DIAGNOSIS

Activity Intolerance

related to:
1. Incisional pain
2. Lymphedema
3. Anxiety

as seen by:
Dyspnea; c/o weakness and fatigue; exertional discomfort

Anxiety

related to:
1. Altered body image and effect on sexuality
2. Life-style changes
3. Diagnosis of cancer
4. Pain
5. Knowledge deficit regarding prescribed treatment regimen

as seen by:
Expressed report of feelings of uncertainty and inadequacy; crying; withdrawn behavior; numerous questions or lack of questions regarding home rehabilitation program

Breathing Pattern, Ineffective

related to:
Incisional pain

as seen by:
Splinted or guarded respirations; dyspnea; c/o pain

Comfort, Alteration in: Pain

related to:
1. Surgical incision
2. Lymphedema of affected arm

as seen by:
Guarding or protective behavior of operative area and affected arm; c/o pain; facial mask of pain

Coping, Ineffective Individual

related to:
1. Depression
2. Feelings of rejection
3. Loss of sense of self-worth
4. Diagnosis of cancer

as seen by:
Feelings of helplessness; overeating or loss of appetite; general irritability; insomnia

Fluid Volume, Alteration in: Excess

related to:
Lymphedema secondary to removal of lymph nodes

as seen by:
Increased swelling of circumference of affected arm; c/o pain or heaviness of arm; inability to move through full ROM; not following prescribed sodium restrictions

Grieving

related to:
1. Altered body image with loss of breast
2. Implication of loss of femininity

as seen by:
Depression; verbalization of distress at loss; anger; isolation; crying

Infection, Potential for

related to:
1. Incisional area, breakdown in body's first line of defense
2. Lymphedema of affected arm

as seen by:
Increased redness and swelling; unusual drainage; pronounced tenderness or pain; elevated temperature

Injury, Potential for: Increased Incidence of Falls and Injuries

related to:
Alteration in balance and mobility as a result of impaired or restricted movement of affected arm

as seen by:
Unsteady gait and balance with ambulation; limited ROM

Knowledge Deficit (Specify)

related to:
1. Prescribed plan of treatment postmastectomy
2. Potential complications, S&S to report to home health nurse or physician

as seen by:
Verbalization of lack of information; inadequate understanding or inability to perform skills necessary to meet health-care needs at home

Mobility, Alteration in

related to:
1. Pain
2. Impaired movement of affected arm secondary to lymphedema and weakness of pectoral muscles
3. Prescribed activity restrictions

as seen by:
Weakness and fatigue; reluctance to attempt movement; limited ROM; imposed medical restrictions on movement

Self-Care Deficit: Feeding, Bathing/Hygiene, Dressing/Grooming, Toileting (Specify)

related to:
1. Activity intolerance
2. Impaired physical mobility
3. Prescribed activity restrictions

as seen by:
Weakness and fatigue; reluctance to attempt movement; limited ROM; imposed medical restrictions on movement

Self-Concept, Disturbance in

related to:
1. Loss of breast

as seen by:
Expressed concern regarding

2. Effect on life-style

femininity; increased dependence on others; signs of grieving, crying, anger, despair, refusal to participate in own care

Sexual Dysfunction

related to:
1. Pain
2. Disturbance in self-concept
3. Depression associated with altered body image

as seen by:
Verbalization of fear of effect of loss of breast on sexuality; altered relationship with significant other

Skin Integrity, Impairment of: Actual/Potential

related to:
1. Surgical incision
2. Skin fragility associated with lymphedema
3. Impaired healing secondary to infection

as seen by:
Increased redness, swelling, and drainage of incisional area; irritation and tissue breakdown; elevated temperature; increased WBC count

LONG-TERM GOAL

To attain optimal physiologic and psychological adjustment following mastectomy.

SHORT-TERM GOALS

The client who has had a mastectomy will be able to:

1. Verbalize nature of disease process, surgical procedure.
2. Verbalize S&S of complications to report to home health nurse or physician.
3. Verbalize importance of well-balanced diet and adequate hydration, prescribed sodium restrictions with lymphedema.
4. Demonstrate compliance with prescribed medication therapy/identify side effects.
5. Identify prescribed measures for pain control management.
6. Demonstrate prescribed wound care management.
7. Demonstrate correct postmastectory exercises/identify activities and procedures that could cause injuries to arm.
8. Verbalize cause of lymphedema/demonstrate good skin care measures to reduce and treat.

9. Identify S&S of cellulitis and lymphangitis of arm on affected side to report to home health nurse or physician.
10. Identify measures to improve body image, various types of prostheses.
11. Demonstrate safety measures with impaired arm movement and loss of balance, to reduce risk of falls and injuries in home environment.
12. Verbalize importance of/demonstrate how to perform monthly self-examination of remaining breast and operative side.
13. Verbalize importance of/wear Medic Alert bracelet.
14. Demonstrate positive adjustment to loss of breast and alterations in life-style.
15. Demonstrate compliance with prescribed home therapy program.

NURSING ACTIONS/TREATMENTS

1. Assess cardiovascular and pulmonary status, sensory and motor functioning of arm on operative side/identify complications.
2. Assess vital signs/identify trends (e.g., elevated temperature).
3. Instruct as to nature of disease process, surgical procedure/instruct about importance of compliance with prescribed postoperative surgical regimen, S&S of complications to report to home health nurse or physician.
4. Assess and evaluate nutritional status, sodium restrictions with lymphedema/ instruct about well-balanced diet, adequate hydration.
5. Observe/instruct to take medications as ordered, purpose and action, side effects/evaluate medication effectiveness.
6. Assess and evaluate cause and level of pain/instruct about prescribed pain control measures (e.g., prescribed use of analgesics, splinting of breast incision with hands or pillow as needed with movement).
7. Assess and evaluate incisional area/instruct about prescribed wound care management, S&S of infection to report to home health nurse or physician.
8. Observe and evaluate functional status of arm on affected side, ability to perform self-care activities/instruct about postmastectomy exercise program with balanced rest periods as ordered, avoiding activities and procedures that could injure arm.
9. Observe and evaluate lymphedema of affected arm/instruct about cause, good skin care, prescribed measures to reduce and treat (e.g., use of elastic bandage on affected arm, diuretics, arm and shoulder exercises, elevation of arm, massage), measures to protect (e.g., avoiding constrictive clothing, cutting of cuticles or hangnails, having blood drawn, having BP taken, receiving an injection).
10. Assess/instruct about S&S of cellulitis and lymphangitis of arm on affected side/report to home health nurse or physician.
11. Assess/instruct about measures to improve body image (e.g., ways to dress), various types of prostheses, proper fit, use of in 2 to 6 months after incision heals.

12. Observe and evaluate impaired arm movement, loss of balance/instruct about safety measures with ambulation and ADL to reduce risk of falls and injuries in home environment.
13. Assess/instruct about importance of and how to perform examination of remaining breast and operative site on a monthly basis, reporting changes to physician.
14. Observe/instruct about importance of wearing Medic Alert bracelet, cautioning not to give injections or tests on arm with lymphedema.
15. Assess level of depression, stage of grieving, associated sexual dysfunction/provide emotional support/refer to social services as ordered to provide counseling regarding altered body image, life-style changes, information on community support groups (e.g., American Cancer Society; Reach for Recovery; prosthetic garments; counseling services).
16. Observe and evaluate alterations in functional status, ADL/refer to rehabilitative services as ordered for evaluation of sensory and motor impairments of affected arm/instruct in prescribed home therapy program (e.g., ROM and strengthening exercises; proper positioning, posture and precautions with self-care; use of adaptive equipment for ADL as needed).

REHABILITATION POTENTIAL

Rehabilitation potential   *excellent   good   fair   guarded   poor*   for   *full partial*   return to a previous level of independent functioning, ability to assume usual patterns of responsibility.

Client's Name _____

Medical Record # _____

ONGOING/DISCHARGE EVALUATION OF TEACHING
The Client Who Has Had a Mastectomy

Teaching Tools:
Printed materials given: _____

Audiovisual aids used: _____

Return Information/Demonstration/Interpretation
_____ Client
_____ Caregiver

OF:	Met	Not Met	Comments
☐ Nature of disease process, surgical procedure.	_____	_____	_____
☐ S&S of complications, actions to take.	_____	_____	_____
☐ Importance of compliance with prescribed treatment regimen.	_____	_____	_____
☐ Importance of well-balanced diet, adequate hydration.	_____	_____	_____
☐ Sodium restrictions with lymphedema.	_____	_____	_____
☐ Medications and administration, purpose and action, side effects.	_____	_____	_____

Client's Name _____

Medical Record # _____

	OF:	**Met**	**Not Met**	**Comments**
☐	Pain control measures.	_____	_____	_____
☐	Wound care management.	_____	_____	_____
☐	Postmastectomy exercise program, balanced rest periods.	_____	_____	_____
☐	Types of breast prostheses.	_____	_____	_____
☐	Skin care measures for arm with lymphedema.	_____	_____	_____
☐	Measures to reduce, treat, and protect arm with lymphedema.	_____	_____	_____
☐	S&S of cellulitis, lymphangitis.	_____	_____	_____
☐	Safety measures with ambulation and ADL.	_____	_____	_____
☐	Monthly self-examination of remaining breast and operative site.	_____	_____	_____
☐	Medic Alert bracelet.	_____	_____	_____

Client's Name _____

Medical Record # _____

OF:	**Met**	**Not Met**	**Comments**
☐ Use of adaptive equipment.	_____	_____	_____

Signature of Home Health Nurse _____

Date _____

■ Cancer Chemotherapy

Chemotherapy is the use of drugs aimed at destroying or suppressing cell development and reproduction of cancer cells with minimal toxicity to healthy cells. These drugs have a systemic effect and may be used in combination with radiation and surgery or used alone as primary treatment for malignant diseases. The various antineoplastic drugs work in different ways to interrupt or alter the cell life cycle. Some affect the cell throughout the entire cell cycle and destroy the cell whether it is in the dividing or resting phase. These are classified as cell-cycle-independent drugs. Other drugs used in chemotherapy affect the cell only during one or more of the phases of the cell life cycle and are classified as cell-cycle-dependent drugs.

Combinations of drugs are designed to complement one another by attacking different cell-cycle phases while avoiding overlapping of toxicities. Also, use of drug combinations allows for the administration of smaller, less toxic doses of each chemotherapeutic agent, which may kill the same number or a greater percentage of cancer cells than is possible with a larger, more toxic single dose.

As well as cancer cells, chemotherapy affects normal cells that have a high rate of cellular proliferation, such as are found in the gastrointestinal mucosa, the oral mucosa, bone marrow, skin, and hair. It is the destruction of these normal cells that results in the toxic effect of antineoplastic drugs. Bone marrow depression is an example of an effect of chemotherapy on rapidly dividing cells. This side effect may seriously compromise the functional capabilities of red blood cells, white blood cells, and platelets and can be life threatening to the client.

Drugs used in chemotherapy generally are classified into five major categories: antimetabolites, alkylating agents, antineoplastic antibiotics, vinca alkaloids, and hormonal therapy. These drugs may be administered by several routes, depending upon the drug and the disease being treated. They include the following: (1) intravenous (most common); (2) intramuscular; (3) oral; (4) intra-arterial; (5) intrathecal (into the cerebrospinal fluid); (6) intracavity (directly into a cavity, e.g., the bladder); and (7) subcutaneous. The focus of this home health-nursing care plan is to assist the client and caregiver in the assessment, treatment, and management of the side effects and toxicities associated with chemotherapy.

POTENTIAL COMPLICATIONS

1. Anemia,
2. thrombocytopenia and hemorrhagic phenomena,
3. leukopenia and infection,
4. fluid and electrolyte imbalances,
5. stomatitis or mucositis,
6. renal toxicity,
7. hyperuricemia,
8. hepatotoxicity,
9. neurotoxicity,
10. cardiotoxicity,

11. alopecia,
12. osteoporosis,
13. extravasation of vesicant drugs with necrosis or phlebitis at IV site,
14. allergic hypersensitivity or anaphylactic reaction,
15. inflammation and fibrosis of lung tissue,
16. ototoxicity,
17. sterility.

TYPES OF CLIENTS/CLINICAL CONDITIONS SEEN BY HOME HEALTH AGENCIES

1. Newly diagnosed with carcinoma: initiation of chemotherapy treatments; instruction in measures to care for and manage central venous catheter, implanted infusion device, implanted infusion pump, or Ommaya reservoir as appropriate; observation, reporting of complications, evaluation of response to treatment.
2. Assessment and instruction in prescribed measures to manage side effects, toxicity of chemotherapy, reporting persistent or unrelieved problems to physician; ongoing assessment of response to chemotherapy.
3. Need for blood studies at specific intervals; changes in ongoing treatment regimen for management of side effects; evaluation of response to changes.
4. Home administration of antineoplastic drugs (drug handling safety that will protect the client, staff, and environment from unnecessary exposure).

RELATED NURSING DIAGNOSIS

Activity Intolerance

related to:
1. Imbalance between oxygen demand and supply as a result of anemia caused by bone marrow depression induced by chemotherapy.
2. Absorption of waste products from rapid destruction of cancerous and normal cells secondary to chemotherapy
3. Poor nutritional status
4. Exhaustion secondary to debilitating side effects of chemotherapy on the body

as seen by:
Extreme fatigue and weakness; abnormal heart and respiratory rate or BP in response to activity; exertional dyspnea; chest pain; dizziness or syncope; changes in normal activity

Airway Clearance, Ineffective

related to:
Pulmonary toxicity:
1. Pneumonitis
2. Pulmonary fibrosis secondary to adverse effects of chemotherapy (e.g., bleomycin, busulfan)

as seen by:
Cough; dyspnea on exertion; shortness of breath; cyanosis; rales, wheezing; ineffective cough; restlessness; irritability; confusion

Anxiety

related to:
1. Lack of knowledge regarding chemotherapy
2. Fear of side effects
3. Altered body image and effect on life-style
4. Knowledge deficit regarding prescribed treatment regimen
5. Fear of death

as seen by:
Verbalization of fears; apprehension; increased tension; facial tension; distress; feelings of increased helplessness; excessive questions regarding home health services or prescribed treatment regimen

Bowel Elimination, Alteration in: Constipation

related to:
1. Effect of antineoplastic drug(s) (e.g., vincristine) on nerve supply to the bowel (paralytic ileus)
2. Inadequate intake of dietary fiber and fluids secondary to dysphagia and anorexia
3. Decreased mobility
4. Bowel obsruction secondary to underlying disease
5. Decreased bowel motility secondary to use of opiates

as seen by:
Straining at stool; c/o of feeling of fullness or pressure in abdomen or rectum; nausea; frequency and amount less than usual pattern; hard, formed stools; abdominal distension

Bowel Elimination, Alteration in: Diarrhea

related to:
1. Irritation and ulceration of rapidly dividing epithelial cells of bowel mucosa secondary to direct stimulation of peristalsis by antineoplastic drugs
2. Fear and anxiety

as seen by:
Loose stools; abdominal pain or cramping; increased frequency of stool; increased bowel sounds

Breathing Pattern, Ineffective

related to:
1. Pulmonary toxicity:
   a. Pneumonitis
   b. Pulmonary fibrosis (e.g., bleomycin, busulfan)
2. Decreased energy or fatigue secondary to anemia, adverse effect of chemotherapy

as seen by:
Changes in breathing; weakness and fatigue; dry cough; cyanosis; tachypnea; shortness of breath; bibasilar fine rales

Cardiac Output, Alteration in: Decreased

related to:
Cardiotoxicity (cardiomyopathy) of specific antineoplastic drugs (e.g., adriamycin, daunomycin)

as seen by:
Fatigue; cold, clammy skin; pale or cyanotic skin; dyspnea; weight gain; swollen ankles; restlessness; decreased peripheral pulses; low BP; variation in pulse rate

Comfort, Alteration in: Pain

related to:
1. Dermatitis, stomatitis, mucositis, perianal and vulvar ulcers, pruritus, abdominal pain secondary to direct effect of antineoplastic drug(s) on rapidly dividing cells of the skin, mucous membranes, and mucosal tissue
2. Local pain secondary to extravasation into tissues surrounding IV site
3. Excoriation of perirectal area secondary to persistent diarrhea, poor hygiene
4. Pain resulting from liver enlargement

as seen by:
Verbalization of pain; facial mask of pain; crying; reluctance to move; oral burning; local inflammation; c/o burning and irritation at the site of drug administration; redness and irritation of perirectal area; pain and tenderness over liver area

Coping, Ineffective Individual

related to:
1. Chemotherapy and side effects (e.g., alopecia)

as seen by:
Verbalization of fears and inability to cope; irritability; insomnia; fatigue;

2. Fear as to effectiveness of chemotherapy
3. Increased dependency on others for care
4. Personality changes caused by drugs

inability to meet basic needs; S&S of grieving; increased emotional lability

Fear

related to:
1. Side effects of chemotherapy, effect on quality of life
2. Uncertainty as to the effectiveness of therapy
3. Dying

as seen by:
Verbalization of feeling of loss of control; increased pulse and respiratory rate; elevated BP; excessive questioning; expressed concern regarding fears

Fluid Volume, Alteration in: Deficit

related to:
1. Dehydration and electrolyte imbalances associated with side effects of chemotherapy (e.g., diarrhea, anorexia)
2. Vomiting secondary to the adverse effects of chemotherapy (e.g., stimulation of the brain's chemoreceptor trigger zone, affecting the vomiting center)

as seen by:
Dry mucous membranes; poor skin turgor; weight loss; low BP; weak, rapid pulse; oliguria; dry skin; lab work indicating electrolyte imbalance and dehydration

Fluid Volume, Alteration in: Excess

related to:
Potential side effects of steroids, androgens, and estrogens

as seen by:
Fluid retention; weight gain

Grieving

related to:
1. Diagnosis of cancer and need for chemotherapy
2. Altered body image
3. Life-style changes
4. Increased dependence on others for care

as seen by:
Sadness; crying; anger; insomnia; depression

Infection, Potential for

related to:
1. Bone marrow depression and depressed immune response system secondary to chemotherapy
2. Debilitated condition secondary to malnutrition and anemic condition
3. Central venous catheter or implanted infusion device; breakdown in body's first line of defense

as seen by:
Malaise; fatigue; elevated temperature and pulse rate; anorexia; skin breakdown; inflammation at intravenous site; sore throat; white patches in mouth; S&S of urinary or respiratory infections; painful, pruritic skin lesions

Injury, Potential for: Increased Risks of Falls and Injuries

related to:
1. Fatigue and weakness secondary to anemia
2. Peripheral neurotoxicity secondary to adverse effects of chemotherapy (e.g., linked with vinca alkaloids)
3. Thrombocytopenia secondary to bone marrow depression

as seen by:
Unsteady gait; c/o severe exhaustion weakness; c/o numbness and tingling of extremities; decreased deep tendon reflexes progressing to foot or wrist drop; decreased sensation of temperature; loss of fine motor control; petechiae of lower extremities; excessive bruising noted following normal daily activities

Knowledge Deficit (Specify)

related to:
1. Prescribed treatment and management of side effects, toxicity caused by chemotherapy
2. Potential complications, S&S to report to home health nurse or physician

as seen by:
Lack of knowledge; inadequate understanding; inability to perform skills necessary to meet health-care needs at home

Mobility, Impaired Physical

related to:
1. Activity intolerance secondary to anemia and poor nutritional status
2. Peripheral neuropathy secondary to direct toxic effect of drugs on nerve cells (e.g., vinca alkaloids)

as seen by:
Weakness and fatigue; loss of deep tendon reflexes, wrist and foot drop; sensory alteration related to paresthesias; gait disturbances; loss of fine motor control, ataxia

3. Cerebellar dysfunction (e.g., floxuridine)
4. Sensory and motor deficits secondary to fluid and electrolyte imbalances
5. Osteoporosis resulting from adverse effect of antineoplastic drugs (e.g., steroids; long-term administration of methotrexate)

Nutrition, Alteration in: Less than Body Requirements

related to:
1. Gastrointestinal disturbances (nausea, vomiting, diarrhea, anorexia) secondary to adverse effects of antineoplastic drugs
2. Taste distortion, stomatitis and mucositis secondary to adverse effects of chemotherapy
3. Anorexia secondary to painful mouth, taste distortion, grieving process and fear
4. Impaired mobility
5. Alteration in gastrointestinal functioning

as seen by:
Body weight 20 percent or more under ideal weight for height, frame, and age; sore, inflamed buccal cavity; c/o nausea and lack of appetite; triceps skin-fold measurement less than normal for build; weakness and fatigue; difficulty swallowing

Oral Mucous Membrane, Alteration in

related to:
1. Bleeding and ulceration of oral mucosa secondary to adverse effects of chemotherapy
2. Diminished response of client to oral flora with predisposition to periodontal disease secondary to altered integrity of oral mucosa
3. Inflammation of oral mucosa caused by inadequate nutritional status and dehydration

as seen by:
Stomatitis; mucositis; erythema; lesions; oral burning and pain; dry mouth; sensitivity to hot, cold, or spicy foods; yellow-white patches of mouth (fungal infection)

Powerlessness, Feelings of

related to:
1. Neoplastic disease requiring chemotherapy

as seen by:
Verbalization of having no control or influence over progress of present

2. Inability to perform ADL
3. Inability to perform role responsibilities

health status, need for chemotherapy; apathy; fear; crying; irritability; depression over physical deterioration

Self-Care Deficit: Feeding, Bathing/Hygiene, Dressing/Grooming, Toileting (Specify)

related to:
1. Activity intolerance secondary to anemia
2. Impaired mobility status
3. Nutritional fluid, and/or electrolyte deficits
4. Prescribed activity restrictions

as seen by:
Inability or decreased ability to participate in daily activities, associated with extreme fatigue and weakness; exertional dyspnea; chest pain; dizziness; motor and sensory deficits; imposed medical restrictions

Self-Concept, Disturbance in

related to:
1. Altered body image (e.g., alopecia, skin pigmentation, nail changes from 5-FU)
2. Low self-esteem
3. Changes in role performance

as seen by:
Increasing dependence on others; signs of grieving; changes in usual patterns of responsibility; self-neglect

Sensory–Perceptual Alteration: Auditory/Visual/Tactile/Taste/Mental Status

related to:
1. Ototoxicity resulting from damage to eighth cranial nerve by antineoplastic drug(s) (e.g., nitrogen mustard, cisplatin)
2. Altered taste distortion (e.g., methotrexate, adriamycin)
3. Sensory alteration related to neuropathies (e.g., vincristine)
4. Invasion of sensory organs by cancer
5. Cerebral hypoxia secondary to anemia
6. Impaired renal function (e.g., asparaginase)
7. Photophobia

as seen by:
Hearing loss, tinnitus; inability to tolerate certain foods; c/o of being able to taste antineoplastic drug; S&S of peripheral neuropathy: decreased sensation, numbness and tingling of extremities, lack of coordination, paresthesias; personality changes, disorientation; apathy; memory loss; decreased level of consciousness, dizziness, and decreased visual acuity with uremia; light sensitivity

Sexual Dysfunction

related to:
1. Adverse effects of certain antineoplastics on ovarian hormone secretion, causing estrogen depletion resulting in premature menopause or amenorrhea, and reduced hormone secretion of the testes, resulting in decreased sperm production (e.g., busulfan)
2. Psychological factors

as seen by:
Verbalization of problem; change of interest in self and others; limitation imposed by illness; therapy; amenorrhea and hot flashes in women; changes in libido; testicular atrophy with gynecomastia and impotence in men

Skin Integrity, Impairment of: Actual/Potential

related to:
1. Abnormal tissue perfusion due to anemia secondary to bone marrow depression
2. Hepatotoxicity secondary to adverse effect of chemotherapy (e.g., methotrexate)
3. Tissue breakdown secondary to inadequate nutritional status; infection; immobilization
4. Tissue damage secondary to extravasation of specific vesicant drugs (e.g., adriamycin, daunomycin)
5. Breakdown in perirectal area secondary to persistent diarrhea
6. Dermal sensitivity to sunlight (e.g., methotrexate)
7. Rash secondary to adverse effect of antineoplastic drugs on skin (e.g., pipobroman)
8. Dry skin secondary to effects of antineoplastic drugs on sebaceous and sweat glands

as seen by:
CBC abnormal; c/o pain and burning at injection site; local abscess at injection site; inflammation; pain; ulceration; necrosis; loss of function; reddened, irritated, tissue breakdown of perirectal area; jaundiced skin; irritation caused by elevated bilirubin

Sleep Pattern Disturbance

related to:
1. Pain and side effects related to chemotherapy
2. High anxiety levels, depression

as seen by:
Frequent yawning; c/o feeling exhausted and not sleeping well; increased irritability; restlessness

Social Isolation

related to:
Cancer and chemotherapy

as seen by:
Expressing feeling of aloneness; sadness; dull affect; feelings of rejection; withdrawn behavior

Urinary Elimination Pattern, Alteration in

related to:
1. Hemorrhagic cystitis secondary to direct irritation of bladder lining by antineoplastic drug(s) (e.g., cyclophosphamide)
2. Renal toxicity caused by damaging effects of antineoplastic drugs on kidney tissue
3. Renal calculi secondary to elevated uric acid levels in the blood. (High cell death releases purines, which convert to uric acid. The uric acid may form obstructive crystals in the kidneys and cause renal parenchymal damage)

as seen by:
S&S of pulmonary congestion; increased serum creatinine and BUN; oliguria; flank pain; hematuria; urinary frequency or urgency; increased BP

LONG-TERM GOAL

To achieve an improved quality of life with optimal physiologic and emotional functioning through control and management of side effects and toxicity of chemotherapy.

SHORT-TERM GOALS

The client on chemotherapy will be able to:

1. Verbalize nature of disease process, purpose and duration of chemotherapy, S&S of complications to report to home health nurse or physician.
2. Demonstrate correct procedure for taking temperature daily or more often as ordered/read a thermometer/record/verbalize importance of not taking a rectal temperature/report elevation to physician.
3. Verbalize knowledge of antineoplastic drug(s) receiving, purpose and action, side effects and toxicity, importance of reporting adverse reactions to physician.
4. Verbalize importance of prescribed, well-balanced, protein- and calorie-enriched diet, increased fluids.
5. Verbalize predisposing factors to decreased oral intake, prescribed measures to improve nutritional status.
6. Verbalize S&S of fluid and electrolyte imbalance with prescribed measures to

treat persistent vomiting and diarrhea, importance of reporting unrelieved problems to physician.

7. Demonstrate correct procedure in measuring and recording daily intake and output.

8. Verbalize importance of taking prescribed nutritional supplements.

9. Verbalize need for/demonstrate correct technique and procedure of prescribed alternative method to provide nutritional support (e.g., enteral or parenteral nutrition).

10. Verbalize importance of reporting excessive weight loss or gain outside parameters set by physician.

11. Demonstrate prescribed pain control measures/report persistent or unrelieved pain to physician.

12. Demonstrate compliance with prescribed medication therapy/identify side effects.

13. Demonstrate compliance with daily skin care program/verbalize importance of reporting S&S of impaired skin integrity, changes in skin pigmentation, and nail changes.

14. Verbalize cause of alopecia, temporary and variable effects, cosmetic management of hair loss.

15. Identify S&S of stomatitis, mucositis, side effect of antineoplastic drugs on GI mucosa, prescribed measures to reduce oral pain, S&S of ulcerations to report to home health nurse or physician.

16. Identify causative factors in alterations in bowel elimination/verbalize understanding of prescribed bowel program, persistent or unrelieved bowel problems to report to home health nurse or physician.

17. Verbalize side effect of antineoplastic drug(s) on tissues, prescribed measures to treat skin impairment of perianal or vulvar area, importance of reporting S&S of infection to home health nurse or physician.

18. Verbalize importance of reporting S&S of hepatotoxicity to physician/demonstrate compliance with prescribed treatment measures.

19. Verbalize side effect of antineoplastic drug(s) on hearing, importance of reporting impaired hearing to physician.

20. Identify S&S of renal toxicity/verbalize knowledge of prescribed treatment measures, importance of reporting excessive weight loss or gain to physician.

21. Verbalize importance of strict compliance with prescribed treatment regimen with elevated serum uric acid levels to reduce risk of urinary calculi formation, complications to report to physician.

22. Verbalize knowledge of S&S to observe with hemorrhagic cystitis, adverse effect of antineoplastic drug on bladder lining, prescribed measures to manage.

23. Verbalize knowledge of S&S of pulmonary toxicity and cardiotoxicity, side effects of antineoplastic drugs, prescribed treatment measures, reporting to physician.

24. Verbalize cause of bleeding tendencies, hemorrhagic precautions, S&S of bleeding to report to home health nurse or physician/demonstrate correct measures to control bleeding.

25. Identify S&S of extravasation at infusion site, prescribed measures to treat, S&S of infection, local necrosis to report to physician.
26. Verbalize understanding of increased susceptibility to infections with bone marrow depression (e.g., side effects and toxicity of chemotherapy)/demonstrate compliance with infection precautions, S&S of infection to report to home health nurse or physician.
27. Identify S&S of anemia and neurotoxicity/demonstrate safety measures to decrease risk of falls and injuries in home environment/report signs of neurologic toxicity to physician.
28. Verbalize S&S of complications of prolonged immobility, S&S to report to home health nurse or physician, prescribed measures to treat, activities to avoid.
29. Demonstrate correct procedure in care and management of central venous catheter, implanted infusion device, implanted infusion pump, or Ommaya reservoir/report complications, S&S of complications and adverse reactions to home health nurse or physician.
30. Verbalize importance of/wear Medic Alert bracelet.
31. Identify risk factors of falls and injuries in home environment/demonstrate safety measures with ambulation and daily activities.
32. Verbalize effects of chemotherapy on functional skills and mobility status/demonstrate ability to perform energy conservation techniques and prescribed exercises to increase and/or maintain function in self-care, ADL, and mobility.
33. Demonstrate effective coping mechanism, setting up of realistic goals, and positive adjustment to altered body image, ability to participate in self-care and daily activities and meet established goals.
34. Explain reasons for sexual changes and appropriate measures to treat, actions to cope.
35. Verbalize purpose of prescribed lab work.

NURSING ACTIONS/TREATMENTS

1. Assess systems of the body/evaluate effects of chemotherapy/identify complications.
2. Assess vital signs/identify trends (e.g., elevated temperature, irregular pulse or tachycardia, hypo- or hypertension).
3. Observe/instruct to take and record oral or axillary temperature daily as ordered, how to read a thermometer, elevation to report to home health nurse or physician.
4. Instruct about nature of disease process/importance of strict compliance with prescribed treatment regimen, purpose and duration of chemotherapy, S&S of complications to report to home health nurse or physician.
5. Assess/instruct about specific antineoplastic drug(s) being received, purpose and action, side effects and toxicity, adverse reactions to report to physician.
6. Assess and evaluate nutritional status (include physical exam, anthropometric measurements, monitoring of biochemical lab determinations)/instruct about

prescribed well-balanced, protein- and calorie-enriched diet, importance of maintaining fluid hydration of 2000 to 4000 ml per day as ordered/obtain dietary consultation as needed.

7. Assess predisposing factors to decreased oral intake/instruct about prescribed measures to improve nutritional intake (e.g., small, frequent meals; antiemetics before meals or as needed; use of artificial saliva; antidiarrheals; good oral hygiene; avoiding highly spiced, gas-forming, difficult-to-chew foods).

8. Assess/instruct about S&S of fluid and electrolyte imbalance with persistant vomiting, diarrhea/monitor and evaluate prescribed lab studies (e.g., electrolyte study results; BUN and serum creatinine levels)/instruct about prescribed measures to treat/report unrelieved problems to physician.

9. Observe/instruct how to measure and record daily intake and output as ordered.

10. Observe/instruct about use of prescribed nutritional supplements.

11. Observe/instruct about prescribed alternative methods to provide nutritional support (e.g., enteral nutrition, parenteral nutrition).

12. Observe and evaluate for weight loss or gain (e.g., steroid or hormonal therapy)/instruct to weigh daily and record as ordered/report weight loss or gain outside parameters set by physician.

13. Assess area and level of pain/instruct about prescribed pain control measures/evaluate for pain relief/report persistent or unrelieved pain to physician.

14. Observe/instruct about prescribed medication therapy, purpose and action, side effects, toxicity/evaluate medication effectiveness.

15. Observe and evaluate understanding of causes of impaired skin integrity, changes in skin pigmentation, and nail changes (usually darkening or transverse ridging)/instruct about prescribed measures to treat/evaluate effectiveness.

16. Observe and evaluate alopecia/instruct about side effects of antineoplastic drug on hair follicles, temporary and variable effects, cosmetic management of hair loss.

17. Observe and evaluate for S&S of stomatitis, mucositis/instruct about direct effect of antineoplastic drugs on cells of GI mucosa, areas of involvement (e.g., eating, speech, ability to rest), prescribed measures to reduce oral pain (e.g., well-fitting dentures; good oral hygiene; avoiding excessively hot or cold foods, spicy foods, hard-bristled toothbrush, toothpicks), S&S of ulcerations to report to home health nurse or physician.

18. Assess and evaluate alteration in bowel elimination (constipation, diarrhea)/instruct about effect of specific antineoplastic drug(s) on bowel functioning, prescribed bowel program (e.g., use of antidiarrheals, laxatives and stool softeners), increase or decrease of dietary fiber as ordered, persistent or unrelieved bowel problems to report to home health nurse or physician.

19. Assess and evaluate S&S of perianal or vulvar inflammation or breakdown/instruct about adverse effect of antineoplastic drugs on skin and mucosal tissue, prescribed measures to treat (e.g., sitz baths; prescribed topical anesthetics, ointments)/S&S of infection to report to home health nurse or physician.

20. Assess/instruct about S&S of hepatotoxicity (e.g., pain or tenderness over liver area, jaundice, pruritus, decreasing level of consciousness)/monitor liver enzymes/report to physician/instruct as to effect of specific antineoplastic drugs on liver, prescribed treatment measures.

21. Assess and evaluate for ototoxicity/instruct about effect of specific antineoplastic drugs on eighth cranial nerve, importance of reporting to physician.

22. Assess/instruct on S&S of renal toxicity/monitor for increasing BUN and serum creatinine levels, daily weights, intake and output/instruct about prescribed diet, restrictions of diet and fluid intake, medications/report changes in urinary pattern, color, and excretion, weight gain or loss outside parameters set by physician.

23. Assess/instruct about prescribed measures to reduce risk of urinary calculi formation with elevated serum uric acid levels (e.g., increased fluids to 2000 to 4000 ml per day as ordered), prescribed diet and dietary restriction (e.g., avoid purines)/instruct about prescribed medications, increased activity levels as tolerated, urine testing to determine degree of acidity or alkalinity of urine, S&S of complications to report to home health nurse or physician.

24. Assess/instruct about S&S to observe for with hemorrhagic cystitis, side effect of specific antineoplastic drug on bladder lining, increasing fluids 2000 to 4000 ml per day as ordered, emptying bladder at least every four hours day and night for two days after chemotherapy as ordered, avoiding substances irritating to the bladder (e.g., caffeine, spicy foods, alcohol).

25. Assess/instruct about S&S of pulmonary toxicity, cardiotoxicity, adverse effects of specific antineoplastic drugs, importance of reporting to physician/instruct about treatment measures as ordered.

26. Assess/instruct about S&S of bleeding with thrombocytopenia (e.g., excessive bruising, nosebleeds, black, tarry stools, bleeding gums)/instruct about hemorrhage precautions (e.g., avoiding trauma with ambulatory and daily activities in the home; avoiding straining, enemas, use of rectal thermometers, use of hard-bristled toothbrush, douches, toothpicks, aspirin or aspirin-containing products), measures to control bleeding (e.g., applying firm manual pressure for ten minutes to bleeding area), reporting to home health nurse or physician.

27. Assess/instruct about S&S of extravasation at infusion site/instruct about prescribed measures to treat, S&S of infection, local necrosis to report to home health nurse or physician.

28. Assess/instruct about S&S of infection, increased susceptibility with bone marrow depression and depressed immune response system/educate about infection precautions (e.g., meticulous oral and body hygiene; adequate nutrition and hydration; sterile or clean technique with procedures as indicated), correct hand-washing technique, avoiding exposure to infection and crowds, washing perianal area well after each BM, reporting S&S of infection to home health nurse or physician.

29. Assess for S&S related to anemia/instruct about safety measures to decrease risk factors of falls and injuries in home environment (e.g., avoiding: sharp

objects, touching hot objects, walking unassisted when gait unsteady), importance of reporting signs of neurologic toxicity to physician (e.g., numbness in hands and feet, lack of coordination).

30. Observe ability to perform self-care and daily activities/evaluate factors that affect activity tolerance (e.g., anemia, malnutrition, exhaustion caused by side effects of chemotherapy/instruct about balanced rest and activity levels, use of self-help devices as needed.

31. Assess and evaluate sexual concerns (e.g., changes in sexual desire, responsiveness, and function)/instruct about reason for sexual changes, appropriate measures to treat or actions to cope (e.g., vaginal lubricant, sexual counseling).

32. Assess systems of the body for S&S of complications related to immobilization, report to home health nurse or physician/instruct about prescribed measures to treat, activities to avoid.

33. Observe/instruct about increased risk factors for falls and injuries in home environment (e.g., severe exhaustion, numbness and tingling of extremities, photophobia), strict safety measures with ambulation and daily activities.

34. Assess/instruct, according to discharge protocol from hospital about physician-prescribed care and management of central venous catheter, implanted infusion device, implanted infusion pump, or Ommaya reservoir (a spongelike plate implanted in the skull that provides direct access to a specific area of the brain), S&S of complications, adverse reactions to report to home health nurse or physician (e.g., redness, pain, unusual drainage at insertion site, fever, headache, stiff neck).

35. Monitor/instruct about purpose of prescribed lab work at specific intervals.

36. Observe/instruct about importance of wearing Medic Alert bracelet.

37. Assess and evaluate effect of disease process and chemotherapy on functional skills and mobility status, toleration of performance of daily activities/refer to rehabilitative services to establish home therapy program, instruct in energy conservation techniques and prescribed exercises to increase and/or maintain function in self-care and ADL and mobility.

38. Assess stage of adaptation, coping mechanisms/provide emotional support/encourage verbalization of feelings/assist with setting realistic goals, meeting spiritual needs/refer to social services to assist with adjustment to altered body image, prescribed treatment regimen/provide information regarding community support groups (e.g., American Cancer Society, National Leukemia Association; counseling services, community support groups).

REHABILITATION POTENTIAL

Rehabilitation potential *excellent good fair guarded poor* for *full partial* return to maximal self-management in personal and therapeutic self-care activities through treatment and control of side effects of chemotherapy.

Client's Name _____

Medical Record # _____

ONGOING/DISCHARGE EVALUATION OF TEACHING
The Client Receiving Chemotherapy

Teaching Tools:
Printed materials given: _____

Audiovisual aids used: _____

Return Information/Demonstration/Interpretation
_____ Client
_____ Caregiver

	OF:	Met	Not Met	Comments
☐	Nature of disease process.	_____	_____	_____
☐	Purpose and duration of chemotherapy.	_____	_____	_____
☐	Antineoplastic drug(s) being received, purpose and action, side effects and toxicity.	_____	_____	_____
☐	S&S of complications, actions to take.	_____	_____	_____
☐	Importance of strict compliance with prescribed treatment regimen.	_____	_____	_____
☐	How to take and record a temperature (oral or axillary),			

Client's Name _____

Medical Record # _____

OF:	**Met**	**Not Met**	**Comments**
read a thermometer.	_____	_____	_____
☐ Well-balanced, protein- and calorie-enriched diet, increased fluids.	_____	_____	_____
☐ S&S of fluid and electrolyte imbalance with persistent vomiting and diarrhea.	_____	_____	_____
☐ Predisposing factors in decreased oral intake; measures to improve nutritional status.	_____	_____	_____
☐ Intake and output.	_____	_____	_____
☐ Nutritional supplements.	_____	_____	_____
☐ Alternative method to provide nutritional support (enteral nutrition or parenteral nutrition).	_____	_____	_____
☐ Pain control measures.	_____	_____	_____

Client's Name ⸻⸻⸻⸻⸻⸻

Medical Record # ⸻⸻⸻⸻⸻⸻

	OF:	**Met**	**Not Met**	**Comments**
☐	Medications and administration, purpose and action, side effects.	⸻	⸻	⸻⸻⸻
☐	Daily skin care program; S&S of impaired skin integrity, infection to report to home health nurse or physician.	⸻	⸻	⸻⸻⸻
☐	Alopecia, temporary and variable effects cosmetic management.	⸻	⸻	⸻⸻⸻
☐	Weighing and recording of weights as ordered; reporting gain or loss outside parameters set by physician.	⸻	⸻	⸻⸻⸻
☐	Measures to reduce oral pain with stomatitis, mucositis/S&S of ulcerations to report to home health nurse or physician.	⸻	⸻	⸻⸻⸻
☐	Alterations in bowel elimination; bowel program.	⸻	⸻	⸻⸻⸻

Client's Name _____

Medical Record # _____

OF:	Met	Not Met	Comments
☐ Measures to treat skin impairment of perianal or vulvar area.	_____	_____	_____
☐ S&S of renal toxicity, prescribed treatment measures.	_____	_____	_____
☐ S&S of hemorrhagic cystitis; prescribed measures to manage.	_____	_____	_____
☐ Measures to reduce risk of urinary calculi.	_____	_____	_____
☐ S&S of pulmonary toxicity; importance of reporting to physician; prescribed treatment measures.	_____	_____	_____
☐ S&S of cardiotoxicity; importance of reporting to physician; prescribed treatment measures.	_____	_____	_____
☐ Bleeding tendencies;			

Client's Name _____

Medical Record # _____

OF:	**Met**	**Not Met**	**Comments**
hemorrhage precautions; measures to control bleeding.	_____	_____	_____
☐ S&S of anemia and neurotoxicity/ safety measures to reduce risk of injuries.	_____	_____	_____
☐ Hepatotoxicity, prescribed treatment measures.	_____	_____	_____
☐ Increased susceptibility to infections with bone marrow depression; infection precautions; S&S to report to home health nurse or physician.	_____	_____	_____
☐ Ototoxicity, importance of reporting to physician.	_____	_____	_____
☐ Balanced rest and activity levels.	_____	_____	_____
☐ Energy-conservation techniques.	_____	_____	_____
☐ Exercise program.	_____	_____	_____

Client's Name _____

Medical Record # _____

OF:	Met	Not Met	Comments
☐ S&S of extravasation, prescribed treatment measures.	_____	_____	_____
☐ Care and management of central venous catheter, implanted infusion device, implanted infusion pump, or Ommaya reservoir.	_____	_____	_____
☐ Medic Alert bracelet.	_____	_____	_____
☐ Effect of kemotherapy on functional skills and mobility.	_____	_____	_____
☐ Measures to manage sexual changes.	_____	_____	_____
☐ Purpose of prescribed lab work.	_____	_____	_____
☐ Risk factors for falls and injuries; safety measures with ambulation and daily activities.	_____	_____	_____

☐ Complications of prolonged immobility;

Client's Name _____

Medical Record #_____

OF: **Met**   **Not Met**   **Comments**
measures to
treat; activities
to avoid.   _____   _____   _____

Signature of Home Health Nurse _____

Date _____

■ Cancer Radiation Therapy

Radiation therapy is currently being used as an important tool in the treatment of malignant disease in approximately one half of all persons with cancer in the United States. Radiation therapy is the use of ionizing radiation (radiation capable of producing ions to damage or destroy malignant cells). Ionizing radiation destroys the cells' ability to reproduce by damaging the cells' DNA. Ionizing radiation consists of two types: electromagnetic (gamma rays or x-rays) or particulate radiation (alpha or beta particles, neutrons). Two modes of treatment can be used: external and internal. With external radiation the ionizing radiation is artificially produced via external beam therapy, using machines or nuclear reactors. With internal radiation, the ionizing radiation that is spontaneously generated by radioactive elements (isotopes) is placed intracavitarily or interstitially.

The goal of radiation therapy is to destroy or deter the proliferation of tumor cells with minimal damage to the surrounding tissue. However, normal cells have a greater ability to repair the DNA damage from irradiation than cancer cells. A radiosensitive tumor is one that is destroyed by irradiation in doses that are well tolerated by tissues in the surrounding area. Sensitivity of tumor cells to radiation varies according to the tumor type. For example, radiosensitivity is greater in cells that are oxygenated (many tumors contain hypoxic cells); cells that rapidly proliferate; and in those cells undergoing mitosis.

Other factors that influence the success of radiation therapy are the location and size of the tumor, the extent of spread, the client's immune and general health status. The very young and the very old have also been found to be more susceptible to the side effects and toxicities of radiation therapy. Local reactions are generally related to the field of treatment (e.g., erythema, edema, and irritation of the area exposed to radiation). Examples of systemic side effects include weakness, fatigue, and GI upset. Radiation therapy may be used as an adjunct to surgery or chemotherapy, as the primary form of treatment, or for palliation of symptoms. The side effects or toxicity of external radiation result from the adverse effect of radiation treatment on normal cells. Radiation exposure alters the cell's capacity to divide and can destroy the cells of the body within a short time, or cellular destruction can occur after a few days, weeks, or months, depending on the type of cell and when the cell attempts division.

The focus of this home health care plan is the care and management of the client receiving external radiation therapy.

POTENTIAL COMPLICATIONS

1. Anemia,
2. thrombocytopenia and hemorrhagic phenomena,
3. leukopenia and infection,
4. fluid and electrolyte imbalances,
5. stomatis or esophagitis,
6. pathologic fractures,
7. radiation sickness,
8. radiation pneumonitis,

9. radiation-induced skin reactions,
10. radiation cystitis,
11. renal calculi,
12. dental caries or periodontal disease,
13. radiation-induced pericarditis.

TYPES OF CLIENTS/CLINICAL CONDITIONS SEEN BY HOME HEALTH AGENCIES

1. Newly diagnosed with carcinoma, initiation of radiation therapy treatments: observation and reporting of complications, instruction and supervision in prescribed measures to manage side effects and toxicity, evaluation of response to treatment.
2. Complications of radiation therapy: changes in prescribed treatment regimen, instruction, supervision, and evaluation of the client's response to new medications, treatments, and ability to participate in self-care and daily activities.

RELATED NURSING DIAGNOSIS

Activity Intolerance

related to:
1. Imbalance between oxygen demand and supply as a result of anemia caused by bone marrow depression (side effect of radiation therapy)
2. Absorption of waste products from rapid destruction of cancerous and normal cells secondary to radiation therapy
3. Poor nutritional status
4. Exhaustion secondary to debilitating side effects of radiation therapy on systems of the body

as seen by:
Extreme fatigue and weakness; abnormal heart and respiratory rate or BP in response to activity; dizziness; syncope; chest pain; exertional dyspnea

Airway Clearance, Ineffective

related to:
Pulmonary toxicity:
1. Pneumonitis
2. Pulmonary fibrosis secondary to radiation treatments to pulmonary system

as seen by:
Cough; dyspnea on exertion; shortness of breath; cyanosis; rales; wheezing; fatigue

Anxiety

related to:
1. Lack of knowledge regarding radiation therapy
2. Fear of side effects
3. Knowledge deficit regarding prescribed treatment regimen
4. Altered body image
5. Life-style changes
6. Fear of death

as seen by:
Verbalization of fears; apprehension; increased tension; facial tension; distress; feeling of increased helplessness; excessive questions regarding home health services, and being able to follow prescribed treatment regimen

Bowel Elimination, Alteration in: Diarrhea

related to:
1. Increased peristalsis secondary to irritability and ulceration of epithelial cells of bowel mucosa as a result of abdominal or pelvic irradiation
2. Fear and anxiety

as seen by:
Frequent, loose stools, abdominal pain and cramping

Breathing Pattern, Ineffective

related to:
1. Pulmonary toxicity:
   a. Pneumonitis
   b. Pulmonary fibrosis secondary to radiation treatments to pulmonary system
2. Decreased energy or fatigue secondary to anemia

as seen by:
Changes in breathing; weakness and fatigue; cough; tachypnea; shortness of breath

Cardiac Output, Alteration in: Decreased

related to:
Radiation-induced pericarditis secondary to mediastinal irradiation

as seen by:
Auscultation of friction rub; chest pain; dyspnea; fever; pulse irregularities

Comfort, Alteration in: Pain

related to:
1. Radiation-induced skin reactions
2. Peripheral neuritis secondary to

as seen by:
Verbalization of pain; irritation and blisters; facial mask of pain;

high doses of external-beam
radiation therapy
3. Oral or esophageal pain secondary
to irradiation of mouth and
oropharynx
4. Excoriation of perirectal area
secondary to persistent diarrhea and
poor hygiene
5. Headache secondary to swelling of
cranial tissue with brain irradiation

guarding of irradiated area; crying;
reluctance to move; oral burning;
local inflammation

Communication, Impaired Verbal

related to:
Stomatitis, mucositis of the
oropharynx secondary to radiation of
the head and neck

as seen by:
Dry lips and mouth; c/o pain and
burning of mouth and pharynx;
bleeding; ulcerations; hoarseness;
c/o headache, pain

Coping, Ineffective Individual

related to:
1. Radiation therapy, effect on life-
style
2. Depression secondary to side
effects (e.g., alopecia)
3. Fear as to effectiveness of therapy
4. Increased dependency on others for
care

as seen by:
Verbalization of fears and inability to
cope; irritability; insomnia; fatigue;
inability to meet basic needs; S&S
of grieving

Fear

related to:
1. Side effects of radiation therapy,
effect on quality of life
2. Uncertainty as to the effectiveness
of therapy
3. Dying

as seen by:
Verbalization of feeling loss of
control; increased pulse and
respiratory rate; elevated BP;
excessive questioning; expressed
concern regarding fears

Fluid Volume Deficit

related to:
Dehydration and electrolyte imbalances
associated with adverse effects of

as seen by:
Poor skin turgor; weight loss; low BP;
weak, rapid pulse; oliguria; dry

radiation therapy (e.g., persistent vomiting, diarrhea, anorexia secondary to effects of irradiation of the brain, mediastinum, stomach, abdominal or pelvic areas)

skin; lab work indicating abnormal electrolytes; blood or mucus in the stools; cramping and pain

Fluid Volume, Alteration in: Excess

related to:
Damage to lymph nodes of arms or legs

as seen by:
Edema of arms and legs; weight gain

Grieving

related to:
1. Diagnosis of cancer and need for radiation therapy
2. Altered body image
3. Life-style changes
4. Increased dependency on others

as seen by:
Sadness; crying; anger; insomnia; depression

Infection: Potential for

related to:
1. Bone marrow depression and depressed immune response system secondary to radiation therapy
2. Debilitated condition secondary to malnutrition and anemic condition
3. Fissuring and infection of dry skin secondary to impaired functioning of sweat glands
4. Perforation and abscess formation secondary to impaired circulation to small bowel caused by radiation therapy

as seen by:
Malaise, fatigue, elevated temperature and pulse rate, anorexia; skin breakdown; sore throat; yellow-white patches in mouth; S&S of urinary or respiratory infections; perirectal or vaginal infections; localized edema or pain; dental infection

Injury, Potential for: Increased Risks of Falls and Injuries

related to:
Fatigue and weakness secondary to anemia, fluid and electrolyte imbalances, debilitated condition

as seen by:
C/o severe exhaustion with unsteady gait; c/o weakness

Knowledge Deficit (Specify)

related to:
1. Prescribed treatment and management of side effects, toxicity caused by radiation therapy
2. Potential complications, S&S to report to home health nurse or physician

as seen by:
Lack of knowledge; inadequate understanding; inability to perform skills necessary to meet health-care needs at home

Mobility, Impaired Physical

related to:
1. Activity intolerance secondary to anemia and poor nutritional status
2. Pathologic fractures secondary to brittle and poorly oxygenated bones as a result of high doses of external-beam radiation
3. Sensory and motor deficits secondary to fluid and electrolyte imbalances
4. Pain and discomfort

as seen by:
Weakness and fatigue; inability to move purposefully within home environment; reluctance to attempt movement; unsteady gait; decreased muscle strength, control, and/or endurance

Nutrition, Alteration in: Less than Body Requirements

related to:
1. Nausea and vomiting; diarrhea, anorexia secondary to adverse effects of radiation therapy
2. Taste distortion or stomatitis and esophagitis secondary to adverse effects of radiation therapy
3. Depression and anxiety

as seen by:
Body weight 20 percent or more under ideal weight for height, frame, and age; sore, inflamed buccal cavity; c/o nausea and lack of appetite; triceps skin-fold measurement less than normal for build; weakness and fatigue; difficulty swallowing

Oral Mucous Membrane, Alteration in

related to:
1. Inflammation of oral mucosa caused by inadequate nutritional status, dehydration
2. Damage to epithelial cells of the oral mucosa caused by adverse effects of radiation therapy on the oral cavity

as seen by:
Stomatitis; mucositis; erythema; lesions; oral burning; sensitivity to hot, cold, or spicy foods; yellow-white patches of mouth (fungal infection); decrease in amount of saliva produced; periodontal disease

3. Decreased salivary gland activity secondary to irradiation of salivary glands

Powerlessness, Feelings of

related to:
Neoplastic disease requiring radiation therapy

as seen by:
Verbalization of having no control or influence over progress of present health status, need for radiation therapy; apathy; fear; crying; irritability; depression over physical deterioration

Self-Care Deficit: Feeding, Bathing/Hygiene, Dressing/Grooming, Toileting (Specify)

related to:
1. Activity intolerance
2. Impaired mobility status
3. Nutritional, fluid, and/or electrolyte deficits
4. Prescribed activity restrictions

as seen by:
Inability or decreased ability to participate in daily activities, associated with extreme fatigue and weakness; exertional dyspnea; chest pain; dizziness; motor and sensory deficits; imposed medical restrictions

Self-Concept, Disturbance in

related to:
1. Altered body image
2. Low self-esteem
3. Changes in role performance

as seen by:
Increasing dependence on others; signs of grieving; changing usual patterns of responsibility; self-neglect

Sensory–Perceptual Alteration: Taste/Visual/Auditory

related to:
1. Taste distortion secondary to damage to epithelial cells of the oral mucosa caused by adverse effects of radiation therapy on oral cavity
2. Conjunctivitis secondary to radiation of the head
3. Otitis secondary to irradiation of the ear area

as seen by:
Inability to tolerate certain foods; bloodshot or burning eyes; tinnitus; earache

Sexual Dysfunction

related to:

1. Temporary or permanent impotence related to possible injury to nerves, blood vessels, and testes if included in the treatment field
2. Alteration in hormonal balance secondary to radiation therapy to gonads
3. Effects of weakness and fatigue, anxiety, fears, and depression on sexual functioning
4. Dryness of vaginal mucosa secondary to direct exposure of the reproductive organs in the treatment field

as seen by:

Verbalization of problem; change of interest in self and others, limitation imposed by illness, therapy; verbalized S&S of sexual dysfunction (e.g., dyspareumia; impotence); menstrual change

Skin Integrity, Impairment of: Actual/Potential

related to:

1. Tissue hypoxia caused by anemia secondary to bone marrow depression
2. Skin reactions secondary to irradiated areas (three stages of skin impairment are (1) erythema; (2) dry disquamation with flaking or moist disquamation; (3) large, open, draining purulent lesions)
   a. Alopecia secondary to destruction of hair follicles
   b. Inhibition or destruction of sweat glands
3. Tissue breakdown secondary to inadequate nutritional status, infection, immobilization, tissue edema secondary to radiation exposure or pruritus over the irradiated field
4. Breakdown in perirectal area secondary to persistent diarrhea

as seen by:

Acute radiation-induced skin reactions: reddening, flaking, scaling, itching, pain, weeping, sloughing, and alopecia; inflammation; pain; ulceration; necrosis; loss of function; reddening, irritation, tissue breakdown of perirectal area; excessive scratching

Sleep Pattern Disturbance

related to:

1. Pain, side effects related to

as seen by:

Frequent yawning; c/o feeling

radiation therapy
2. High anxiety levels, depression

exhausted and not sleeping well;
increased irritability; restlessness

Social Isolation

related to:
Cancer and radiation therapy

as seen by:
Expressing feeling of aloneness;
sadness; dull affect; feelings of
rejection; withdrawal

Tissue Integrity, Impaired

related to:
1. Cancer
2. Radiation therapy

as seen by:
Warmth; redness; dry scaling; pruritus;
moistness; blistering; ulceration

Urinary Elimination Pattern, Alteration in

related to:
1. Hemorrhagic cystitis secondary to
   pelvic irradiation
2. Renal failure secondary to high-
   dose radiation on kidney tissue (end
   result of radiation nephritis and
   chronic hemorrhagic cystitis)
3. Renal calculi secondary to elevated
   uric acid levels in the blood. (High
   cell death releases purines, which
   convert to uric acid. The uric acid
   may form obstructive crystals in the
   kidneys and cause renal
   parenchymal damage.)

as seen by:
Increased serum creatinine and BUN;
dysuria; oliguria; flank pain;
hematuria; nausea and vomiting;
urinary frequency or urgency;
increased BP

LONG-TERM GOAL

To achieve an improved quality of life with optimal physiologic and emotional functioning through control and management of side effects and toxicity of radiation therapy.

SHORT-TERM GOAL

The client receiving radiation therapy will be able to:

1. Demonstrate correct procedure to take and record temperature daily or more

often as needed/read a thermometer/verbalize importance of not taking a rectal temperature/report elevation to physician.

2. Verbalize nature of disease process, purpose and duration of radiation therapy, S&S of complications to report to home health nurse or physician.

3. Verbalize importance of prescribed well-balanced, protein- and calorie-enriched diet, increased fluids.

4. Identify predisposing factors in decreased oral intake, prescribed measures to improve nutritional status.

5. Verbalize S&S of fluid and electrolyte imbalance with persistent vomiting and diarrhea, prescribed measures to treat, importance of reporting unrelieved problems to physician.

6. Demonstrate correct procedure in measuring and recording daily intake and output.

7. Verbalize need for/demonstrate correct technique and procedures in prescribed alternative measures to provide nutritional support (e.g., enteral nutrition, parenteral nutrition).

8. Verbalize importance of reporting weight loss or gain outside parameters set by physician.

9. Demonstrate prescribed pain control measures, report persistent or unrelieved pain to physician.

10. Demonstrate compliance with prescribed medication therapy/identify side effects.

11. Identify predisposing factors in impaired skin integrity/demonstrate ability to perform daily skin care program, activities to avoid breakdown, S&S of infection to report to home health nurse or physician.

12. Verbalize cause of alopecia, temporary and variable effects, cosmetic management of hair loss.

13. Demonstrate prescribed measures to promote healing and enhance comfort of irradiated skin areas, S&S of infection to report to home health nurse or physician.

14. Demonstrate prescribed measures to reduce pain with stomatitis and esophagitis, verbalize knowledge of S&S of ulcerations or infection to report to home health nurse or physician.

15. Identify causative factors of alterations in bowel elimination (diarrhea)/demonstrate compliance with prescribed bowel program/report persistent or unrelieved bowel problems to physician.

16. Verbalize importance of strict compliance with prescribed treatment regimen with elevated serum uric acid levels, complications to report to physician.

17. Verbalize S&S of hemorrhagic cystitis to report to home health nurse or physician/demonstrate compliance with prescribed measures to treat.

18. Verbalize cause of bleeding tendencies, knowledge of hemorrhagic precautions, S&S of bleeding to report to home health nurse or physician/demonstrate correct measures to control bleeding.

19. Verbalize factors that affect activity tolerance/demonstrate balanced rest and activity levels, energy conservation techniques.

20. Verbalize S&S of pulmonary toxicity, cardiotoxicity/demonstrate compliance with prescribed measures to treat/report continued or unrelieved problems to physician.
21. Verbalize side effects of radiation therapy to head and neck on teeth and gums/demonstrate measures to treat/report S&S of dental infection or gum ulcerations to home health nurse or physician.
22. Verbalize understanding of increased susceptibility to infections with bone marrow depression, S&S to report to home health nurse or physician/demonstrate compliance with infection precautions.
23. Identify risk factors of falls and injuries in home environment/demonstrate safety measures with ambulation and daily activities.
24. Verbalize complications of prolonged immobility, S&S to report to home health nurse or physician, prescribed measures to treat, activities to avoid.
25. Verbalize importance of/wear Medic Alert bracelet.
26. Verbalize knowledge of effects of radiation therapy on sexual functioning and prescribed measures to treat.
27. Demonstrate effective coping mechanisms and positive adjustment to management of side effects, altered body image, changes in life-style, meeting realistic goals.
28. Verbalize purpose of prescribed lab work.

NURSING ACTIONS/TREATMENTS

1. Assess systems of the body for side effects related to radiation therapy/identify complications.
2. Assess vital signs/identify trends (e.g., elevated temperature, rapid pulse and respiratory rate, hypo- or hypertension).
3. Observe/instruct to take (oral or axillary) temperature daily as ordered or more often as needed, how to read a thermometer and record, elevation to report to physician.
4. Instruct as to nature of disease process, purpose of radiation therapy, importance of strict compliance with prescribed treatment regimen, planned radiation therapy schedule, S&S of complications to report to home health nurse or physician.
5. Assess and evaluate nutritional status (include physical exam, anthropometric measurements, monitoring biochemical lab determinations)/instruct about prescribed well-balanced protein- and calorie-enriched diet, importance of fluid hydration of 2000 to 4000 ml per day as ordered/obtain dietary consultation as needed.
6. Assess and evaluate predisposing factors in decreased oral intake/instruct about prescribed measures to improve nutritional status (e.g., small, frequent meals; antiemetics before meals or as needed; semisoft or pureed foods; use of artificial saliva, good oral hygiene, flavorings and spices to client's taste, vitamin and mineral nutritional supplements; avoiding highly spiced, gas-forming, difficult-to-chew foods).

7. Observe/instruct about S&S of fluid and electrolyte imbalance with persistent vomiting or diarrhea/monitor electrolyte study results and other prescribed lab studies/instruct about prescribed measures to treat/report persistent or unrelieved problems to physician.

8. Observe/instruct how to measure and record daily intake and output as ordered.

9. Observe/instruct about prescribed alternative methods to provide nutritional support (e.g., enteral nutrition, parenteral nutrition).

10. Assess and evaluate for weight loss or weight gain/instruct to weigh daily and record as ordered/report weight loss or gain outside parameters set by physician.

11. Assess area and level of pain, factors that aggravate or alleviate, prescribed pain control measures (e.g., good oral hygiene, avoiding substances that irritate stomatitis or esophagitis, skin care measures for pruritus, perianal care with diarrhea, use of prescribed analgesics)/report persistent or unrelieved pain to physician.

12. Observe/instruct about prescribed medication therapy, purpose and action, side effects, toxicity/evaluate medication effectiveness.

13. Assess and evaluate skin integrity, predisposing factors to breakdown (e.g., prolonged immobility, pruritus, persistent diarrhea, poor nutritional status)/instruct about daily skin care program as prescribed, activities to avoid, S&S of infection to report to home health nurse or physician.

14. Assess factors contributing to hair loss (e.g., radiation treatment, hormonal changes, protein malnutrition)/instruct that effects usually temporary and variable, about measures to cope with altered body image (e.g., hairpiece, wig).

15. Assess and evaluate irradiated skin areas for impairment of skin integrity and sweat gland destruction/instruct about prescribed measures to promote healing, enhance comfort (e.g., avoiding rubbing treatment area; avoiding constrictive clothing, temperature extremes, tape, lotions or cosmetics, emollient-based lotions with sweat gland destruction, shaving area, lying on areas for prolonged periods of time; exposure to sun)/instruct about washing gently as prescribed, use of mild lubricants, antiseptics, steroid creams, topical antibiotics for treatment of skin reactions as ordered, importance of not removing treatment markings, S&S of infection to report to home health nurse or physician.

16. Assess and evaluate for S&S of stomatitis or esophagitis, dry mouth, effect on eating, speech, ability to rest/instruct about good oral hygiene, prescribed measures to reduce pain (e.g., use of artificial saliva; mouthwashes; prescribed medications to reduce pain with eating and swallowing; soft toothbrush; well-fitting dentures; avoiding irritating foods and fluids), S&S of infection to report to home health nurse or physician.

17. Assess alterations in bowel elimination diarrhea/instruct about causative factors (e.g., abdominal or pelvic irradiation, poor nutritional status)/instruct about prescribed bowel program (e.g., use of antidiarrheals, avoiding poorly digested and irritating food and fluids)/evaluate effectiveness of bowel program/report persistent or unrelieved bowel problems to physician.

18. Assess/instruct about prescribed measures to reduce risk of urinary calculi

formation with elevated serum uric acid levels (e.g., minimum intake of fluids of 2000 to 4000 ml per day as ordered, prescribed diet and dietary restrictions (e.g., avoiding purines)/instruct about medications as ordered (e.g., allupurinol to reduce purine metabolism alkinization of urine when indicated), increased activity levels as tolerated, urine testing to determine degree of acidity or alkalinity of urine, reporting to physician.

19. Assess/instruct about S&S of hemorrhagic cystitis, adverse effects of radiation therapy to pelvic area/instruct about minimum intake of fluids as ordered: 2000 to 4000 ml per day, avoiding substances irritating to the bladder (e.g., caffeine, spicy foods, alcohol), prescribed treatment measures, reporting continued bleeding to physician.

20. Assess/instruct about S&S of bleeding with thrombocytopenia (e.g., excessive bruising, nosebleeds, black, tarry stools, bleeding gums), hemorrhage precautions (e.g., avoiding trauma with ambulatory and daily activities in the home, avoiding straining, enemas, rectal thermometer, use of hard-bristled toothbrush, douches, toothpicks, aspirin or aspirin-containing products), measures to control bleeding (e.g., applying firm manual pressure to bleeding area for ten minutes), reporting to physician.

21. Observe ability to perform self-care and daily activities/evaluate factors that affect activity tolerance (e.g., anemia, malnutrition, exhaustion caused by side effects of radiation therapy)/instruct about balanced rest and activity levels, energy conservation techniques, use of self-help devices as needed.

22. Assess/instruct about S&S of pulmonary toxicity, cardiotoxicity, adverse effects of radiation therapy to the pulmonary system and heart/instruct about importance of reporting to physician/educate about treatment measures as ordered.

23. Assess and evaluate oral cavity for periodontal disease, excessive tooth decay, dental infection (side effect of radiation therapy to head and neck)/instruct about good oral hygiene, use of a fluoridated toothpaste, soft toothbrush, prescribed mouth rinses/report S&S of dental infection or gum ulcerations to physician.

24. Assess/instruct about S&S of infection (increased susceptibility with bone marrow depression), infection precautions (e.g., meticulous oral and body hygiene, sterile or clean technique with procedures as indicated, correct handwashing technique, adequate nutrition and hydration, avoiding exposure to infection and crowds, washing perianal area well after each BM)/report S&S of infection to home health nurse or physician.

25. Observe/instruct about increased risk factors for falls and injuries in home environment (e.g., severe exhaustion with unsteady gait; conjunctivitis; otitis media)/instruct about safety measures with ambulation and daily activities.

26. Assess systems of the body for S&S of complications related to immobilization/report to home health nurse or physician/instruct about prescribed measures to treat, activities to avoid.

27. Observe/instruct about importance of wearing Medic Alert bracelet.

28. Assess for S&S of sexual dysfunction (e.g., verbalization of inability to engage

in sexual functioning, inability to express sexual concerns and show feelings to significant other)/instruct about effects of radiation therapy on sexual functioning and prescribed measures to treat (e.g., dyspareumia and use of a water-based lubricant for dry vaginal mucosa; hormonal replacement)/encourage to verbalize feelings and discuss sexual changes/obtain counseling services as ordered.

29. Assess effect of disease process and radiation therapy on functional skills and mobility status, tolerance to perform daily activities/refer to rehabilitative services as ordered to establish home therapy program/instruct in energy conservation techniques, exercises to increase and/or maintain function in self-care, ADL, and mobility.

30. Monitor/instruct about purpose of prescribed lab work at specific intervals.

31. Assess stage of adaptation, coping mechanisms/provide emotional support, meeting of spiritual needs/encourage verbalization of feelings/assist with realistic goals/refer to social services as ordered to assist with adjustment to altered body image, prescribed treatment regimen/provide information regarding community services (e.g., American Cancer Society, National Leukemia Association; counseling services, community support groups, transportation services).

REHABILITATION POTENTIAL

Rehabilitation potential *excellent good fair guarded poor* for *full partial* return to maximal self-management in personal and therapeutic self-care activities through treatment and control of side effects of radiation therapy.

Client's Name _____

Medical Record # _____

ONGOING/DISCHARGE EVALUATION OF TEACHING
The Client Receiving Radiation Therapy

Teaching Tools:
Printed materials given: _____

Audiovisual aids used: _____

Return Information/Demonstration/Interpretation
_____ Client
_____ Caregiver

OF:	Met	Not Met	Comments
☐ Nature of disease process.	_____	_____	_____
☐ Purpose of radiation therapy, planned radiation therapy schedule.	_____	_____	_____
☐ S&S of complications, actions to take.	_____	_____	_____
☐ Importance of strict compliance with prescribed treatment regimen.	_____	_____	_____
☐ How to take and record a temperature/ read a thermometer.	_____	_____	_____
☐ Well-balanced protein- and calorie-enriched diet, increased fluids.	_____	_____	_____

Client's Name _____

Medical Record # _____

OF:	Met	Not Met	Comments
☐ Predisposing factors in decreased oral intake; measures to improve nutritional status.	_____	_____	_____
☐ Intake and output.	_____	_____	_____
☐ S&S of fluid and electrolyte imbalance with persistent vomiting and diarrhea.	_____	_____	_____
☐ Alternative methods to provide nutritional support (enteral nutrition, parenteral nutrition).	_____	_____	_____
☐ Weighing and recording of weights as ordered; reporting weight gain or loss outside parameters set by physician.	_____	_____	_____
☐ Pain control measures.	_____	_____	_____
☐ Medications and administration; purpose and			

Client's Name _____

Medical Record #_____

OF:	Met	Not Met	Comments
action; side effects.	____	____	_____
☐ Daily skin care program, S&S of impaired skin integrity, infection to report to home health nurse or physician.	____	____	_____
☐ Measures to promote healing, enhance comfort of irradiated skin areas.	____	____	_____
☐ Alopecia, cosmetic management.	____	____	_____
☐ Management of stomatitis, esophagitis.	____	____	_____
☐ Bowel program.	____	____	_____
☐ Measures to reduce risk of urinary calculi.	____	____	_____
☐ S&S of hemorrhagic cystitis to report to home health nurse or physician, measures to treat.	____	____	_____
☐ Bleeding tendencies;			

Client's Name _____

Medical Record #_____

OF:	**Met**	**Not Met**	**Comments**
hemorrhagic precautions; measures to control bleeding.	_____	_____	_____
☐ Balanced rest and activity levels.	_____	_____	_____
☐ Exercise program.	_____	_____	_____
☐ Energy conservation techniques.	_____	_____	_____
☐ S&S of pulmonary toxicity, cardiotoxicity, to report to home health nurse or physician, measures to treat.	_____	_____	_____
☐ Periodontal disease, excessive tooth decay, prescribed measures to treat.	_____	_____	_____
☐ Increased susceptibility to infections; infection precautions.	_____	_____	_____
☐ Risk factors for falls and injuries; safety			

Client's Name _____

Medical Record # _____

OF:	**Met**	**Not Met**	**Comments**
measures with ambulation and daily activities.	_____	_____	_____
☐ Complications of prolonged immobility, measures to treat, activities to avoid.	_____	_____	_____
☐ Medic Alert bracelet.	_____	_____	_____
☐ Effects of radiation therapy on sexual functioning, measures to treat.	_____	_____	_____
☐ Purpose of prescribed lab work.	_____	_____	_____

Signature of Home Health Nurse _____

Date _____

DISORDERS OF THE
IMMUNE SYSTEM

■ Acquired Immune Deficiency Syndrome (AIDS)

Acquired Immune Deficiency Syndrome (AIDS) is a disease that impairs the body's immune system and interferes with its ability to protect itself from various diseases.

The causative agent of the AIDS virus and related clinical manifestations is a retrovirus known as the human immunodeficiency virus (HIV).

The virus has been found in the blood, bone marrow, and lymph nodes, as well as semen, urine, vaginal cervical secretions, saliva, and tears. It has also been cultured in plasma in the absence of lymphocytes. Semen and blood are found to be the most abundant source of the AIDS virus. Only a small percentage of infected clients actually harbor the virus in the saliva and tears.

HIV has been shown to be spread by sexual contact; by parenteral exposure to blood (most often through intravenous [IV] drug abuse), and rarely by other exposures to blood; and from an infected woman to her fetus or infant. Tears and saliva are not considered to be an effective source of transmission.

To understand the profound acquired immunodeficiency that occurs in clients with AIDS and the clinical diseases that can result from an infection with the virus, it is essential to have a working knowledge and understanding of the functioning of the normal human immune system.

The building blocks of the immune system are the lymphocytes (Band T cells), which fight viral and intracellular infections. Another major component of the immune system is the macrophage, which is called a monocyte when in the bloodstream and a macrophage when secreted into the tissues. They originate in the hematopoietic system and are distributed throughout the peripheral lymphoid organs, with the principal concentration in the lymph nodes and spleen.

The first defenders to arrive to combat invading antigens are the macrophages. They do not react to a specific antigen but rather, through phagocytosis, engulf, ingest, and destroy anything suspicious found in the bloodstream, tissues, or lymphatic system.

T lymphocytes are responsible for what is called cell-mediated immunity (that taking place inside or on the surface of the cell). The T lymphocytes are the actual cells involved in fighting antigens that are physically or structurally inaccessible to antibody attack. When an antigen binds with an antigen receptor on the surface of the T lymphocyte, the antigen-activated T cells proliferate and form various kinds of T cells: killer cells, which directly destroy antigens; helper cells, which stimulate B cells; suppressor cells, which control the extent of T-cell help for B cells; lymphokine-producing T cells, which are chemical messengers involved in delayed hypersensitivity and other immune reactions that increase the function of phagocytic activity, induce the inflammatory process, enhance vascular reactivity, and alter the coagulation of blood; and memory cells, which are stored and later recognize and attack the same antigen at other times.

Humoral immunity (that occurring in the blood and tissue fluid outside the cells)

A case of AIDS is defined by the Centers for Disease Control (CDC) as an illness characterized by one or more "indicator diseases" (diseases that are indicative of immunodeficiencies) dependent on the status of laboratory evidence of HIV infection (as outlined by the CDC for surveillance purposes).

involves B cells, which differentiate into plasma cells and produce specific antibodies (immunoglobulins); these antibodies bind to specific antigens and thus neutralize them. These antigen-antibody reactions then activate the complement system to remove the antigen from the body. Complement normally circulates in the bloodstream as a series of inactive proteins that, once activated, destroy antigens.

In the AIDS client, the virus selectively strikes helper T cells (T_4) and impairs their ability to recognize antigens. This allows the AIDS virus to proliferate within the T cells, gradually depleting their number and impairing their function. This results in an inverse ratio of the T_4 helper cells to T_8 suppressor cells, which profoundly impairs cell-mediated immunity. In addition, findings indicate that there are evidences of excessive B cell proliferation and activation. This includes excessive specific production or turnover of B lymphocytes, with decreased response to specific antigens.

Persons exposed to HIV usually develop detectable levels of antibody against the virus within 6 to 12 weeks of infection. The presence of antibody indicates current infection, though many infected persons may have minimal or no clinical evidence of the disease for years.

Once an individual is infected, he or she may remain well but is able to infect others. Others may develop a disease that is less serious than AIDS, referred to as AIDS-related complex (ARC). ARC is a condition caused by the AIDS virus in which the person tests positive for AIDS and has a specific set of clinical symptoms. However, the symptoms are often less severe than those with the disease of AIDS. Signs and symptoms include loss of appetite, weight loss, fever, night sweats, skin rashes, diarrhea, tiredness, lack of resistance to infection, and swollen lymph nodes. In other individuals, the protective immune system may be destroyed by the virus, allowing other organisms that ordinarily would never get a foothold to cause "opportunistic diseases," using the opportunity of lowered resistance to infect and destroy. Some of the most common are *Pneumocystis carinii* pneumonia and tuberculosis.

Individuals infected with the AIDS virus may also develop certain types of cancers such as Kaposi's sarcoma. Evidence also shows the AIDS virus may infect the nervous system, resulting in damage to the brain and causing neurologic changes that vary in severity depending on the involvement of the central nervous system.

There is at present no vaccine or cure for AIDS. Management of the AIDS client is aimed at supportive measures to treat clinical manifestations associated with existing infections and malignancies as well as provide emotional, psychological, and spiritual support.

The home health nurse has the responsibility of establishing and coordinating a plan of care specifically designed to the client's current health status. In addition, the home health nurse must be knowledgeable in current concepts and guidelines for infection control practices in order to help paraprofessionals, clients, and caregivers cope with this illness at home.

POTENTIAL COMPLICATIONS

Opportunistic Diseases

I. AIDS-Related Complications: Infections
1. Herpes simplex virus,
2. *Pneumocystis carinii* pneumonia,

3. Lymphoid pneumonia or hyperplasia,
4. tuberculosis,
5. other mycobacteriosis,
6. toxoplasmosis,
7. candidiasis,
8. Cryptosporidiosis,
9. Cytomegalovirus,
10. coccidioidomycosis,
11. cryptococcosis,
12. histoplasmosis,
13. salmonellosis,
14. progressive multifocal leukoencephalopathy,
15. HIV encephalopathy.
16. HIV wasting syndrome,
17. isosporiasis,
18. other bacterial infection.

II. AIDS-Related Complications: Malignant

1. Kaposi's sarcoma,
2. non-Hodgkin's B cell lymphoma,
3. primary lymphoma of the brain.

TYPES OF CLIENTS/CLINICAL CONDITIONS SEEN BY HOME HEALTH AGENCIES

1. Diagnosed with AIDS or ARC: treatment, management of existing infections, malignancies.
2. Instruction on etiology of AIDS, method of transmission, and infection control.
3. Instruction, supervision of client and caregiver of prescribed treatment regimen: including chemotherapeutics, antibiotics, radiation therapy, immunomodulating agents.
4. Terminal care.

RELATED NURSING DIAGNOSIS

Activity Intolerance

related to:
Imbalance between oxygen supply and demand secondary to respiratory infections from opportunistic infection

as seen by:
Exertional dyspnea with ADL; c/o fatigue and weakness; abnormal heart rate or BP in response to activity

Anxiety

related to:
1. Diagnosis of AIDS, related complications
2. Threat of premature death
3. Knowledge deficit regarding prescribed treatment regimen
4. Transmission of disease to significant other

as seen by:
Increased helplessness; uncertainty; fearfulness; distress; regretfulness

Airway Clearance, Ineffective

related to:
Difficulty in mobilization of tracheobronchial secretions secondary to pneumonia from opportunistic infection

as seen by:
Dyspnea, cough, adventitious breath sounds, tachypnea

Bowel Elimination, Alterations in: Diarrhea

related to:
Infectious process secondary to effect of AIDS virus on immune system

as seen by:
Persistent, loose stools; abdominal cramping; urgency

Breathing Pattern, Ineffective

related to:
Decreased energy or fatigue

as seen by:
Exertional dyspnea; shortness of breath, cyanosis, cough, tachypnea, abnormal blood gases, anxiety

Comfort, Alteration in: Pain

related to:
1. Mouth sores
2. Perioral or perirectal herpes lesions

as seen by:
Verbalization of pain; oral burning; redness and irritation of perirectal area

Coping, Ineffective Individual

related to:
1. Stigma attached to diagnosis of AIDS

as seen by:
Depression; alienation secondary to fear of rejection; inability to meet

2. Alteration in body image
3. Life-style changes
4. Changes in relationships

physical needs; general hostility; anger

Fluid Volume Deficit

related to:
1. Diarrhea
2. Dehydration
3. Poor nutritional status

as seen by:
S&S of dehydration; decreased skin turgor; poor fluid intake; weight loss; increased heart rate; hypotension; dry mucous membranes

Grieving

related to:
1. Altered body image
2. Changes in life-style (includes sexual and personal relationships)
3. Diagnosis of AIDS
4. Threat of premature death
5. Loss of self-esteem

as seen by:
Changes in eating and sleeping patterns; anger; sorrow; denial; noncompliance; depression

Hopelessness

related to:
1. Deteriorating, failing condition
2. Poor prognosis

as seen by:
Decreased communication; frequent sighing; lack of involvement in care; decreased appetite; increased sleep

Infection, Potential for

related to:
1. Inverse ratio of helper T cells to suppressor T cells ($T_4 : T_8$).
2. Reduced number of T lymphocytes
3. Net decrease of T helper cells
4. Altered humoral immune response
5. Leukopenia

as seen by:
Weight loss; constant fatigue; dry cough; sore throat; fever; night sweats; persistent diarrhea; generalized lymphadenopathy; white spots on tongue; other S&S related to malignancies or opportunistic infections

Injury, Potential for: Increased Risk of Falls and Injuries

related to:
1. Cognitive and/or motor dysfunction secondary to encephalopathy

as seen by:
Constant fatigue; confusion; apathy; memory loss; partial paralysis;

2. Neurologic changes caused by neurologic diseases seen in AIDS
3. Generalized weakness

impaired gait, balance, and muscle strength

Knowledge Deficit (Specify)

related to:
1. Lack of information and adequate understanding of disease process, related S&S, and transmissibility
2. Prescribed plan of treatment for management of condition
3. Potential complication, S&S to report to home health nurse or physician

as seen by:
Verbalization of lack of information; inadequate understanding; inability to perform skills necessary to meet health-care needs at home

Nutritional Status, Alteration in: Less than Body Requirements

related to:
1. Anorexia secondary to fatigue, fear, grieving; depression
2. Stomatitis; pharyngitis; esophagitis

as seen by:
Loss of body weight, 20 percent or more under ideal weight for height and frame; repeated inadequate oral intake; caloric intake inadequate to meet increased metabolic needs

Oral Mucous Membrane, Alteration in

related to:
Stomatitis secondary to *Candida* infection associated with deficient immune system

as seen by:
Inflammation or ulcerations of oral mucosa; leukoplakia; dysphagia

Powerlessness, Feelings of

related to:
1. Isolation from family and friends
2. Discouraging prognosis associated with the diagnosis of AIDS

as seen by:
Verbalization of no control over present condition; apathy; anger; hostility; passivity; grieving; increased dependence on others to meet personal and daily needs

Self-Care Deficit: Feeding, Bathing/Hygiene, Dressing/Grooming, Toileting (Specify)

related to:
1. Intolerance of activities

as seen by:
Fatigue; weakness; exertional dyspnea

2. Prescribed activity restrictions
3. Depression
4. Loss of memory
5. Neurologic impairment

noted when attempting self-care activities; medically imposed restrictions; apathy, with decreased participation in daily activities and self-care; confusion; changes in gait, balance, and strength

Sexual Dysfunction

related to:
1. Weakness and fatigue
2. Depression, fear, and anxiety
3. Impotence secondary to fear of rejection by desired partner or transmitting AIDS to others
4. Effect of medically imposed restrictions on sexual activities
5. Loss of sexual drive secondary to neurological involvement

as seen by:
Alteration in relationship with desired partner(s); change of interest in self and others; verbalization of problem; actual or perceived limitation imposed by disease and/or medical restrictions

Skin Integrity, Impairment of: Potential for

related to:
1. Inadequate nutritional status
2. Prolonged inactivity
3. Dehydration
4. Persistent excretion and secretions secondary to disease process
5. Kaposi's sarcoma lesions
6. Perioral herpes simplex

as seen by:
Reddened, irritated skin; edema; breakdown of skin surface; extensive ulcerations; pink, red, or violet macules, papules, or nodules on skin

Self-Concept, Disturbance in

related to:
1. Altered body image
2. Changes in life-style
3. Loss of self-esteem

as seen by:
Anxiety; depression; noncompliance; verbalized fear of losing independence, dependence on others for physical needs

Sensory-Perceptual Alteration: Mental Status

related to:
Neurologic changes secondary to neurologic diseases seen in the AIDS client

as seen by:
Symptoms of dull perception; confusion; apathy; hallucinations; short- and long-term memory loss

Social Isolation

related to:
1. AIDS diagnosis
2. Fear of transmitting disease to others

as seen by:
Withdrawn behavior; lack of communication; verbalized feelings of rejection; aloneness

Thermoregulation, Ineffective

related to:
Infectious process associated with oportunistic infection

as seen by:
Fever; chills; diaphoresis; flushing; tachycardia

LONG-TERM GOAL

To maintain an optimum quality of life, reduce the risk of opportunistic infections through treatment of the disease manifestations and supportive care.

SHORT-TERM GOALS

The client with AIDS will be able to:

1. Verbalize nature of disease process, altered immune functioning in AIDS or ARC, increased susceptibility to opportunistic disease.
2. Verbalize S&S of complications to report to home health nurse or physician.
3. Demonstrate how to take a temperature, read a thermometer, record, report elevations as directed.
4. Demonstrate prescribed measures to decrease or reduce risk of contracting opportunistic infections.
5. Identify factors of decreased oral intake/verbalize importance of well-balanced diet with increase in protein and calories, measures to improve eating.
6. Verbalize importance of/demonstrate compliance with prescribed vitamin and mineral supplements.
7. Demonstrate compliance with prescribed medication therapy/identify complications.
8. Verbalize importance of weighing daily, recording/reporting excessive weight loss to physician.
9. Verbalize importance of low-fat and -fiber, lactose-reduced diet with persistent diarrhea, medications ordered, S&S of fluid and electrolyte imbalance to report to home health nurse or physician.
10. Verbalize cause of stomatitis, esophagitis, pharyngitis/identify prescribed measures to relieve oral discomfort and treat ulcerations.
11. Verbalize importance of adequte rest and sleep in combating infectious process, reducing risk of contracting additional infections.

12. Demonstrate energy conservation techniques.
13. Demonstrate prescribed daily skin care program, prescribed measures to treat lesions, S&S of infection to report to home health nurse or physician.
14. Demonstrate adherence to prescribed measures to improve respiratory status.
15. Verbalize measures to prevent transmission of AIDS, safe sexual practices.
16. Verbalize knowledge of/demonstrate adherence to Universal Precautions in providing care to AIDS client.
17. Verbalize knowledge of S&S of inflammation of meninges, importance of reporting to physician immediately/demonstrate adherence to prescribed antibiotic therapy and measures to manage neurologic changes.
18. Verbalize purpose, importance of prescribed lab work.
19. Demonstrate involvement in self-care and daily activities, effective measures to manage stress levels associated with altered body image and life-style changes and attain realistic goals.

NURSING ACTIONS/TREATMENTS

1. Assess systems of the body for disease manifestations, associated conditions seen with AIDS and ARC/identify complications.
2. Assess vital signs/identify trends (e.g., elevated temperature, tachycardia, increased respiratory rate and depth, hypotension)/instruct how to take temperature, read thermometer, record, report elevation as directed.
3. Instruct about body's normal immune system, altered immune functioning with AIDS virus, increased susceptibility to opportunistic infections and malignancies, S&S of complications or the development of new opportunistic infections to report to home health nurse or physician.
4. Assess and evaluate for infection daily/Instruct about importance of strict compliance with prescribed treatment regimen to resolve current infectious process and to decrease risk of contracting additional infections (e.g., good handwashing technique, avoiding exposure to others with infections or crowds, multiple sex partners, unclean home environment, poor nutritional status).
5. Assess and evaluate nutritional status (e.g., S&S of malnutrition, caloric intake and anthropometric measurements, causative factors in decreased oral intake)/instruct about well-balanced diet as tolerated with prescribed increase in protein and calories, adequate hydration (1500 to 2000 ml per day), measures to improve appetite (e.g., appropriate food textures for dysphagia, resting before meals; small, frequent meals), prescribed measures to reduce discomfort with oral lesions (e.g., good oral hygiene, need for soft diet).
6. Obtain dietary consultation as needed.
7. Assess/instruct about prescribed vitamin, mineral, nutritional supplements.
8. Observe/instruct about prescribed medication therapy, purpose and action, side effects, toxicity, and other treatment modalitities specific to condition (e.g., antibiotics, analgesics, antipyretics, chemotherapeutic agents, radiation)/evaluate effectiveness of prescribed treatment.

9. Assess for continued weight loss/instruct to weigh and record daily/to report weight loss outside parameters set by physician.

10. Assess bowel elimination, problems with persistent diarrhea/instruct about prescribed diet (e.g., low-fat and -fiber, lactose-reduced), medications as ordered, S&S of electrolyte imbalance/monitor results of lab work ordered and report to physician.

11. Assess and evaluate oral mucous membrane for S&S of stomatitis, pharyngitis, esophagitis/instruct about cause, prescribed measures to relieve discomfort and treat ulcerations (e.g., good oral hygiene, topical antifungal, antibacterial medications; daily oral rinsing with prescribed mouth washes; antacids; topical anesthetics; no smoking; soft toothbrush; nonirritating foods and fluids).

12. Observe and evaluate activity tolerance and quality and quantity of sleep/instruct about importance of adequate rest and sleep in combating the infectious process, reducing the risk of contracting additional infections, energy conservation techniques, activities as tolerated with frequent rest periods.

13. Assess skin for lesions and breakdown (e.g., perioral or perianal lesions)/instruct about daily skin care program and measures to treat lesions as prescribed (e.g., local anesthetic agents, compresses, sitz bath)/evaluate healing and effectiveness of comfort measures.

14. Assess respiratory status/evaluate sputum production and ability to effectively clear secretions/instruct about proper positioning to improve ventilation, breathing exercises to strengthen respiratory muscles, keeping the environment free of irritants (e.g., aerosols, smoke, dust) and use of oxygen therapy as prescribed.

15. Observe/instruct about Universal Precautions (CDC guidelines for infection control practices) in providing care for an AIDS client.

16. Assess and evaluate neurologic status/observe for signs of inflammation of meninges (e.g., Kernig's sign, Brudzinski's sign) and report to physician immediately/instruct about prescribed antibiotic therapy, measures to manage neurologic changes.

17. Assess concerns about sexual dysfunction in relationship to AIDS/instruct about measures to prevent disease transmission, safe sexual practices.

18. Monitor/instruct about purpose, importance of prescribed lab work.

19. Assess effects of disease process on functional skills and mobility status, toleration of performance of daily activities/refer to rehabilitative services as ordered to establish home therapy program/instruct in energy conservation techniques and activities, exercises to increase or maintain function in performing self-care, ADL, and mobility activities.

20. Assess stress levels, isolation, and sadness associated with altered body image and feelings of powerlessness with diagnosis/give the client as much control over activities as possible/encourage social or group activities as tolerated/answer questions/refer to social services to provide counseling and support to client and caregiver, assist with grieving process, setting realistic goals/meeting spiritual needs/provide information about AIDS support groups

(e.g., Local Gay Lesbian Community Service; National Gay Task Force; Centers for Disease Control; AIDS Action Council; Gay Rights National Lobby; National Institute of Allergy and Infectious Disease; Public Health Service; Lambda Legal Defense and Education Fund; National Coalition of Gay STD Services; National Lesbian and Gay Health Foundation).

REHABILITATION POTENTIAL

Rehabilitation potential *excellent* *good* *fair* *guarded* *poor* for *full* *partial* achievement of an improved level of well-being and functional status, participation in self-care and daily activities.

Client's Name _____

Medical Record # _____

ONGOING/DISCHARGE EVALUATION OF TEACHING
The Client with AIDS

Teaching Tools:
Printed materials given: _____

Audiovisual aids used: _____

Return Information/Demonstration/Interpretation
_____ Client
_____ Caregiver

OF:	Met	Not Met	Comments
☐ Normal immune functioning.	_____	_____	_____
☐ Nature of disease process, altered immune functioning in AIDS.	_____	_____	_____
☐ S&S of complications, actions to take.	_____	_____	_____
☐ Importance of strict compliance with prescribed treatment regimen.	_____	_____	_____
☐ How to take a temperature, read a thermometer, record daily, report elevations.	_____	_____	_____
☐ Infection precautions against			

Client's Name _____

Medical Record # _____

OF:	**Met**	**Not Met**	**Comments**
contacting opportunistic infections.	_____	_____	_____
☐ Well-balanced, protein- and calorie-enriched diet, adequate hydration.	_____	_____	_____
☐ Measures to increase oral intake.	_____	_____	_____
☐ Vitamin and mineral supplements.	_____	_____	_____
☐ Medications and administration, purpose and action, side effects.	_____	_____	_____
☐ Weighing and recording as ordered, report excessive weight loss to physician.	_____	_____	_____
☐ Low-fat and -fiber, lactose-reduced diet with persistent diarrhea.	_____	_____	_____
☐ S&S of fluid and electrolyte imbalance to report to home health nurse or physician.	_____	_____	_____

Client's Name _____

Medical Record # _____

OF:	**Met**	**Not Met**	**Comments**
☐ Measures to reduce oral discomfort, treat ulcerations.	_____	_____	_____
☐ Balanced rest and activity levels, importance of rest in combating infections.	_____	_____	_____
☐ Skin care program.	_____	_____	_____
☐ Respiratory therapy program.	_____	_____	_____
☐ Measures to manage neurologic change.	_____	_____	_____
☐ Energy conservation techniques.	_____	_____	_____
☐ Measures to prevent transmission of the AIDS virus; safe sexual practices.	_____	_____	_____
☐ Universal precautions in providing care for AIDS client.	_____	_____	_____

Client's Name _____

Medical Record # _____

OF:	Met	Not Met	Comments
☐ Purpose of prescribed lab work.	_____	_____	_____

Signature of Home Health Nurse _____

Date _____

NUTRITIONAL/PARENTERAL THERAPY

■ Home Enteral Nutrition

Delivery of nutrients by means of the gastrointestinal tract rather than the oral route is often a feasible and desirable method of nutritional support to restore and maintain metabolic function. Clients may be discharged home in need of total or supplemental nutritional support, depending on their clinical situation and indications for nutritional therapy. Some examples of the types of clinical situations in which enteral administration of nutrients is indicated are: chronic illnesses, neoplasms, cerebrovascular accidents, central nervous system disorders, and in conjunction with and following parenteral hyperalimentation.

Route of administration is dependent on the clinical situation of the client and may be by nasogastric (NG) tube, orogastric tube, esophagostomy, gastrostomy, duodenostomy, or jejunostomy. The functional status of the client's gastrointestinal tract and the size and location of the tube are factors that are considered in the choice of the formula and the delivery of the feeding. Delivery may be by bolus administration or intermittent or continuous feeding.

Clients who receive total enteral nutrition at home require careful monitoring to ensure both effective nutritional therapy and a low incidence of related complications.

POTENTIAL COMPLICATIONS

Mechanical
1. Aspiration pneumonia,
2. tube displacement,
3. obstruction of feeding tube,
4. nasopharyngeal irritation or breakdown,
5. sinusitis.

Gastrointestinal Function
1. Abdominal distension,
2. diarrhea or constipation,
3. cramping,
4. nausea and vomiting.

Metabolic and Fluid and Electrolyte Imbalances
1. Glucose intolerance,
2. hypertonic dehydration,
3. hyperosmolar nonketotic coma,
4. edema.

TYPES OF CLIENTS/CLINICAL CONDITIONS SEEN BY HOME HEALTH AGENCIES

1. Initiation of home enteral nutrition: inclusive teaching plan in daily care and management routines for tube feeding.

2. Complications related to home enteral nutrition: changes in prescribed plan of treatment, increased home health nursing visits to instruct and supervise in changes and observe response to treatment, report to physician.

RELATED NURSING DIAGNOSES

Airway Clearance, Ineffective

related to:
Aspiration of feeding secondary to:
1. Tube displacement
2. Impaired gag reflex
3. Overfeeding

as seen by:
Changes in rate or depth of respirations; cyanosis; dyspnea; coughing; presence of abnormal breath sounds

Anxiety

related to:
1. Insertion of feeding tube
2. Inability to eat and oral deprivation
3. Discomfort from tube
4. Knowledge deficit regarding prescribed treatment regimen in care and management of tube and enteral feeding at home

as seen by:
Oral cravings for food and eating; distress and apprehension associated with debilitated condition and need for tube feedings; irritability; fearfulness regarding management of tube feedings at home, increased dependence on others for care; changes in bowel functioning

Bowel Elimination, Alteration in: Constipation

related to:
1. Sensitivity to solution
2. Dehydration
3. Immobility

as seen by:
Hard, formed stools; reported feeling of abdominal or rectal fullness; c/o feeling constipated; straining at stool; frequency and amount less than usual pattern

Bowel Elimination, Alteration in: Diarrhea

related to:
1. Infusion rate too rapid
2. Anxiety
3. Temperature of feeding too cold
4. Contamination of feeding
5. High osmolality of feeding

as seen by:
Abdominal pain and cramping; increased frequency and loose, liquid stools; increased frequency of bowel sounds

Comfort, Alteration in: Pain

related to:
1. Nasal skin irritation or breakdown
2. Excessive irritation of peristomal skin secondary to gastric juice leakage
3. Dry mucous membranes from mouth breathing and dehydration
4. Poor oral hygiene
5. Tape irritation

as seen by:
Increased mucous secretions; c/o nasal skin discomfort; reddened, irritated peristomal skin; cracked corners of the mouth and dry lips; skin irritation and breakdown of taped areas

Coping, Ineffective Individual

related to:
Altered body image with changes from usual manner of eating, effect on life-style

as seen by:
Inability to meet basic needs; poor self-esteem; depression; general irritability; withdrawn behavior

Fluid Volume, Alteration in: Excess

related to:
Retaining of fluids associated with:
1. Too rapid infusion
2. Too-frequent feeding or too large a volume

as seen by:
Changes in mental status; edema; weight gain; intake greater than output

Fluid Volume Deficit

related to:
1. Hypertonic dehydration secondary to hyperosmolar nutrient preparations
2. Vomiting
3. Diarrhea
4. Inadequate intake

as seen by:
Decreased urine output; elevated temperature; low BP; increased pulse rate; lethargy; weight loss; poor skin turgor; skin coolness

Infection, Potential for

related to:
Contaminated formula

as seen by:
Diarrhea; abdominal cramps; generalized weakness; nausea and vomiting

Knowledge Deficit (Specify)

related to:
1. Prescribed plan of treatment for management and maintenance of home enteral nutrition
2. Potential complications, S&S to report to home health nurse or physician

as seen by:
Verbalization of lack of information; inadequate understanding or inability to perform skills necessary to meet health-care needs at home

Mobility, Impaired Physical

related to:
Limitation of physical movement secondary to infusion equipment and tubing with enteral nutrition

as seen by:
Inability to move because of imposed restrictions

Nutrition, Alteration in: Less than Body Requirements

related to:
1. Diarrhea and vomiting associated with intolerance of feedings
2. Clogging of feeding tube, not receiving amounts prescribed

as seen by:
Continual weight loss; weakness and fatigue; pale conjunctiva and mucous membranes; bloating; abdominal distension, cramping; glycosuria

Oral Mucous Membrane, Alteration in

related to:
1. Dry mucous membranes secondary to mouth breathing and dehydration
2. Poor oral hygiene

as seen by:
Dry mouth; c/o oral pain and discomfort; oral lesions; coated tongue; halitosis

Self-Care Deficit: Feeding, Bathing/Hygiene, Dressing/Grooming, Toileting (Specify)

related to:
1. Inability to meet basic needs secondary to depression and ineffective coping mechanisms
2. Debilitated condition and need for total assistance

as seen by:
Withdrawn behavior; lack of interest or participation in self-care; increased dependency on others; inability to physically carry out self-care activities

Self-Concept, Disturbance in

related to:
1. Changes in life-style and role performance secondary to altered body image
2. Loss of self-esteem

as seen by:
Lack of participation in personal care and feeding regimen; withdrawal from social contacts; avoiding looking at feeding tube

Skin Integrity, Impairment of: Potential

related to:
1. Gastric juice leakage from gastrostomy tube
2. Sensitivity of skin to tape
3. Repeated removal of tape
4. Nasal skin secondary to NG tube

as seen by:
Redness and irritation of peristomal skin; pronounced tenderness at insertion site; encrusted secretions; tissue irritation and breakdown of taped areas

Social Isolation

related to:
Altered body image because of feeding tube

as seen by:
Withdrawn behavior; staying in bedroom; refusing visitors

LONG-TERM GOAL

To improve nutritional status and meet daily metabolic requirements through receiving of essential nutrients by enteral feedings.

SHORT-TERM GOALS

The client receiving enteral nutrition will be able to:

1. Verbalize nature of clinical condition, need for and purpose of enteral nutrition, S&S of complications to report to home health nurse or physician.
2. Demonstrate proper hand-washing technique.
3. Verbalize type of feeding tube, how to insert, prescribed formula, method of delivery.
4. Demonstrate how to check position and patency of tube prior to feedings.
5. Verbalize S&S of reactions to observe for with feedings, importance of reporting to physician.
6. Verbalize purpose of elevating head with feedings.

7. Verbalize purpose of aspirating for gastric residual prior to each feeding, when to hold feeding and report to home health nurse or physician.
8. Verbalize purpose/demonstrate how to irrigate feeding tube with water following feeding and at prescribed times during day.
9. Demonstrate how and when to remove and change feeding tube and container, mark day and time changed.
10. Demonstrate current procedure for weighing daily, recording/verbalize importance of reporting weight gain or loss outside parameters set by physician.
11. Demonstrate correct measuring, recording of daily intake and output.
12. Demonstrate correct fractional urinary testing/instruct to report 3+ or 4+ sugar or acetone to physician.
13. Demonstrate compliance with prescribed medication therapy/identify side effects, how to give medications via feeding tube.
14. Demonstrate safe use and care of infusion pump and equipment, checking of flow rate as ordered.
15. Demonstrate correct procedure of suctioning and use of equipment.
16. Verbalize where to obtain feeding formulas and supplies.
17. Demonstrate good peristomal skin care/verbalize S&S of irritation or breakdown to report to home health nurse or physician.
18. Demonstrate good oral hygiene, cleaning of nares/verbalize S&S of irritation or breakdown to report to home health nurse or physician.
19. Demonstrate activity levels within prescribed levels.
20. Verbalize purpose of prescribed lab work.
21. Verbalize prescribed measures to treat constipation or diarrhea.
22. Demonstrate decreased level of anxiety with use of effective coping mechanisms for positive adaptation to altered body image and need for enteral feedings.
23. Identify names and phone numbers to call for assistance with home enteral feeding.
24. Verbalize importance of/wear Medic Alert bracelet.

NURSING ACTIONS/TREATMENTS

1. Assess cardiorespiratory and GI status, evaluate response to nutrient feedings/identify S&S of complications.
2. Assess vital signs/identify trends (e.g., elevated temperature, increased pulse and respiratory rate, BP changes).
3. Instruct about nature of clinical condition, need for and purpose of enteral nutrition, importance of strict compliance with prescribed treatment regimen, S&S of complications to report to home health nurse or physician.
4. Assess and evaluate nutritional status (include physical exam, anthropometric measurements, results of biochemical laboratory determinations)/obtain dietary consultation as needed.
5. Observe/instruct about proper hand-washing technique.

6. Observe/instruct about type of feeding tube, insertion as ordered, prescribed formula (e.g., preparation, amount, feeding schedule, temperature of feeding formula at room temperature), avoiding bacterial overgrowth at room temperature (e.g., filling feeding bag only with prescribed amounts to be used, storing and reusing as directed), delivery of feeding (e.g., bolus, intermittent, continuous).

7. Assess/instruct how to check position and patency of tube prior to feeding (e.g., injecting air into nasogastric tube and listening over stomach; aspirating any gastric residual feeding)/evaluate tube placement.

8. Assess/instruct to evaluate respiratory status and bowel functioning prior to and during feeding and every hour for next 2 hours for adverse reactions to feeding/report to physician (e.g., respiratory distress, nausea and vomiting, restlessness).

9. Observe/instruct to elevate head to high or semi-Fowler's position during feeding and to keep elevated 30 minutes after feeding (to promote digestion and avoid gastric reflux and aspiration).

10. Observe/instruct to aspirate for gastric residual prior to each feeding, hold feeding and report to home health nurse or physician if 100 ml or more.

11. Observe/instruct about purpose and how to irrigate feeding tube with 30 to 50 ml water following feeding and at prescribed times as ordered.

12. Observe/instruct how to remove and change feeding tube and container at frequency ordered, mark day and time changed.

13. Assess and evaluate for fluid volume excess or deficit/instruct to daily weigh and record at the same time of day on the same scale with same clothing, record, report weight gain or loss outside parameters set by physician.

14. Observe/instruct how to measure and record intake and output.

15. Observe/instruct about purpose, procedure, schedule for fractional urine testing for sugar and acetone/evaluate urine test results/report to physician 3+/4+ sugar or acetone.

16. Observe/instruct about prescribed medication therapy, purpose and action, side effects, how to give prescribed oral medications via feeding tube/evaluate ability to give medications as ordered.

17. Observe/instruct about safe use and care of infusion pump and equipment, checking flow rate every 30 minutes to 1 hour.

18. Observe/instruct about suctioning procedure and use of suctioning equipment as prescribed.

19. Observe/instruct how to obtain feeding formula and supplies.

20. Evaluate skin integrity/instruct about good peristomal skin care (e.g., cleaning and use of skin care products, changing dressing with use of precut drain sponges), S&S of irritation, breakdown, or blood around tube to report to home health nurse or physician.

21. Assess and evaluate oral mucosa and nares/instruct about good oral hygiene and cleaning of nares/report S&S of breakdown or blood in nares to home health nurse or physician.

22. Observe and evaluate degree of self-care/instruct about activity levels and limitations as prescribed.
23. Monitor/instruct about purpose of prescribed lab work.
24. Assess and evaluate alteration in bowel elimination: diarrhea or constipation/instruct about prescribed measures to treat (e.g., stool softeners, enemas as ordered for constipation; correction of causative factor of diarrhea).
25. Assess level of anxiety, coping mechanisms, readiness to learn/provide emotional support/encourage to verbalize feelings/refer to social services to assist client to a positive adaptation to condition and home enteral feedings/provide information of needed community resources (e.g., financial assistance; homemaker chore application; attendant services).
26. List names and phone numbers of pharmacy, home health agency, physician beside client's phone and/or on home enteral instruction sheet/instruct about importance of calling with S&S of complications, adverse reactions, concerns or questions.
27. Observe/instruct about importance of wearing Medic Alert bracelet listing medical condition and current treatment.

REHABILITATION POTENTIAL

Rehabilitation potential   *excellent   good   fair   guarded   poor*   for   *full partial*   achievement of an improved state of metabolic functioning following enteral feedings, ability to independently take care of personal and daily needs.

Client's Name _____

Medical Record # _____

ONGOING/DISCHARGE EVALUATION OF TEACHING
The Client Receiving Home Enteral Nutrition

Teaching Tools:
Printed materials given: _____

Audiovisual aids used: _____

Return Information/Demonstration/Interpretation
_____ Client
_____ Caregiver

	OF:	Met	Not Met	Comments
☐	Nature of clinical condition; purpose and need for enteral nutrition.	_____	_____	_____
☐	S&S of complications, actions to take.	_____	_____	_____
☐	Importance of compliance with prescribed treatment regimen.	_____	_____	_____
☐	Proper hand-washing technique.	_____	_____	_____
☐	Type of feeding tube, how to insert.	_____	_____	_____
☐	Feeding formula, method of administration.	_____	_____	_____

Client's Name _____

Medical Record # _____

OF:	Met	Not Met	Comments
☐ Checking position and patency of tube.	_____	_____	_____
☐ Adverse reactions with feeding to report to physician.	_____	_____	_____
☐ Correct positioning to receive feeding.	_____	_____	_____
☐ Aspirating for residual prior to feedings.	_____	_____	_____
☐ Irrigation of feeding tube with water.	_____	_____	_____
☐ Frequency and procedure for removal and changing of feeding tube and container.	_____	_____	_____
☐ Weighing and recording of weights as ordered, reporting weight gain or loss outside parameters set by physician.	_____	_____	_____
☐ Daily recording of intake and output.	_____	_____	_____

Client's Name _____

Medical Record #_____

OF:	Met	Not Met	Comments
☐ Fractional urine testing.	_____	_____	_____
☐ Oral medications and administration via feeding tube, purpose and action, side effects.	_____	_____	_____
☐ Suctioning procedure; use of suction equipment.	_____	_____	_____
☐ Use and care of infusion pump and equipment.	_____	_____	_____
☐ Peristomal skin care.	_____	_____	_____
☐ Oral hygiene; care of nares.	_____	_____	_____
☐ Purpose of prescribed lab work.	_____	_____	_____
☐ Measures to treat alterations in bowel elimination: diarrhea or constipation.	_____	_____	_____
☐ Review of emergency situations, procedures and			

Client's Name _____

Medical Record # _____

OF:	**Met**	**Not Met**	**Comments**
phone numbers to call when needing assistance.	_____	_____	_____
☐ Medic Alert bracelet.	_____	_____	_____

Signature of Home Health Nurse _____

Date _____

■ Home Parenteral Nutrition

Hyperalimentation or total parenteral nutrition (TPN) involves infusing a hypertonic solution of nutrients in amounts substantially in excess of basal requirements to meet the body's metabolic needs. The major constituents of a solution of hyperalimentation include glucose, water, amino acids, electrolytes, minerals, and trace elements. With these constituents, the composition of the hyperalimentation solution is individualized to meet the nutrient requirements of the client.

Parenteral hyperalimentation fluids are indicated when adequate nutrition cannot be maintained through the gastrointestinal tract. This may be seen in such conditions as intractable vomiting, cerebrovascular accident, cancer, chemotherapy, radiation, anorexia nervosa, in situations in which oral or nasogastric intubation may not be effective, and when silent aspiration is a constant threat.

TPN may also be indicated in those clients with an impaired or diseased gastrointestinal tract, which interferes with the absorption of essential nutrients needed to maintain a positive nitrogen balance and nutrition equilibrium. Hyperalimentation fluids allow the gastrointestinal tract to rest and thereby decrease gallbladder, pancreatic, and small-intestinal activity. Decreasing peristatlic and secretory activities involved with the digestive process promotes healing and tissue synthesis of the affected portion of the alimentary tract, as well as improves metabolic functioning. Severe inflammatory bowel disease, radiation enteritis, and short-bowel syndrome following major bowel resection are all clinical conditions that benefit from placing the bowel at complete rest.

Generally most clients are able to resume oral feedings after a course of TPN in the hospital. However, those groups of individuals that require prolonged intravenous nutritional support after discharge will need instruction in specialized skills to manage hyperalimentation at home (home parenteral nutrition, HPN).

The hyperalimentation solution may be administered either through a direct central line into the client's subclavian vein or a central line through a peripheral vein or the jugular vein. The advantage of direct central lines is that they are easily dressed, allow greater movement, and because of the longer veins and high blood flow and rapid dilution permit administration of a solution with high osmolality. This reduces the risk of phlebitis, venous thrombosis, and sclerosing of the vein wall.

Intravenous fat emulsion (lipids), consisting of soybean and safflower oils with added water, phospholipids, and glycerol, are usually administered adjunctive to TPN solutions to provide a source of essential fatty acids. Fat emulsions also provide twice the caloric value of glucose and may be given to a client whose body's nutritional requirements are greatly increased, requiring extra calories. Fat emulsions may be piggybacked into the TPN tubing or administered simultaneously via a Y-connector. Since fat emulsions are isotonic, they may also be administered through a peripheral vein.

IV fat emulsion may be indicated for clients with severe nutritional disorders occurring with reduced oral intake, such as a result of anorexia, nausea and vomiting, and severe mucositis secondary to chemotherapy and radiation therapy. It may also be given to clients with an impaired or diseased gastrointestinal tract, or in any other condition in which the client is in need of essential fatty acids.

POTENTIAL COMPLICATIONS

1. Catheter maintenance complications:
   a. catheter sepsis (e.g., infection from contaminated solution, infection at insertion site or IV apparatus),
   b. venous thrombosis (e.g., local trauma from vein puncture, irritation of intima of vessel from hyperosmolar solution, catheter sensitivity, infection),
2. air embolism,
3. circulatory overload and dehydration,
4. metabolic complications:
   a. glucose imbalances (e.g., hyperglycemia, hypoglycemia, hyperosmolar nonketotic coma),
   b. fluid and electrolyte abnormalities,
   c. amino-acid-related problems,
5. parenteral nutritional deficiencies:
   a. essential fatty acid deficiency (EFAD),
   b. trace element deficiency,
6. skin sensitivity or ulceration from sensitivity to iodine or tape,
7. cardiac arrhythmias,
8. adverse reaction to intralipid infusion.

TYPES OF CLIENTS/CLINICAL CONDITIONS SEEN BY HOME HEALTH AGENCIES

1. Initiation of HPN: inclusive teaching plan in daily care and management routines necessary for HPN (e.g., dressing changes, specialized skills needed for daily infusion, observation for complications)/evaluation of competence in all areas of training associated with HPN.
2. Complications related to hyperalimentation: changes in prescribed plan of treatment; increased home health nursing visits to instruct and supervise in changes, evaluate response to treatment changes; report to physician.

RELATED NURSING DIAGNOSES

Anxiety

related to:
1. Inability to eat and oral deprivation
2. HPN as a foreign means of life support
3. Fear of potential complications

as seen by:
Oral cravings and food-related hallucinations; apprehension; fearfulness; increased dependency on others; expressed concern about

associated with HPN
4. Knowledge deficit regarding specialized skills to manage HPN
5. Fear of death

having skills necessary to manage hyperalimentation at home

Comfort, Alteration in: Pain

related to:
1. Nutritional deficiencies
2. Restricted oral intake
3. Poor oral hygiene
4. Extravasation from dislodged catheter

as seen by:
Oral lesions; glossitis; dry mucous membranes; edema and pain at catheter site

Coping, Ineffective Individual

related to:
Effect of hyperalimentation on body image, life-style, and usual manner of eating

as seen by:
Verbalization of inabilty to cope; inability to meet basic needs and role expectations; general irritability

Fluid Volume, Alteration in: Excess

related to:
Pulmonary edema resulting from circulatory overload o´ hyperalimentation solution

as seen by:
Dyspnea; moist respirations; neck vein distension; elevated BP

Fluid Volume Deficit

related to:
Hyperglycemia, osmotic diuresis; dehydration; hyperosmolar nonketotic acidosis associated with fluid running too rapidly, intolerance of glucose

as seen by:
Glycosuria; headache; nausea; lethargy; hypotension; poor skin turgor; rapid weight loss

Infection, Potential for

related to:
1. Catheter maintenance complications
2. Contaminated solution

as seen by:
Swelling; drainage at catheter site; chills; temperature spikes; worsening of condition; purulent drainage; ulceration

Knowledge Deficit (Specify)

related to:
1. Prescribed plan of treatment for management and maintenance of HPN
2. Potential complications, S&S to report to home health nurse or physician

as seen by:
Verbalization of lack of information; inadequate understanding; inability to perform skills necessary to manage HPN

Mobility, Impaired Physical

related to:
Limitation of physical movement secondary to infusion equipment and tubing with HPN

as seen by:
Inability to move because of imposed restrictions

Oral Mucous Membrane, Alteration in

related to:
1. Dry mucous membranes secondary to inability to ingest food or fluids
2. Poor oral hygiene

as seen by:
Discomfort, and dry mouth; c/o oral pain, coated tongue; oral lesions; halitosis

Self-Care Deficit: Feeding, Bathing/Hygiene, Dressing/Grooming, Toileting (Specify)

related to:
1. Impaired physical mobility secondary to HPN and equipment
2. Prescribed activity restrictions

as seen by:
Decreased ability to meet personal and daily needs, requiring assistance; imposed medical restrictions

Self-Concept, Disturbance in

related to:
1. Changes in life and role performance associated with altered body image
2. Lack of self-esteem and confidence

as seen by:
Increasing dependence on others; signs of grieving; withdrawn behavior

Skin Integrity, Impairment of: Potential

related to:
1. Extravasation of hyperalimentation solution

as seen by:
Erythema; edema; pain; pallor and coldness; crusting at insertion site;

2. Sensitivity to iodine or tape
3. Infection at catheter insertion site

drainage; chills and fever; tissue
breakdown

LONG-TERM GOAL

To maintain a positive nitrogen balance and nutritional equilibrium by an intravenous route to meet anabolic needs.

SHORT-TERM GOALS

The client who is receiving home parenteral nutrition will be able to:

1. Demonstrate how to take and record vital signs, what alterations to report to home health nurse or physician.
2. Verbalize knowledge of clinical condition, need and purpose for HPN, catheter insertion site, type of solution.
3. Verbalize S&S of complications to report to home health nurse or physician.
4. Verbalize type and amount of oral foods allowed.
5. Demonstrate compliance with prescribed medications/identify complications.
6. Verbalize importance of strict hand-washing technique.
7. Verbalize importance of maintaining aseptic technique with all activities and procedures concerned with HPN.
8. Demonstrate step-by-step procedure for daily setting up of infusion pump with solution and tubing, all needed supplies.
9. Verbalize how to obtain and store supplies.
10. Verbalize importance of/inspect all supplies, equipment, and parenteral solution prior to use for damage to equipment and supplies, contamination of solutions.
11. Verbalize purpose, type, operation of infusion pump, filter, and tubing, power source and maintenance.
12. Demonstrate how to attach tubing to infusion pump, clean catheter insertion site, connect tubing to catheter.
13. Demonstrate following of schedule for infusion/verbalize importance of not changing rate without specific order.
14. Demonstrate measures to protect IV site.
15. Verbalize importance of/demonstrate tapering of HPN solution as ordered.
16. Demonstrate how to disconnect infusion.
17. Verbalize purpose/demonstrate correct procedure for drawing up normal saline and heparin and flushing of catheter, application of heparin cap.
18. Demonstrate changing of injection cap.
19. Demonstrate correct procedure for prepping and changing of dressing over skin exit site at frequency ordered.
20. Verbalize purpose, frequency, procedure for changing of IV tubing and filter.

21. Demonstrate correct procedure for weighing daily, recording/verbalize importance of reporting weight gain or loss outside parameters set by physician.
22. Demonstrate correct measuring, recording of daily intake and output.
23. Demonstrate correct fractional urine testing/reporting 3+ or 4+ sugar or acetone to physician.
24. Verbalize importance/demonstrate good oral hygiene.
25. Demonstrate fat emulsion setup and infusion process as ordered/verbalize S&S of adverse reactions/actions to take.
26. Verbalize effect of oral deprivation on hunger sensation.
27. Verbalize purpose and need for prescribed lab work.
28. Verbalize importance of/wear Medic Alert bracelet.
29. Demonstrate activities within prescribed levels.
30. Describe actions to handle infusion equipment problems.
31. Identify names and phone numbers to call when in need of assistance with HPN.
32. Describe actions to handle emergency situations (e.g., catheter complications).
33. Demonstrate decreased level of anxiety with use of effective coping mechanisms for positive adaptation to altered body image and need for HPN.

NURSING ACTIONS/TREATMENTS

1. Assess cardiovascular, respiratory status, response to nutrient solution/identify S&S of complications.
2. Assess vital signs/identify trends (e.g., elevated temperature, cardiac arrhythmias, tachycardia, labored respirations)/instruct how to take and record vital signs every four hours or more often as prescribed, what alterations to report to home health nurse or physician.
3. Instruct about clinical indication, need, purpose for HPN, catheter insertion site, type of solution, importance of strict compliance with prescribed treatment regimen.
4. Observe/instruct about S&S of complications to report to home health nurse or physician.
5. Assess and evaluate on an ongoing basis nutritional status (include physical exam, anthropometric measurements, results of biochemical lab determinations)/instruct about amount and type of oral foods, fluids allowed/obtain dietary consultation as needed.
6. Observe/instruct about taking medications as ordered, purpose and action, side effects/evaluate medication effectiveness.
7. Observe/instruct about importance of strict hand-washing technique, importance of maintaining aseptic technique with all activities and procedures concerned with HPN.
8. Observe/instruct about importance of following a step-by-step procedure for

daily setting up the infusion pump with solution and tubing, medications and supplies (including additives, vials, ampules).

9. Observe/instruct how to obtain and store needed supplies.

10. Observe/instruct about importance of inspecting all supplies and parenteral solutions prior to use for cracks, punctures, leakage, discolored tubing, contaminated solution.

11. Observe/instruct about purpose, type, operation of infusion pump and filter ordered, tubing, power source and maintenance, manufacturer's instructions for operation.

12. Observe/instruct how to attach tubing to infusion pump, clean catheter insertion site, connect to catheter.

13. Observe/instruct about schedule for infusion, importance of continuously infusing parenteral solution at a constant rate over ordered time, not to ''catch up'' or slow down without specific instruction from physician, to check flow rate at least every 30 minutes to 1 hour.

14. Observe/instruct about protection of IV site (e.g., avoiding tension on catheter; not touching area of catheter insertion).

15. Observe/instruct to taper HPN solution as ordered to avoid glucose intolerance and rebound hypoglycemia, how to disconnect infusion.

16. Observe/instruct as to purpose and procedure for preparing and drawing up of normal saline and heparin for flushing of catheter, sterile application of heparin cap.

17. Observe/instruct how to change injection cap.

18. Observe/instruct about frequency, purpose, and procedure for prepping and changing of dressing over skin exit site, use of solutions, ointments as ordered (e.g., acetone, alcohol, povidone-iodine, iodine, iodophor), dressing changes every 24 hr/48 hr/72 hr, depending on agency policy and as required when dressing is wet, contaminated, or loose, marking date of change, importance of taping of all tubing connections.

19. Observe/instruct about purpose, frequency, procedure in changing of tubing and filter (e.g., 24 hr/48 hr) depending on agency policy and as required, marking date of change, importance of taping of all tubing connections.

20. Assess and evaluate for fluid volume excess or deficit/instruct to weigh daily at the same time of day on the same scale with same clothing, record, report weight gain or loss outside parameters set by physician.

21. Assess/instruct about strict intake and output, how to measure, record.

22. Observe/instruct about purpose, procedure, schedule for fractional urine testing for sugar and acetone, reporting to physician 3+ or 4+ sugar or acetone as ordered.

23. Observe/instruct about fat emulsion setup and infusion process as ordered, S&S of adverse reactions, actions to take.

24. Assess/instruct about effect of oral deprivation on hunger sensation.

25. Observe/evaluate oral mucosa/instruct importance of good oral hygiene; S&S of breakdown report to home health nurse or physician.

26. Monitor/instruct about purpose of prescribed lab testing to assess progress of HPN therapy and assess for impending complications and imbalances.
27. Observe and evaluate degree of self-care/instruct about activity levels and limitations as prescribed.
28. Evaluate equipment functioning/instruct about infusion equipment problems that may arise while on HPN, measures to correct (e.g., air in tubing and battery alarms, occlusion alarms, pump not working, accidental tubing disconnection), actions to take, persons to contact.
29. Evaluate for complications/instruct about handling emergency situations (e.g., catheter complications: air embolism, signs of infection, catheter clotting, catheter break or leaking), persons to contact, actions to take.
30. Assess level of anxiety, coping mechanisms, readiness to learn/provide emotional support/encourage to verbalize feelings and concerns/refer to social services as ordered to assist the client to a positive adaptation to condition and HPN therapy program/provide information of needed community resources (American Cancer Society, financial assistance; attendant services).
31. Observe/instruct about importance of wearing Medic Alert bracelet with information on medical condition and current treatment.
32. List names and phone numbers of pharmacy, home health agency, physician beside client's phone and/or home HPN instruction sheet/instruct about importance of calling with S&S of complications, adverse reactions, concerns or questions.

REHABILITATION POTENTIAL

Rehabilitation potential   *excellent   good   fair   guarded   poor*   for   *full partial*   achievement of an improved state of metabolic functioning and quality of life, ability to independently manage self-care and daily activities.

Client's Name _____

Medical Record # _____

ONGOING/DISCHARGE EVALUATION OF TEACHING
The Client Receiving Home Patenteral Nutrition

Teaching Tools:
Printed materials given: _____

Audiovisual aids used: _____

Return Information/Demonstration/Interpretation
_____ Client
_____ Caregiver

OF:	Met	Not Met	Comments
☐ Nature of clinical condition; purpose and need for HPN.	_____	_____	_____
☐ S&S of complications, actions to take.	_____	_____	_____
☐ Importance of strict compliance with prescribed treatment regimen.	_____	_____	_____
☐ How to take and record vital signs, what alterations to report to physician.	_____	_____	_____
☐ Type and amount of oral foods allowed.	_____	_____	_____
☐ Medications and administration,			

Client's Name _____

Medical Record #_____

OF:	Met	Not Met	Comments
purpose and action, side effects.	_____	_____	_____
☐ Proper hand-washing technique.	_____	_____	_____
☐ Aseptic technique.	_____	_____	_____
☐ Step-by-step procedure for daily setting up of infusion pump with solution, tubing, medications, supplies.	_____	_____	_____
☐ How to obtain and store supplies.	_____	_____	_____
☐ Inspecting of all supplies, equipment, and parenteral solutions for damage or contamination prior to use.	_____	_____	_____
☐ Use and care of infusion pump, filter, or tubing.	_____	_____	_____

Preparation of Hyperalimentation Infusion

☐ Connect new tubing solution container	_____	_____	_____

Client's Name _____

Medical Record # _____

OF:	Met	Not Met	Comments
☐ Running fluid through tubing;	_____	_____	_____
☐ attach tubing to infusion pump; regulate rate	_____	_____	_____
☐ cleaning catheter insertion site;	_____	_____	_____
☐ connecting tubing to central venous tubing catheter;	_____	_____	_____
☐ starting parenteral infusion;	_____	_____	_____
☐ infusing solution at constant rate over ordered time, importance of not changing rate;	_____	_____	_____
☐ Protection of IV site: avoiding tension on catheter, not touching area of catheter insertion.	_____	_____	_____
☐ checking flow rate every 30 min to 1 hr.	_____	_____	_____

Client's Name _____

Medical Record #_____

OF:	Met	Not Met	Comments
☐ discontinuing parenteral infusion;	_____	_____	_____
☐ tapering of HPN solution;	_____	_____	_____
☐ Correct procedure for drawing up of heparin and saline and flushing catheter; of heparin lock.	_____	_____	_____
☐ Sterile application of heparin cap.	_____	_____	_____
☐ Changing injection cap.	_____	_____	_____
☐ Prepping and changing of dressing over skin exit site at frequency ordered.	_____	_____	_____
☐ Purpose, frequency, procedure of changing IV tubing, filter.	_____	_____	_____
☐ Daily weighing recording, reporting weight loss or gain outside parameters set by physician.	_____	_____	_____

Client's Name _____

Medical Record # _____

	OF:	Met	Not Met	Comments
☐	Daily recording of intake and output.	_____	_____	_____
☐	Fractional urine testing.	_____	_____	_____
☐	Fat emulsion setup and infusion process.	_____	_____	_____
☐	Oral deprivation on hunger sensations.	_____	_____	_____
☐	Oral hygiene.	_____	_____	_____
☐	Purpose of prescribed lab work.	_____	_____	_____
☐	Prescribed activity levels.	_____	_____	_____
☐	Infusion equipment problems, actions to handle.	_____	_____	_____
☐	Emergency situations, procedures, names and phone numbers to call when needing assistance.	_____	_____	_____
☐	Medic Alert bracelet.	_____	_____	_____

Signature of Home Health Nurse _____

Date _____

■ Intravenous Therapy

Intravenous therapy (IV) is a means of administering fluids, electrolytes, and other nutrients through the veins in those clients who are unable to maintain an adequate intake by mouth and/or when the digestive system cannot maintain an adequate nutritional status. The intravenous route also serves as medium for administering systemic medications and restoring and maintaining acid–base balance and blood volume when clinically indicated.

POTENTIAL COMPLICATIONS

1. Speed shock (medications administered too quickly or bolus infused improperly),
2. catheter embolism,
3. circulatory overload,
4. air embolism,
5. thrombophlebitis,
6. infection, local or systemic,
7. infiltration,
8. hematoma,
9. blood loss from inadvertant disconnection of catheter,
10. allergic reaction to tape, solution, or ointment.

TYPES OF CLIENTS/CLINICAL CONDITIONS SEEN BY HOME HEALTH AGENCIES

1. Initiation of IV therapy: inclusive teaching program for prescribed management of home IV therapy in those clients placed on intravenous medications, including antibiotics, chemotherapy, and others specific to clinical condition and needs of the client.
2. Local reactions and/or systemic complications associated with IV therapy: changes in ongoing plan of treatment, evaluation of response to therapy changes.

RELATED NURSING DIAGNOSIS

Anxiety

related to:
1. IV therapy at home
2. Potential complications related to intravenous therapy

as seen by:
Frequent questions; frequent calling of home health nurse and/or IV team for reassurance; restlessness; lack of

3. Knowledge deficit regarding prescribed treatment regimen for management of IV

questions after teaching

Comfort, Alteration in: Pain

related to:
1. Infiltration
2. Thrombophlebitis
3. Hematoma formation
4. Infection of venipuncture site
5. Rapid infusion
6. Certain types of medications

as seen by:
Edema; acute tenderness, redness, and soreness at IV site or along the vein

Fluid Volume, Alteration in: Excess

related to:
1. Too much fluid
2. IV solution delivered too fast

as seen by:
Increased BP; shortness of breath; tachypnea; dilation of veins

Infection, Potential for

related to:
1. Venipuncture, breakdown in body's first line of defense
2. Failure to keep IV site clean
3. Failure to perform IV site care, change tubing as prescribed
4. Poor aseptic or hand-washing technique

as seen by:
Redness, swelling, and tenderness at IV site; foul-smelling drainage; elevated temperature

Knowledge Deficit (Specify)

related to:
1. Prescribed plan of treatment for home IV therapy
2. Associated potential complications, adverse reactions to report to home health nurse or physician

as seen by:
Verbalization of lack of knowledge; inadequate understanding; inablility to perform skills necessary to manage IV at home

Mobility, Impaired Physical

related to:
Limitation of physical movement

as seen by:
Reluctance to attempt movement;

secondary to infusion equipment and tubing with intravenous therapy

restriction of movement

Self-Care Deficit: Feeding, Bathing/Hygiene, Dressing/Grooming, Toileting (Specify)

related to:
1. Impaired physical mobility
2. Prescribed activity restrictions

as seen by:
Limitations in mobility status secondary to IV equipment, needing assistance to meet personal needs (e.g., dressing/bathing); medically imposed restrictions

Self-Concept, Disturbance in

related to:
Change in body functioning

as seen by:
Inability to care for self; inability to meet role expectations; verbalized feelings of not being able to eat in normal manner

Skin Integrity, Impairment of: Potential

related to:
1. Infection at venipuncture site
2. Infiltration

as seen by:
Chills and fever; erythema; edema; pain; pallor; coldness along needle site; drainage

LONG-TERM GOAL

To restore fluid and electrolyte balance and nutritional status of the client through the safe administration of water, electrolytes, and other nutrients through intravenous therapy.

SHORT-TERM GOALS

The client on a home intravenous therapy program will be able to:

1. Verbalize the purpose of IV therapy, principle of gravity and air, type of catheter, limitations and movement allowed.
2. Verbalize S&S of complications to report to home health nurse or physician.
3. Demonstrate how to accurately take and record vital signs/identify alterations to report to home health nurse or physician.

4. Demonstrate good hand-washing technique, aseptic technique in handling of IV site and sterile areas of IV setup.
5. Verbalize importance of inspecting container and IV solution, all equipment and supplies prior to use to ensure safety: disposing of contaminated materials safely.
6. Identify the type and amount of solution ordered, factors that may interfere with proper infusion/demonstrate correct technique for regulating and maintaining flow rate.
7. Verbalize purpose and type of infusion pump ordered/demonstrate correct usage and care of equipment.
8. Demonstrate IV site care as prescribed, dressing changes.
9. Verbalize frequency and purpose of changing IV site and tubing by home health nurse or IV team, importance of labeling IV bag or bottle with date, time, and IV medication.
10. Verbalize type of IV piggyback medications ordered/demonstrate correct procedure in administration, adverse reactions to report.
11. Identify S&S of potential complications, actions to take, how and when to stop or discontinue IV and seek medical attention.
12. Verbalize knowledge of/demonstrate how to check placement of heparin lock and correct procedure for preparing and flushing heparin lock with normal saline and heparin as ordered.
13. Verbalize dietary and fluid amounts prescribed.
14. Demonstrate compliance with prescribed medication therapy/identify side effects.
15. Verbalize prescribed activities allowed while on intravenous therapy.
16. Demonstrate how to measure and record intake and output.
17. Verbalize importance of weighing daily and recording/report weight gain outside parameters set by physician.
18. Verbalize purpose of prescribed laboratory testing.
19. Identify health professional(s) to call regarding assistance with intravenous therapy.
20. Demonstrate effective coping mechanisms for positive adjustment in management of home intravenous therapy program.

NURSING ACTIONS/TREATMENTS

1. Assess cardiovascular and respiratory status, venipuncture site and surrounding area/identify complications.
2. Assess vital signs/identify trends (e.g., bounding or weak pulse, increased BP, elevated temperature)/instruct how to take and record vital signs, what alterations to report to home health nurse or physician.

3. Instruct about purpose of intravenous therapy, principles that govern flow of IV fluids, continuous or intermittent, type of catheter (limitations and movement allowed), gravity drip or infusion pump, importance of compliance with prescribed treatment regimen, S&S of complications to report to home health nurse or physician.

4. Observe/instruct about proper hand-washing technique, aseptic technique in handling of IV site and sterile areas of IV setup (e.g., inside of IV bag or bottle; connections of tubing; IV solution).

5. Observe/instruct in the following: inspecting bottle or bags for cracks, puncture, leakage; solution and tubing for discoloration, solution expiration date; storage requirements of solutions, medications, and supplies as directed; disposing of contaminated materials safely.

6. Observe/instruct as to amount and type of solution ordered, calculation and technique of regulating and maintaining of flow rate, factors that may interfere with proper infusion and flow rate (e.g., kinking or clogging of tubing; position of client's extremity; solution hanging too low; defect in control clamp; pressure over IV insertion site; needle moved against vein wall; defective solution bag or bottle).

7. Observe/instruct about purpose, type, operation, care of infusion pump ordered, changing of bag or bottle, alarm system, special tubing, photoelectric sensor, power source and maintenance, manufacturer's instructions for maintenance.

8. Observe/instruct about inspecting skin at or near veinipuncture site for redness, swelling, drainage; frequency of dressing changes, including cleaning of area site with prescribed skin preparations (e.g., iodine, povidone-iodine, alcohol) and application of bacteriostatic ointment.

9. Observe/instruct about importance of labeling IV bag or bottle with date, time, and IV medication.

10. Instruct about frequency and purpose of changing IV site and tubing by home health nurse or IV team (e.g., 24 hours, 48 hours/72 hours) depending on agency policy and as required, labeling date of change.

11. Observe/instruct about prescribed "piggyback" medication(s); dose, type, and amount of diluent; how often administered; adverse reactions to report.

12. Assess/instruct about how to check placement of heparin lock, purpose, how to flush with normal saline and heparin as ordered.

13. Observe/instruct about S/S of complications, actions to take, how and when to stop or discontinue IV and seek medical attention.

14. Assess and evaluate nutritional status/instruct about dietary and fluid amounts as prescribed.

15. Observe/instruct about prescribed medication therapy, purpose and action, side effects/evaluate medication effectiveness.

16. Assess/instruct as to prescribed activity levels while on intravenous therapy.

17. Observe/instruct about purpose and how to measure and record daily intake and output while on intravenous therapy.

18. Assess/instruct to weigh daily and record/report weight gain outside parameters set by physician.
19. Monitor/instruct about purpose of prescribed lab testing/confer with physician on all lab results.
20. List names and phone numbers of pharmacy, home IV team, physician beside client's phone and/or on home IV instruction sheet/instruct about importance of calling about S&S of complications, adverse reactions, or with any concerns or questions regarding intravenous therapy.
21. Assess level of coping with home intravenous therapy/provide emotional support/encourage verbalization of concerns and feelings/refer to social services to provide counseling to assist with positive adjustment to home intravenous therapy, modification in life-style.

REHABILITATION POTENTIAL

Rehabilitation potential *excellent good fair guarded poor* for *full partial* achievement of an improved state of well-being and independence in self-care activities, after completion of home intravenous therapy.

Client's Name _____

Medical Record # _____

ONGOING/DISCHARGE EVALUATION OF TEACHING
The Client on Intravenous Therapy

Teaching Tools:
Printed materials given: _____

Audiovisual aids used: _____

Return Information/Demonstration/Interpretation
_____ Client
_____ Caregiver

OF:	Met	Not Met	Comments
☐ Purpose of intraveneous therapy.	_____	_____	_____
☐ S&S of complications, actions to take.	_____	_____	_____
☐ Type of IV catheter, limitations and movement allowed.	_____	_____	_____
☐ Importance of compliance with prescribed treatment regimen.	_____	_____	_____
☐ How to take and record vital signs, what alterations to report to physician.	_____	_____	_____
☐ Hand-washing technique.	_____	_____	_____

Client's Name _____

Medical Record # _____

OF:	Met	Not Met	Comments
☐ Aseptic technique in handling of IV site and sterile areas of IV setup.	_____	_____	_____
☐ Importance of inspecting all IV solutions and related supplies prior to use.	_____	_____	_____
☐ Disposing of contaminated materials safely.	_____	_____	_____
☐ Amount and type of solution ordered.	_____	_____	_____
☐ Regulating and maintaining of flow rate; factors that interfere with rate of infusion.	_____	_____	_____
☐ Using gravity drip method.	_____	_____	_____
☐ IV infusion pump, tubing, changing of bag or bottle; alarm system, photoelectric sensor, power source and maintenance.	_____	_____	_____
☐ IV site care, dressing changes.	_____	_____	_____

Client's Name _____

Medical Record #_____

OF:	**Met**	**Not Met**	**Comments**
☐ How to check placement of heparin lock.	_____	_____	_____
☐ Preparing and flushing heparin lock with normal saline and heparin.	_____	_____	_____
☐ Frequency and purpose of changing IV site and tubing; labeling IV bag or bottle with date, time, and IV medication.	_____	_____	_____
☐ Piggyback medications.	_____	_____	_____
☐ How and when to discontinue IV and seek medical attention.	_____	_____	_____
☐ Intake and output.	_____	_____	_____
☐ Weighing and recording of weight as ordered/ reporting weight gain outside parameters set by physician.	_____	_____	_____
☐ Purpose of prescribed lab work.	_____	_____	_____

Client's Name _____

Medical Record #_____

OF:	**Met**	**Not Met**	**Comments**
☐ Emergency situations, procedures, and names and phone numbers to call when needing assistance.	_____	_____	_____
☐ How and when to discontinue an IV.	_____	_____	_____
☐ Dietary and fluid amounts allowed.	_____	_____	_____
☐ Medications and administration, purpose and action, side effects.	_____	_____	_____
☐ Daily activity levels while on IV therapy.	_____	_____	_____

Signature of Home Health Nurse _____

Date _____

APPENDICES

■ Appendix A. Health History at a Glance

Identification (ID)
Name, address, telephone number, age, sex, race, nationality, marital status, occupation, Social Security number, informant, reliability.

Current Complaint (CC)
Reason seeking health care. Duration.

History of Present Illness (HPI)
Onset date, situation, mode, precipitating events; symptom location, quality, severity, how relieved, duration, association, relation to habits; order of symptom development, recurrence, treatment effect, effect of change in situation; current symptoms, location, severity; client's idea of cause and effect; reason problem of concern; reason for seeking help at present.

Past Medical History (PMH)
Medical, surgical, psychiatric illnesses, hospitalizations, childhood illnesses, immunizations, injuries or disabilities, allergies, current medications, transfusions.

Family History (FH)
Age and health status, or age of death of parents, siblings, children; familial diseases.

Personal/Social History (P/SH)
Type of work, exposure to harmful agents, years schooling, military history, hobbies, finances, effect of illness; location of family members, number dependents, who lives in home, type of housing; marital status, age and health of spouse, satisfaction with relationship, effect of illness on marriage and family; sexual education, orientation, performance, satisfaction, effect of illness, birth control; social satisfaction, group membership, religion, effect of illness; use of tobacco, alcohol, other drugs; client or family under psychiatric care, duration, name of psychiatrist, type of care; activities of daily life (ADL); diet.

Review of Symptoms (ROS)

General:
Overall state of health, ability to carry out ADL, weight changes, fatigue, exercise tolerance, fever, night sweats, repeated infections.

Integument:
Change in skin pigmentation, texture, moisture, eruptions, rashes, pruritus, pain, unusual hair growth or loss, deformities of nails.

Head, Face, Scalp:

Headache, trauma, sinus pain, scalp itching, scalp infestations.

Eyes:

Visual problems, diplopia, scotomata, use of glasses, date of last examination, eye pain, eye itching, lid edema, excessive tearing, tests for glaucoma, photophobia.

Ears:

Mastoiditis, pain, discharge, tennitus, dizziness, vertigo, hearing problem, sensitive to certain types of noise.

Nose, Mouth, Throat:

Smell, sinusitis, epistaxis, nasal obstruction, pain, discharge, head colds, trauma; fit of dentures, last visit to dentist, dental problems, pain, lesions, soreness of tongue, bleeding or swelling of gums, brush teeth regularly, fluoride treatments, change in taste sense, difficulty swallowing, hoarseness.

Neck:

Stiffness, pain, masses.

Breasts, axillae:

Discharge, bleeding, masses, changes with menses, breast self-examination.

Respiratory:

Chest x-ray (date, result), wheezing, cough, hemoptysis, expectoration, dyspnea, night sweats, sneezing, rhinorrhea.

Cardiovascular:

Dyspnea on exertion, orthopnea, paroxysmal nocturnal dyspnea, hypertension, claudication, varicose veins, thrombophlebitis, Raynaud's Disease, syncope, chest pain, palpitations, tachycardia, heart murmur, peripheral edema.

Gastrointestinal:

Dietary habits, appetite, food intolerance, use of antacids, indigestion, nausea, vomiting, distension, abdominal pains, abdominal masses, jaundice, hematemesis, bowel habits, use of laxatives, constipation, melena, mucus in stools, acholic stools, diarrhea, hemorrhoids, incontinence, abdominal surgery.

Genitourinary:

Male and female: Sexual habits, venereal disease, potency, dysuria, polyuria, oliguria, hematuria, pyuria, calculi, force of stream, retention, frequency, hesitancy, nocturia, incontinence, discharge. Male: Prostatitis, hernia.

Gynecologic:

Menarche, duration, amount, interval, catamenia, menorrhagia, metrorrhagia, date last menstrual period, amenorrhea, type of contraception, infertility, dyspareunia, postcoital bleeding, vaginal discharge, pruritus, date and result of last Pap smear, vaginal or uterine surgery.

Obstetrical:

Pregnancies, full-term deliveries, premature deliveries, abortions, living children, complications of pregnancies.

Musculoskeletal:

Muscle weakness, pain, aches, cramps, atrophy, back or joint stiffness, pain, deformity, dislocation, fractures, radicular pain.

Neurologic:

Headache, nervousness, sleep disturbance, vertigo, syncope, sensory or motor disturbance, paralysis or paresis, paresthesia, hyperesthesia, hypesthesia, memory loss, nightmares, twitching, convulsions, tremors, dysphagia, handwriting changes, loss of consciousness, disorientation.

Psychiatric:

Disorientation, irritability, depression, mood swings, suicidal or homicidal attempts, delusions, hallucinations, feelings of persecution, ideas of reference, paranoia, anxiety, phobias, indecision, preoccupation, obsessive rumination.

Endocrine:

Change in skin color or texture, hair distribution, sexual vigor, voice, goiter, polydipsia, polyphagia, polyuria, growth change, intolerance of temperature, sugar in blood or urine, excessive sweating.

Lymphatic and Hematologic:

Lymph node swellings, excessive bleeding, bruising, anemia, blood transfusions.

(From Berger, K., Fields, W. *Pocket Guide to Health Assessment,* Reston, Va.: Reston Publishing Co., 1980.)

■ Appendix B. Physical Examination at a Glance

Measurements
Height, weight, BP, temperature, pulse, respirations, tonometry, visual acuity, audiometry.

General Survey
Mental status; appearance; apparent sex, race, age, nutrition; body development, proportions; station, posture; movement, gait; dominance; energy; speech; odors.

Integument
Skin color, texture, temperature, turgor, hygiene, veins, lesions, masses, edema; hair; nails.

Head, Skull, Scalp, Face
Size, contour, hygiene, proportions, pigmentation, expression, movement, sensation, edema, masses, lesions, lymph nodes, tenderness.

Eyes
Brows and lashes; lid conformation position, blinking, inflammation, lesions, tearing, eyeball and orbit; conjunctiva color, moisture, lesions, sclera color; cornea color, contour, depth, sensitivity; iris color, shape; pupil shape, size, reactivity; eye alignment; extraocular movement; red reflex; disk shape, size, margins, color, cup-to-disk ratio; retinal vessels; ocular tension, compressibility; visual acuity, color visions, near vision, visual fields.

Ear
Pinna shape, position, tenderness; mastoid tenderness; auditory canal malformation, cerument, foreign body, lesion; Tympanic Membrane landmarks; hearing voice, watch tick, tuning-fork tests.

Nose, Mouth, Throat
Turbinates, septal deviation; mucosal moisture, lips movement, condition; teeth; gum condition; tongue texture, size, movement; sublingual veins; oral mucosal texture; salivary duct patency; palate contour, movement; uvula; tonsil size, contour, membrane; posterior pharyngeal wall edema, discharge, movement; sinus tenderness; smell; taste; voice quality; color and lesions of all tissues.

Neck
Symmetry, curvature, range of motion, head movement, pulsation, lymph nodes, venous distension, thyroid enlargement, masses; tracheal position; muscle strength.

Breasts, axillae
Breasts: size, symmetry, color, contour, hair pattern, venous pattern, edema, lesions, scars, rashes, masses, retractions, premenstrual changes, tenderness; areola:

color; nipple: lesions, discharge, retractions; axilla: hair distribution, rashes, ulcers, masses, tenderness.

Chest
Contour, dimensions, rib angle, movement; skin color, moisture, scars; respiratory rate, rhythm, depth, quality, type, ratio to heart rate; fremitus; crepitations; tenderness; masses, swelling; lung borders; diaphragm excursion; breath sounds.

Cardiovascular
Precordial bulges, retractions, pulsations, thrills, lifts; point of maximum impulse (PMI); left cardiac border; suprasternal thrill; pulse rate, rhythm, amplitude; arterial elasticity; heart sounds, extra sounds, murmurs, BP; neck pulsations, venous distension; arm, groin, leg, foot pulses; bruits; nail, skin color; leg hair distribution.

Abdomen
Skin; venous pattern; hair pattern; contour, pulsations; fluid wave; umbilical hernias; peristaltic sounds; bruits; organ borders; gaseous distension; shifting dullness; friction rub; succession splash; tenderness, rigidity, guarding; masses; skin reflexes.

Anus, rectum
Perianal area: color, hair, lesions, rashes, anal lumps, fistulas, hemorrhoids, prolapse, rectal polyps, masses, nodules, fissures, prolapse, tenderness, sphincter tone, stricture, internal hemorrhoids, pilonidal dimples, drainage; prostate: enlargement, tenderness, consistency, mobility; cervix: location, shape; fecal color, consistency, smear.

Gynecologic Genitourinary Female (GU)
Pubic hair pattern; perineal lesions, scars, masses, edema, inflammation, discharge, incontinence, prolapse; cervical color, diameter, position, mobility, discharge erosion, ulcers, masses, tenderness, inflammation; os size, shape, eversion, erosion, polyps; vaginal texture, color, discharge, bulging; uterine size, position, consistency, contour, mobility, tenderness; ovary size, contour, mobility, tenderness, cul de sac bulging, tenderness, masses.

Male GU
Pubic hair distribution; penis size, foreskin retraction, location of meatus, inflammation, scars, masses, discharge, tenderness; scrotal inflammation, scars, rashes, nodules, ulcers, discharge; testicular presence, mobility, size, shape, tenderness; epididymal tenderness; spermatic cord masses, tenderness, hernias.

Musculoskeletal
Body symmetry, formation, posture; thoracic contour; spinal ROM, tenderness; straight leg raising; scapular position; chest expansion, extremity length, diameter, mass, muscle condition, bone and joint formation, ROM; hip ROM; muscle tone,

tenderness, fasciculations, masses; joint crepitation, tenderness, masses, temperature; costrovertebral angle tenderness; muscle strength size.

Neurologic-Psychiatric

Level of consciousness (LOC), orientation, mood and behavior, knowledge and vocabulary, judgment and abstraction, memory, calculation; speech, language; stereognosis, cranial nerves; balance, gait, Romberg test, finger-to-toe, heel-to-shin, alternating motion; involuntary movement; sensation; superficial skin and deep tendon reflexes, Babinski reflex.

(From Berger, K., Fields, W. *Pocket Guide to Health Assessment,* Reston, Va.: Reston Publishing Co., 1980.)

■ Appendix C. Nutrition, Weight, and Stature

NUTRITIONAL ASSESSMENT CHART

Client's Name _____
Medical Record # _____
Date of Admission _____

NUTRITIONAL ASSESSMENT

Objective Data

Age: _____   Sex: _____   Primary Diagnosis: _____
Height: _____   Weight: _____   Diet Order: _____
Pertinent Diagnostic Lab Work _____   Ideal Body Weight: _____   Recent Weight Change _____
     Body Type: Small ___   Medium ___   Large ___

Subjective Data

	Yes	No
1. Diet understood by client/caregiver?		
If no, explain.		
2. Is diet followed?		
If no, explain.		
3. Eats at least 75 percent of each meal?		
If no, why not?		
4. Resides alone?		
5. Prepares own food?		
If no, who prepares?		
6. Has adequate funds for food?		
7. Follows three-meal pattern daily?		
8. Client is a vegetarian?		

If yes, will client eat:
___ Poultry   ___ Cheese   ___ Eggs
___ Fish   ___ Milk   ___ Yogurt

	Yes	No
13. Needs between-meal nourishments?		
14. Uses nutritional supplements?		
Identify.		
15. Is client a diabetic? If yes, type of therapy:		
___ Oral hypoglycemic		
___ Diet control		
___ Insulin-dependent		
16. Nutritional problems caused by treatment and/or medication therapy? If yes, specify.		

(e.g., Taste alteration and change in sense of smell secondary to radiation therapy to head and neck; stomatitis

9. Food preferences (includes culture factors)? ___
   If yes, specify. ___

10. Needs assistance eating? ___
    If yes, explain. ___

11. Wears dentures? ___
    Fit? ___

12. Client has chewing or swallowing problems? ___
    If yes, please explain? ___
    What texture of food is needed?
    — Regular — Soft — Pureed — Liquid

resulting from chemotherapy or electrolyte imbalance with use of diuretics). ___

17. Psychological factors. If yes, specify (e.g., grief, anxiety, fear, depression, ineffective coping mechanisms: eats/doesn't eat; depression). ___

18. Client eats from which of the following food groups?
    ___ Group I: Milk, cheese
    ___ Group II: Meat, fish, poultry
    ___ Group III: Eggs, nuts, seeds, peanut butter
    ___ Group IV: Beans
    ___ Group V: Fruits and vegetables
    ___ Group VI: Breads and cereals

19. Activity level:
    ___ Immobile   ___ Sedentary   ___ Moderate   ___ Active

20. Physical conditions that may affect nutritional requirements:
    ___ Ulcer: ___ Fever   ___ Diarrhea   ___ Surgery
    ___ Decubitus or ___ Nausea and vomiting   ___ Constipation   ___ Anorexia
    ___ Stasis   ___ Burns   ___ Obesity   ___ Other

Comments ___

Assessment of Nutritional Status:

Weight:

☐ Weight is within range of ideal weight.
☐ Weight is 20 percent or more under ideal weight.
☐ Weight is 10 percent or more over ideal weight.
☐ Nutritional support program may be indicated.

Food Intake:

___ Adequate food intake (no significant nutritional problems).
___ Inadequate food intake (specify food group(s) or nutrients deficient in diet).
___ Low financial resources resulting in inadequate food selection.
___ Needs nutritional supplements.

Diet Information:

___ Client is complying with a modified diet or dietary restrictions as ordered by physician.
___ Client does not follow a modified diet or dietary restrictions as ordered by physician and needs diet instruction.

Plan:

___ Consult with physician regarding diet instructions
___ Give/instruct about prescribed diet or dietary restrictions.
___ Consult with social worker.
___ Perform calorie count to determine food intake and fluid volume.
___ Consult with dietitian.
___ Consult with physician regarding necessity of nutritional supplements.

Signature of Home Health Nurse _____
Date _____

FRAME SIZE APPROXIMATION

Extend your arm and bend the forearm upward at a 90 degree angle. Keep fingers straight and turn the inside of your wrist toward your body. If you have a caliper, use it to measure the space between the two prominent bones on either side of your elbow. Without a caliper, place thumb and index finger of your other hand on these two bones. Measure the space between your fingers against a ruler or tape measure. Compare it with these tables that list elbow measurements for medium-framed men and women. Measurements lower than those listed indicate you have a small frame. Higher measurements indicate a larger frame.

Men		Women	
Height in 1" Heels	*Elbow Breadth*	*Height in 1" Heels*	*Elbow Breadth*
5'2"–5'3"	2 1/2"–2 7/8"	4'10"–4'11"	2 1/4"–2 1/2"
5'4"–5'7"	2 5/8"–2 7/8"	5'0"–5'3"	2 1/4"–2 1/2"
5'8"–5'11"	2 3/4"–3"	5'4"–5'7"	2 3/8"–2 5/8"
6'0"–6'3"	2 3/4"–3 1/8"	5'8"–5'11"	2 3/8"–2 5/8"
6'4"	2 7/8"–3 1/4"	6'0"	2 1/2"–2 3/4"

(*How You Can Control Your Weight.* Metropolitan Life Insurance Company, 1984. Used with permission.)

1983 METROPOLITAN HEIGHT AND WEIGHT TABLES[a]

Men					Women				
Height		*Small Frame*	*Medium Frame*	*Large Frame*	*Height*		*Small Frame*	*Medium Frame*	*Large Frame*
Feet	*Inches*				*Feet*	*Inches*			
5	2	128–134	131–141	138–150	4	10	102–111	109–121	118–131
5	3	130–136	133–143	140–153	4	11	103–113	111–123	120–134
5	4	132–138	135–145	142–156	5	0	104–115	113–126	122–137
5	5	134–140	137–148	144–160	5	1	106–118	115–129	125–140
5	6	136–142	139–151	146–164	5	2	108–121	118–132	128–143
5	7	138–145	142–154	149–168	5	3	111–124	121–135	131–147
5	8	140–148	145–157	152–172	5	4	114–127	124–138	134–151
5	9	142–151	148–160	155–176	5	5	117–130	127–141	137–155
5	10	144–154	151–163	158–180	5	6	120–133	130–144	140–159
5	11	146–157	154–166	161–184	5	7	123–136	133–147	143–163
6	0	149–160	157–170	164–188	5	8	126–139	136–150	146–167
6	1	152–164	160–174	168–192	5	9	129–142	139–153	149–170
6	2	155–168	164–178	172–197	5	10	132–145	142–156	152–173
6	3	158–172	167–182	176–202	5	11	135–148	145–159	155–176
6	4	162–176	171–187	181–207	6	0	138–151	148–162	158–179

[a]Weights at ages 25–59 based on lowest mortality. Weight in pounds according to frame (in indoor clothing weighing 5 lbs. for men and 3 lbs. for women; shoes with 1 inch heels).

(*1979 Build Study.* Society of Actuaries and Association of Life Insurance Medical Directors of America, 1980. [Taken from How You Can Control Your Weight. Metropolitan Life Insurance Company, 1984]).

PERCENTILES FOR STATURE OF ELDERLY WOMEN in cm (and inches)

Age (years)	95%	50%	5%
65	171.6(67.6)	161.6(63.4)	153.1(60.3)
70	169.8(66.9)	159.1(62.6)	151.3(59.6)
75	167.9(66.1)	157.3(61.9)	149.4(58.8)
80	166.1(65.4)	155.4(61.2)	147.6(58.1)
85	164.2(64.6)	153.6(60.5)	145.7(57.4)
90	162.4(63.9)	151.7(59.7)	143.9(56.6)

PERCENTILES FOR STATURE OF ELDERLY MEN in cm (and inches)

Age (years)	95%	50%	5%
65	181.6(71.5)	170.3(67.0)	159.1(62.6)
70	181.6(71.5)	169.9(66.9)	158.7(62.5)
75	181.2(71.3)	169.5(66.7)	158.4(62.4)
80	180.9(71.2)	169.1(66.6)	158.0(62.2)
85	180.5(71.1)	168.8(66.5)	157.7(62.1)
90	180.2(70.9)	168.5(66.3)	157.3(61.9)

PERCENTILES FOR WEIGHT OF ELDERLY WOMEN in kg (and lb)

Age (years)	95%	50%	5%
65	87.1(192.0)	66.8(147.3)	51.2(112.9)
70	84.9(187.2)	64.6(142.4)	49.0(108.0)
75	82.8(182.5)	62.4(137.6)	46.8(103.2)
80	80.6(177.7)	60.2(132.7)	44.7(98.5)
85	78.4(172.8)	58.0(127.9)	42.5(93.7)
90	76.2(168.0)	55.9(123.2)	40.3(88.8)

PERCENTILES FOR WEIGHT OF ELDERLY MEN in kg (and lb)

Age (years)	95%	50%	5%
65	102.0(224.9)	79.5(175.0)	62.6(138.0)
70	99.1(218.5)	76.5(168.7)	59.7(131.6)
75	96.3(212.3)	73.6(162.3)	56.8(125.2)
80	93.4(205.9)	70.7(155.9)	53.9(118.8)
85	90.5(199.5)	67.8(149.5)	51.0(112.4)
90	87.6(193.1)	64.9(142.8)	48.1(106.0)

Tables contain reference data by 95th, 50th, and 5th percentiles for men and women at ages 65, 70, 75, 80, 85, and 90. The 50th percentile represents the value that half the population is above and half below; the 95th and 5th percentiles are the upper and the lower limits of the normal range of values.

(*Nutritional Assessment of the Elderly Through Anthropometry.* Columbus, Ohio: Ross Laboratories, 1987. Used with permission.)

DIETARY CONSIDERATIONS FOR THE CLIENT WITH A GASTROINTESTINAL STOMA

High Fiber, Bulk-Forming Foods That May Cause Blockage	Gas-Producing Foods	Odor-Producing Foods	Foods that May Cause Loose Stools
Celery	Melons	Cabbage	Raw vegetables and fruits
Bean sprouts	Cabbage	Cheese	Highly seasoned foods
Nuts	Beans	Eggs	Some high-fiber cereals
Foods with seeds or kernels	Broccoli	Fish	
Chinese vegetables	Cauliflower	Onions	
Dried fruits	Brussel sprouts	Broccoli	
Popcorn	Fried foods	Beans	
Granola	Highly seasoned foods	Garlic	
Raw carrots	Onions	Turnips	
Fruit skins	Corn	Asparagus	
	Dairy products		
	Carbonated beverages and beer		
	Radishes		

EXCELLENT DIETARY SOURCE OF POTASSIUM (LOW IN SODIUM)

The following foods provide 400 mg (10 mEq) of potassium or more in the serving amounts listed

	Milligrams of Sodium
Fruits	
Apricots, dried: 10 halves	3
Avocado (Calif): 1/2	8
Banana, raw: medium	1
Cantaloupe: 1/2 cup	23
Nectarine, raw: 1	0.1
Orange juice: 1 cup	2
Prunes, dried: 10 pitted	3
Vegetables	
Potato, baked (flesh and skin): 1 medium	15
Potatoes peeled, boiled (flesh): 1/2 cup	4
Soybeans, cooked: 1/2 cup	13

(From Watt, B. K., & Merril A. L. *USDA Revised Handbook 8*, December 1963. Consumer and Food Economics Research Division Agricultural Research Service—U.S. Department of Agriculture, Washington, D.C.)

SODIUM-RESTRICTED EXCHANGE LISTS

Milk Exchanges
(1 cup [8 oz] contains 120 mg sodium)

Whole milk	Evaporated milk
Skim milk	Unsalted buttermilk
	6 oz plain yogurt

Meat Exchanges
(Each ounce, cooked, contains 25 mg sodium)

Fresh or frozen meat

Beef	Tongue
Lamb	Liver
Pork	Rabbit
Veal	

Fresh or Frozen Poultry
Chicken
Cornish hens
Duck
Turkey

Fresh or Dietetic Canned Fish

Cod	Tuna
Flounder	Bass
Haddock	Perch (lake)
Halibut	Pike
Perch (ocean)	Whitefish
Salmon	

Egg Exchange
(1 egg contains 70 mg sodium)

Vegetable Exchanges
(1 serving [½ cup] contains about 9 mg sodium)

Fresh, frozen without any sodium compound, and low-sodium canned dietetic vegetables or vegetable juices

Asparagus	Onions
Broccoli	Peas, green
Brussels sprouts	Peppers
Cabbage	Pumpkin
Cauliflower	Radishes
Chicory	Rutabagas
Cucumbers	String beans
Eggplant	Squash, summer
Escarole	Squash, winter
Green beans	Tomatoes
Lettuce	Tomato juice
Mushrooms	Wax beans
Okra	

Fruit Exchanges
(Each serving contains about 2 mg sodium)

Fresh, frozen, canned, or dried fruit and fruit juices

Bread Exchanges
(Each serving contains about 5 mg sodium)

Low-sodium bread, 1 slice
Low-sodium rolls, 1 medium
Crackers
  Low-sodium dietetic melba toast, 4 slices
Cereals, long cooking, ½ cup
  Farina
  Hominy grits
  Oatmeal
  Rolled wheat
  Wheat meal
Dry cereals, ¾ cup
  Puffed rice
  Puffed wheat
Pasta and other cereal products, ½ cup cooked
  Macaroni
  Noodles
  Spaghetti
  Barley
Flour, white or whole wheat, 1 cup
Dried beans and peas, ½ cup cooked
Corn, ⅓ cup cooked
Potato, white, 1 small or ½ cup, cooked
Sweet potatoes, ¼ cup cooked

Fat Exchanges
(1 tsp contains practically no sodium)

Unsalted butter and margarine
Vegetable oils
Shortenings
Low-sodium mayonnaise and salad dressings

Miscellaneous Foods
The following foods contain no sodium

Coffee, noninstant	Limes
Tea, noninstant	Gelatin
Sugar, white	Vinegar
Honey	Sodium-free
Calcium saccharin	baking powder
Lemons	Yeast

(From Anderson, L., Dibble, M. V., Turkki, P. R., Mitchell, H. S., Rynbergen, H. J., *Nutrition in Health and Disease,* (17th ed), Philadelphia: Lippincott, 1982.)

■ Appendix D. Diabetes

TYPES OF INSULIN

Insulin	Action	Onset	Peak	Duration
Regular insulin	Rapid	30–60 min	2–4 hr	6–8 hr
Prompt insulin zinc suspension (semilente)	Rapid	1–2 hr	4–8 hr	10–16 hr
Isophane insulin suspension (NPH)	Intermediate	1.5–2 hr	4–12 hr	18–24 hr
Insulin zinc suspension (lente)	Intermediate	2–4 hr	6–12 hr	18–26 hr
Protamine zinc insulin suspension (PZI)	Long-acting	4–8 hr	14–24 hr	28–36 hr
Extended insulin zinc suspension (ultralente)	Long-acting	4–8 hr	14–24 hr	28–36+

■ Appendix E. Aids

Recommendations for the Individual with Aids

An individual judged most likely to have an HIV infection should be provided the following information and advice:

1. The prognosis for an individual infected with HIV over the long term is not known. However, data available from studies conducted among homosexual men indicate that most persons will remain infected.
2. Although asymptomatic, these individuals may transmit HIV to others. Regular medical evaluation and follow-up is advised, especially for individuals who develop signs or symptoms suggestive of AIDS.
3. Refrain from donating blood, plasma, body organs, other tissue, or sperm.
4. There is a risk of infecting others by sexual intercourse, sharing of needles, and possibly exposure of others to saliva through oral–genital contact or intimate kissing. The efficacy of condoms in preventing infection with HIV is unproved, but the consistent use of them may reduce transmission.
5. Toothbrushes, razors, or other implements that could become contaminated with blood should not be shared.
6. Women with a seropositive test, or women whose sexual partner is seropositive, are themselves at increased risk of acquiring AIDS. If they become pregnant, their offspring are also at risk of acquiring AIDS.
7. After accidents resulting in bleeding, contaminated surfaces should be cleaned with household bleach freshly diluted 1 : 10 in water.
8. Devices that have punctured the skin, such as hypodermic and acupuncture needles, should be steam sterilized by autoclave before reuse or safely discarded. Whenever possible, disposable needles and equipment should be used.
9. When seeking medical or dental care for intercurrent illness, these persons should inform those responsible for their care of their positive antibody status so that appropriate evaluation can be undertaken and precautions taken to prevent transmission to others.
10. Testing for HIV antibody should be offered to persons who may have been infected as a result of their contact with seropositive individuals (e.g., sexual partners, persons with whom needles have been shared, infants born to seropositive mothers).

(Reported by Centers for Disease Control; Food and Drug Administration; Alcohol, Drug Abuse, and Mental Health Administration; National Institutes of Health; Health Resources and Services Administration. *Morbidity and Mortality Weekly Report.* Centers for Disease Control, *34*:1, 1985.)

RECOMMENDATIONS BY THE CENTERS FOR DISEASE CONTROL (CDC) FOR PREVENTION OF HIV TRANSMISSION

Universal Precautions

Since medical history and examination cannot reliably identify *all* clients infected with HIV or other blood-borne pathogens, blood and body-fluid precautions should be consistently used for all clients. This approach, previously recommended by the CDC, and referred to as "universal blood and body-fluid precautions" or "universal precautions," should be used in the care of *all* clients, including those in emergency-care settings in which the risk of blood exposure is increased and the infection status of the client is usually unknown. Universal precautions are intended to prevent parenteral, mucous membrane, and nonintact exposure of health-care workers to blood borne pathogens.

1. All health-care workers should routinely use appropriate barrier precautions to prevent skin and mucous-membrane exposure when contact with blood or other body fluids of any client is anticipated. Gloves should be worn for touching blood and body fluids, and for performing venipuncture and other vascular access procedures. Gloves should be changed after contact with each client. Masks and protective eyewear or face shields should be worn during procedures that are likely to generate droplets of blood or other body fluids to prevent exposure of mucous membranes of the mouth, nose, and eyes. Gowns or aprons should be worn during procedures that are likely to generate splashes of blood or other body fluids.

2. Hands and other skin surfaces should be washed immediately and thoroughly if contaminated with blood or other body fluids. Hands should be washed immediately after gloves are removed.

3. All health-care workers should take precautions to prevent injuries caused by needles, scalpels, and other sharp instruments or devices during procedures, when cleaning used instruments, during disposal of used needles, and when handling sharp instruments after procedures. To prevent needlestick injuries, needles should not be recapped, purposely bent or broken by hand, removed from disposable syringes, or otherwise manipulated by hand. After they are used, disposable syringes and needles, scalpel blades, and other sharp items should be placed in puncture-resistant containers for disposal; the puncture resistant containers should be located as close as practical to the use area. Large-bore reusable needles should be placed in a puncture-resistant container for transport to the reprocessing area.

4. Although saliva has not been implicated in HIV transmission, to minimize the need for emergency mouth-to-mouth resuscitation, mouthpieces, resuscitation bags, or other ventilation devices should be available for use in areas in which the need for resuscitation is predictable.

5. Health-care workers who have exudative lesions or weeping dermatitis should refrain from all direct care of client and from handling equipment used in the care of the client until the condition resolves.

6. Pregnant health-care workers are not known to be a greater risk of contacting HIV infection than health-care workers who are not pregnant; however, if a health-care worker develops HIV infection during pregnancy, the infant is at risk of infection resulting from perinatal transmission. Because of this risk, pregnant health-care workers should be especially familiar with and strictly adhere to precautions to minimize the risk of HIV transmission.

Isolation precautions (e.g. enteric, ''AFB'') should be used as necessary if associated conditions, such as infectius diarrhea or tuberculosis, are diagnosed or suspected.

Selection of Gloves

Medical gloves include those marketed as sterile surgical or nonsterile examination gloves made of vinyl or latex. General purpose utility (''rubber'') gloves are also used in health-care settings, but they are not regulated by the FDA since they are not promoted for medical use. There are no reported differences in barrier effectiveness between intact latex and intact vinyl used to manufacture gloves. Thus the type of gloves selected should be appropriate for the task being performed.

The following general guidelines are recommended:

1. Use sterile gloves for procedures involving contact with normally sterile areas of the body.
2. Use examination gloves for procedures involving contact with mucous membranes, unless otherwise indicated, and for other patient care or diagnostic procedures that do not require the use of sterile gloves.
3. Change gloves between patient contacts.
4. Do not wash or disinfect surgical or examination gloves for reuse. Washing with surfectants may cause ''wicking'', e.g. the enhanced penetration of liquids through undetected holes in the glove. Disinfecting agents may cause deterioration.
5. Use general-purpose utility gloves (e.g. rubber household gloves) for housekeeping chores involving potential blood contact and for instrument cleaning and decontamination procedures. Utility gloves may be decontaminated and reused but should be discarded if they are peeling, cracked, or discolored, or if they have punctures, tears, or other evidence of deterioration.

Body Fluids to which Universal Precautions Apply

Universal precautions apply to blood and to other body fluids containing visible blood. Blood is the single most important source of HIV and other blood borne pathogens in the occupational setting. Infection control efforts for HIV and other blood borne pathogens must focus on preventing exposures to blood.

Universal precautions also apply to semen and vaginal secretions. Although both of these fluids have been implicated in the sexual transmission of HIV, they have not been implicated in the occupational transmission from client to health-care worker. This observation is not unexpected, since exposure to semen in the usual health-care setting is limited, and the routine practice of wearing gloves for performing vaginal examinations protects health-care workers from exposure to potentially infectious vaginal secretions.

Universal precautions also apply to tissues and to the following fluids: cerebrospinal fluid (CSF), synovial fluid, pleural fluid, peritoneal fluid, pericardial fluid, and amniotic fluid. The risk of transmission of HIV from these fluids is unknown; epidemiologic studies in the health-care and community setting are currently inadequate to assess the potential risk to health care workers from occupational exposures to HIV.

Body Fluids to which Universal Precautions Do Not Apply
Universal precautions do not apply to feces, nasal secretions, sputum, sweat, tears, urine, and vomitus unless they contain visible blood. The risk of transmission of HIV from these fluids and materials is extremely low or nonexistent.

Precautions for Other Body Fluids in Special Settings
Human breast milk has been implicated in perinatal transmission of HIV, and HB$_s$Ag has been found in milk of mothers infected with HIV. However, occupational exposure to human breast milk has not been implicated in the transmission of HIV infection to health-care workers. Moreover, the health-care worker will not have the same type of intensive exposure to breast milk as the nursing neonate. Whereas universal precautions do not apply to human breast milk, gloves may be worn by health-care workers in situations where exposures to breast milk might be frequent.

Universal precautions do not apply to saliva. General infection control practices already in existence—including the use of gloves for digital examination of mucous membranes and endotracheal suctioning, and handwashing after exposure to saliva—should further minimize the minute risk, if any, for saliva transmission of HIV. Gloves need not be worn when feeding clients and when wiping saliva from skin.

Waste Management
The most practical approach to the management of infective waste is to identify those wastes with the potential for causing infection during handling and disposal and for which some special precautions appear prudent. While any item that has had contact with blood exudates or secretions may be potentially infective, it is not usually considered practical or necessary to treat all such waste as infective. Infective waste in general should either be incinerated or should be autoclaved before disposal in a sanitary landfill. Bulk blood, suctioned fluids, excretions, and secretions may be carefully poured down a drain connected to a sanitary sewer. Sanitary sewers may also be used to dispose of other infectious wastes capable of being ground and flushed into the sewer.

Morbidity and Mortality Weekly Report. Centers for Disease Control, 36:25, 1987.
Morbidity and Mortality Weekly Report. Centers for Disease Control, 37:24, 1988.

■ Appendix F. Specimens: Blood and Urine

SPECIMEN CONTAINERS FOR COLLECTING BLOOD

Red Top Tubes: blood clots normally in this tube and produces serum. These tubes are used for a variety of chemistry studies, serology tests, and blood banking. Draw-volume may be 9.5–10 ml.

Speckled Top Tubes contain a gel that, when centrifuged, forms a layer between serum and packed red blood cells. They contain no anticoagulants and are used for various chemistries. If the test is also to determine glucose, the blood should not be allowed to set more than 45 minutes since glycolysis will occur leading to low glucose values and an invalid result.

Lavender Top Tubes contain EDTA (an anticoagulant). Draw volume may be 2–10 ml. These tubes are used for tests performed on whole blood samples. Each tube should be inverted immediately at least 10 times to ensure adequate mixing of blood and anticoagulant.

Gray Top Tubes contain a glycolytic inhibitor. Draw volume may be 3–10 ml. These tubes are used most often for glucose determinations in serum or plasma samples. Invert at least 10 times to ensure adequate mixing of the blood and anticoagulant.

Blue Top Tubes contain sodium citrate and citric acid. Draw volume may be 2.7 or 4.5 ml. These tubes are used for coagulation studies requiring plasma samples. The tube should be filled to obtain a proper ratio of blood to anti-coagulant and immediately inverted at least 10 times.

Green Top Tubes contain heparin. Draw volume may be 2–15 ml. These tubes are used for tests performed on plasma samples.

Adapted from Humphrey, Carolyn, J. *Home Care Nursing Handbook*. Norwalk, Conn.: Appleton-Century-Crofts, 1986.

■ Appendix G. Values & Measures

REFERENCE FOR LABORATORY VALUES

Men	Women
Hematocrit	
38–54%	35–47%
Hemoglobin	
14–18 g/100 mL	12–16 g/100 mL
Sedimentation Rate	
<20 mm/hr	<30 mm/hr

Constituent	Normal Values	Deviations
Blood cells		
Red blood cells		Increase
		Acute poisoning
Men	4,600,000–6,200,000/nm³	Bone marrow hyperplasia
Women	4,200,000–5,400,000/nm³	Dehydration
		Diarrhea
		Polycythemia
		Pulmonary fibrosis
		Decrease
		Anemias
		Hemorrhage
		Hypothyroidism
		Thalassemia
		Toxicity
White blood cells	5000–10,000/nm³	Increase
		Acute bacterial infection
		Leukemia
		Polycythemia
		Decrease
		Acute alcohol ingestion
		Acute viral infection
		Agranulocytosis
		Bone marrow depression
Neutrophils	50–70% of total WBC count	Increase
		Acute hemorrhage
		Bacterial infections
		Carcinoma
		Cushing's disease
		Diabetes mellitus
		Gout
		Hemolytic anemia
		Increased corticosteroids

(continued)

Constituent	Normal Values	Deviations
		Lead poisoning
		Pancreatitis
		Rheumatic fever
		Rheumatoid arthritis
		Thyroiditis
		Stress
		Decrease
		Acute viral infection
		Bone marrow damage
		Folic acid deficiency
		Vitamin B_{12} deficiency
Eosinophils	1–4% of total WBC count	Increase
		Allergy
		Colitis
		Collagen diseases
		Eosinophilic
		granulomatosis
		Eosinophilic leukemia
		Parasitosis
Basophils	0–1% of total WBC count	Increase
		Myelofibrosis
		Polycythemia vera
		Decrease
		Anaphylactic reaction
Lymphocytes	20–40% of total WBC count	Increase
		Cushing's disease
		Infectious diseases
		Leukemia
		Thyrotoxicosis
Monocytes	0–6% of total WBC count	Increase
		Malaria
		Subacute bacterial
		endocarditis
		Tuberculosis
		Typhoid fever
Platelets	200,000–350,000/nm³	Increase
		Chronic granulocytic
		leukemia
		Hemoconcentration
		Polycythemia
		Splenectomy
		Decrease
		Acute leukemia
		Aplastic anemia
		Bone marrow
		depression
		Chemotherapy
		Thrombocytopenic pur-pura
Blood chemistry		
Bilirubin, total	0.1–1.2 mg/100 ml	Increase
		Liver disease
		Hemolysis post-transfusion

(*continued*)

Constituent	Normal Values	Deviations
		Pernicious anemia (jaundice present when bilirubin level exceeds 1.5 mg/100 ml)
		Decrease
		Carcinoma
		Chronic renal disease
Calcium	9–11 mg/100 ml (4.5–5.5 mEq/L)	Increase
		Addison's disease
		Hyperparathyroidism
		Malignant bone tumors
		Decrease
		Chronic renal disease
		Hypoparathyroidism
		Vitamin D deficiency
Bicarbonate	24–32 mEq/L	Increase
		Alkalosis
		Intestinal obstruction
		Respiratory disease
		Tetany
		Vomiting
		Decrease
		Acidosis
		Diarrhea
		Nephritis
Chloride	350–390 mg/100 ml (95–105 mEq/L)	Increase
		Renal tubular acidosis
		Decrease
		Diuretics that save potassium
		Hypokalemic alkalosis
		Ingestion of potassium without chloride
		Loss of gastric secretions
Cholesterol		Increase
Total	150–250 mg/100 ml	Chronic renal disease
Free	40–50 mg/100 ml	Diabetes mellitus
Esterified	75–210 mg/100 ml	Hypothyroidism
		Liver disease with jaundice
		Pancreatic dysfunction
		Decrease
		Fasting state
		Hemolytic anemia
		Hypermetabolic states
		Hyperthyroidism
		Intestinal obstruction
		Liver disease
		Malnutrition
		Pernicious anemia
		Tuberculosis
Creatinine	0.6–1.2 mg/100ml	Increase
		Chronic glomerulonephritis

(*continued*)

Constituent	Normal Values	Deviations
		Nephrosis
		Pyelonephritis
		Other renal dysfunctions
Fibrinogen	150–300 mg/100ml	Increase
		Infection
		Decrease
		Liver disease
		Malnutrition
Glucose	70–120 mg/100ml	Increase
		Cerebral lesions
		Cushing's disease
		Diabetes mellitus
		Emotional stress
		Exercise
		Hyperthyroidism
		Infections
		Pancreatic dysfunctions
		Steroid therapy
		Thiazide diuretic therapy
		Decrease
		Addison's disease
		β-cell neoplasm
		Hyperinsulinism
		Hypothyroidism
		Starvation
Iodine, protein-bound	4–8 μg/100ml	Increase
		Hyperthyroidism
		Decrease
		Hypothyroidism
Iron	65–170 μg/100ml	Increase
		Aplastic anemia
		Hemolytic anemia
		Hemochromatosis
		Hepatitis
		Pernicious anemia
		Decrease
		Iron deficiency anemia
Lead	$\leq$40 μg/100ml	Increase
		Lead poisoning
Lipids, total	400–1000 mg/100ml	Increase
		Diabetes mellitus
		Glomerulonephritis
		Hypothyroidism
		Nephrosis
		Decrease
		Hyperthyroidism
$Paco_2$	35–45 mmHg	Increase
		Metabolic alkalosis
		Respiratory acidosis
		Decrease
		Metabolic acidosis
		Respiratory alkalosis
pH (arterial)	7.35–7.45	Increase
		Fever
		Hyperpnea

(*continued*)

Constituent	Normal Values	Deviations
		Intestinal obstruction
		Vomiting
		Decrease
		Diabetic acidosis
		Hemorrhage
		Nephritis
		Uremia
Phosphatase		Increase
Acid	0.5–3.5 units	Bony metastasis
Alkaline	0.2–4.5 units	Carcinoma of the prostate
Pao_2	95–100 mmHg	Increase
		Administration of pure O_2
		Decrease
		Circulatory disorders
		Decreased hemoglobin
		Decreased O_2 supply
		High altitudes
		Poor O_2 uptake and utilization
		Respiratory exchange problems
Potassium	18–22 mg/100 ml (3.5–5.5 mEq/L)	Increase
		Addison's disease
		Anuria
		Bronchial asthma
		Burns
		Renal disease
		Tissue breakdown
		Trauma
		Decrease
		Cirrhosis
		Cushing's disease
		Diabetic acidosis
		Diarrhea
		Diuretic therapy
		Potassium-free intravenous therapy
		Steroid therapy
		Vomiting
Protein, total	6–8 g/100ml	Increase
		Infections
		Decrease
		Intestinal tract disease
		Liver disease
		Malnutrition
		Renal disease
Albumin	3.2–4.5 g/100ml	Increase
		Multiple myeloma
		Decrease
		Acute stress
		Chronic infection
		Chronic liver disease
		Loss of plasma
		Malabsorption of protein

(continued)

Constituent	Normal Values	Deviations
		Malnutrition
		Nephrotic syndrome
Globulin	2.3–3.5 g/100 ml	Increase
		Chronic hepatitis
		Chronic infections
		Collagen disease
		Leukemia
		Liver disease
		Multiple myeloma
		Sarcoidosis
		Decrease
		Proteinuria
Sodium	310–340 mg/100ml	Increase
	(135–145 mEq/L)	Cardiac disease
		Cushing's disease
		Excessive water loss
		Insufficient water intake
		Renal disease
		Decrease
		Addison's disease
		Chronic renal
		insufficiency
		Cirrhosis
		Congestive heart failure
		Dehydration
		Diabetic acidosis
		Diarrhea
		Diuretic therapy
		Excessive ingestion of
		water
		Overhydration
		(intravenous)
		Starvation
Urea nitrogen (BUN)	10–18 mg/100ml	Increase
		Acute
		glomerulonephritis
		Burns
		Dehydration
		Gastrointestinal
		hemorrhage
		High protein intake
		Intestinal obstruction
		Mercury poisoning
		Prostatic hypertrophy
		Protein catabolism
		Renal disease
		Decrease
		Cirrhosis
		Liver disease
		Low protein intake
		Starvation
Uric acid		Increase
Men	2.1–7.8 mg/100ml	Chronic lymphocytic and
Women	2–6.4 mg/100ml	granulocytic leukemia
		Chronic renal failure
		Fasting

(*continued*)

Constituent	Normal Values	Deviations
		Gout
		High salicylate intake
		Leukemia
		Multiple myeloma
		Pneumonia
		Thiazide diuretic therapy
		Decrease
		Allopurinol therapy
Urine Chemistry		
Acetone; Acetoacetate	0	Increase
		Starvation
		Uncontrolled diabetes
Creatine	0–200 mg/24 hr	Increase
		Fever
		Hyperthyroidism
		Liver cancer
Creatinine	0.8–2.0 g/24 hr	Increase
		Salmonella infections
		Tetanus
		Typhoid fever
		Decrease
		Anemia
		Leukemia
		Muscular atrophy
		Renal failure
Creatinine clearance	100–150 ml/min	Decrease
		Renal disease
Glucose	Negative (1+ not unusal finding in older adults)	Increase
		Diabetes mellitus
		Increased intracranial pressure
		Pituitary disorder
Lead	≤150 μg/24 hr	Increase
		Lead poisoning
pH	4.6–8.0	Increase
		Metabolic alkalemia
		Proteus infections
		Stale specimen
Phenolsulfonphthalein (PSP)	25% excreted: 15 min 40% excreted: 30 min 60% excreted: 120 min	Decrease
		Congestive heart failure
		Renal disease
Protein	0.1 g/24 hr	Increase
		Fever
		Infection
		Kidney disease
		Strenuous exercise
Specific gravity	1.001–1.035	Increase (Urine more concentrated)
		Dehydration
		Decrease (Urine less concentrated)
		Diuretic therapy
		Renal tubular dysfunction

(*continued*)

Constituent	Normal Values	Deviations

Urea nitrogen	9–16 g/24 hr	Increase
		  Excessive protein
		    catabolism
		Decrease
		  Renal disease

Uric acid	250–750 mg/24 hr	Increase
		  Gout
		Decrease
		  Nephritis

(From Eliopoulos, C. *Health Assessment of the Older Adult,* Menlo Park, Calif: Addison-Wesley, 1984.)

HOUSEHOLD TO METRIC CONVERSIONS

Standard Household Measure	Apothecary	Metric Volume	Metric Weight
1/8 teaspoon (t)	7–8 gtts/ 1/48 oz	0.6 ml	0.6g
1/4 teaspoon	15 gtts/ 1/24 oz	1.25 ml	1.25 g
1/2 teaspoon	30 gtts/ 1/12 oz	2.5ml	2.5 g
1 teaspoon	60 gtts/ 1/6 oz	5 ml	5 g
1 tablespoon (T)/3 teaspoons	1/2 oz	15 ml	15 g
2 tablespoons/6 teaspoons	1 oz	1/4 dl/30 ml	30 g
1/4 cup/4 tablespoons	2 oz	1/2 dl/60 ml	55 g
1/3 cup/5 tablespoons	2 1/2 oz	3/4 dl/75 ml	75 g
1/2 cup	4 oz	1 dl/120 ml	110 g
1 cup	8 oz	1/4 L/240–250 ml	225 g
1 pint	16 oz	1/2 L/480–500 ml	
1 quart	32 oz	1 L/1000 ml	
2 quarts/ 1/2 gallon	64 oz	2 L/2000 ml	
1 gallon	128 oz	3 3/4 L/3840–4000 ml	

Kee, J. L., and Marshall, S. M. *Clinical Calculations with Applications with General and Specialty Areas*. Philadelphia, PA: W. B. Saunders Co., 1988.

EQUIVALENTS AND CONVERSIONS

APPROXIMATE WEIGHT EQUIVALENTS: METRIC AND APOTHECARY SYSTEMS

Apothecary	Metric	Apothecary	Metric
1 ounce(8 drams)	30 g	1/150 grain	0.4 mg
15 grains	1 g	1/200 grain	0.3 mg
1 grain	60 mg	1/250 grain	0.25 mg
1/60 grain	1 mg	1/300 grain	0.2 mg
1/80 grain	0.8 mg	1/400 grain	0.15 mg
1/100 grain	0.6 mg	1/500 grain	0.12 mg
1/120 grain	0.5 mg	1/600 grain	0.1 mg

WEIGHT CONVERSIONS

Weight		Weight	
lb	kg	kg	lb
1	0.5	1	2.2
2	0.9	2	4.4
4	1.8	3	6.6
6	2.7	4	8.8
8	3.6	5	11.0
10	4.5	6	13.2
20	9.1	8	17.6
30	13.6	10	22
40	18.2	20	44
50	22.7	30	66
60	27.3	40	88
70	31.8	50	110
80	36.4	60	132
90	40.9	70	154
100	45.4	80	176
150	66.2	90	198
200	90.8	100	220

LENGTH CONVERSIONS

Length		Length	
in	cm	cm	in
1	2.5	1	0.4
2	5.1	2	0.8
4	10.2	3	1.2
6	15.2	4	1.6
8	20.3	5	2.0
12	30.5	6	2.4
18	46	8	3.1
24	61	10	3.9
30	76	20	7.9
36	91	30	11.8
42	107	40	15.7
48	122	50	19.7
54	137	60	23.6
60	152	70	27.6
66	168	80	31.5
72	183	90	35.4
78	198	100	39.4

1 lb = 0.454 kg   1 kg = 2.204 lb   1 in = 2.54 cm   1 cm = 0.3937 in

Saxton, D. F., Pelikan, P. K., Nugent, P. M., Hyland, P. A. *The Addison-Wesley Manual of Nursing Practice*, Menlo Park, Calif: Addison-Wesley, 1983.

■ Appendix H. Clinical Characteristics of Pressure Sores

Decubitus, stage 1	Skin redness that disappears on pressure.
Decubitus, stage 2	Redness, edema, and induration with epidural blistering and desquamation.
Decubitus, stage 3	The skin is necrotic with exposure of fat.
Decubitus, stage 4	Necrosis extends through the skin and fat to muscle.
Decubitus, stage 5	Extended fat and muscle necrosis.

(From *Medicare Home Health Agency Manual*, Health Care Financing Administration, Transmittal No. 203, December 1987.)

REFERENCES AND INDEX

■ References

Abernathy, E. (1987). Immunology—How the immune system works. *American Journal of Nursing*: *87:* 455.

Abrams, D.I. (1986). AIDS Update: Part I. *California Nursing Review, 53,* 4.

Abrams, D.I. (1986). AIDS: Battling a retroviral enemy. *California Nursing Review, 8*(6), 10.

Abrams, D.I. (1987). AIDS: In search of hope. *California Nursing Review, 9*(1), 5.

Aminoff, M.J. (1987). Parkinson's disease in the elderly: Current management strategies. *Geriatrics, 42*(7), 31.

Arnell, I. (1983). Testing decubitus ulcers. *Nursing '83, 13*(6), 50.

Anderson, L., Dibble, M.V., Junkki, P.R., Mitchel, H.J., Rynbergen, H.J. (1982). *Nutrition in Health and Disease* (17th ed.). Philadelphia: Lippincott.

Atkins, J.M., Oakly, C.W. (1986). A nurse's guide to TPN. *RN, 49*(6), 20.

Ballentine, R. (1983). Cancer chemotherapy. *Nursing '83, 13*(7), 17.

Bates, S., Ahern, J.A. (1986). Tight control: What does it mean? *American Journal of Nursing, 86*(11): 1256.

Baum, P. (1983). Carotid endarterectomy: One strike against stroke. *Nursing '83, 13*(3), 50.

Baum, R.M. (1987). The molecular biology. *Chemical and Engineering News, Nov.:* 14.

Bayer, L.M., Scholl, D.E., Ford, E.G. (1983). Tube feeding at home. *American Journal of Nursing, 83*: 1321.

Bayley, E.W., Smith, G.A. (1987). The three degrees of burn care. *Nursing '87, 17*(3): 34.

Begg, E., LeBlanc, D. (1975). Cancer chemotherapy. *Nursing '75, 5*(11): 22.

Beland, I.L., Passos, J.Y. (1981). *Clinical Nursing: Pathophysiological and Psychosocial Approaches* (4th ed.). New York: Macmillan.

Bennett, J.A. (1985). HTLV–III AIDS link. *American Journal of Nursing, 85*(10): 1086.

Bennett, J.A., Christman, C. (1984). Diabetes: New names, new test, new diet. *American Journal of Nursing, 87*: 34.

Berger, K., Fields, W. (1980). *Pocket Guide to Health Assessment.* Reston, Va.: Reston Publishing.

Beyers, M., Durburg, S., Werner, J. (1984). *Complete Guide to Cancer Nursing.* Oradell, N.J.: Medical Economics Books.

Biggs, C. (1987). The cancer that can cost a patient his voice. *RN, 50*(4): 44.

Brunner, L.S., Suddarth, D.S. (Eds.). (1984). *Textbook of Medical–Surgical Nursing* (5th ed.). Philadelphia: Lippincott.

Brunner, L.S., Suddath, D.S. (Eds.). (1982). *The Lippincott Manual of Nursing Practice* (3rd ed.). Philadelphia: Lippincott.

Byrne, N., Feld, M. (1984). Preventing and treating decubitus ulcers. *Nursing '84, 14*(4): 55.

Cahill, K.M. (1983). *The AIDS Epidemic.* New York: St. Martin's Press.

Carey, K.W. (Ed.). (1984). *Cardiac Crisis.* Springhouse, Penn.: Springhouse.

Carey, K.W. (Ed.). (1985). *Respiratory Emergencies.* Springhouse, Penn.: Springhouse.

Carlson, J.H., Craft, C.A., McGuire, A.D. (1982). *Nursing Diagnosis.* Philadelphia: Saunders.

Carpenito, L.J. (1983). *Nursing Diagnosis.* Philadelphia: Lippincott.

Carver, J.A. Cataract care made plain. *American Journal of Nursing, 87*: 626.

Catanzaro, M. (1980). MS: Nursing care of the person with MS. *American Journal of Nursing, 80*: 286.

Centers for Disease Control. (1982). Diffuse, undifferentiated non-Hodgkins lymphoma among homosexual males: United States. *Morbidity and Mortality Weekly Report, 31*: 277.

Centers for Disease Control. (1982). Persistent generalized lymphadenopathy among homosexual males. *Morbidity and Mortality Weekly Report, 31*(19): 249.

Centers for Disease Control. (1985). Provisional public health service, inter-agency recommendations for screening donated blood and plasma for antibody to the virus causing Acquired Immunodeficiency Syndrome. *Morbidity and Mortality Weekly Report, 34*: 1.

Centers for Disease Control. (1981). Reports on AIDS. *Morbidity and Mortality Weekly Report*, June 1981–May 1986.

Centers for Disease Control. (1987). Recommendations for prevention of HIV transmission in health-care settings. *Morbidity and Mortality Weekly Report, 36*: 2S.

Centers for Disease Control. (1987). Revision of the CDC surveillance case definition for Acquired Immunodeficiency Syndrome. *Morbidity and Mortality Weekly Report, 36*: 1s.

Christman, C., Bennett, J. (1987). Diabetes. *Nursing '87, 17*(1): 34.

Chumela, W.C., Roche, A.F., Mukherjee, D. (1987). *Nutritional Assessment of the Elderly through Anthropometry*. Columbus, Oh: Ross Laboratories.

Clark, N., O'Connell, P. (1984). Prostatectomy. *Nursing '84, 14*(4): 48.

Coping with neurological problems proficiently. (1979). Horsham, Penn.: Intermed Communications.

Cress, S.S., Taylor, C.M. (1987). *Nursing Diagnosis Cards–Nursing '87*. Springhouse, Penn.: Springhouse.

Cromwell, V., Huey, R., Korn, R., Weiss, J., Woodley, R. (1980). Understanding the needs of your coronary artery bypass patient. *Nursing '80, 10*: 34.

Dellefield, M.E. (1986). Caring for the elderly patient with cancer. *Oncology Nursing Forum, 13*(3): 19.

Denis, M.E., Baumann, A. (1982). Alzheimer's disease: The silent epidemic. *The Canadian Nurse, 78*(7): 32.

Department of Health and Human Services. (1987). *Medicare Home Health Agency Manual.* Baltimore: Health Care Financing Administration. Transmittal #203.

Diseases. (1983). Springhouse, Penn.: Intermed Communications.

Donehower, M.G. (1987). Malignant complications of AIDS. *Oncology Nursing Forum, 14* (1): 57.

Drugs. (1982). Springhouse, Penn.: Intermed Communications.

Eggland, E.T. (1987). Teaching the ABC's of C.O.P.D. *Nursing '87, 17*(1): 61.

Elliott, C.S. (1976). Radiation therapy: How you can help. *Nursing '76, 6*: 34.

Eliopoulos, C. (1987). Geroentological Nursing. Philadelphia: Lippincott.

Eliopoulos, C. (1984). *Health Assessment of the Older Adult*. Menlo Park, Cal.: Addison-Wesley Co.

Felicetta, J.V. (1987). Thyroid changes with aging: Significance and management. *Geriatrics, 42*(1): 86.

Fredette, S.L., Gloriant, F.S. (1981). Nursing diagnosis in cancer chemotherapy. *American Journal of Nursing, 81*: 2013.

Gettrust, K.V., Ryan, S.C., Engelman, D.S. (1985). *Applied Nursing Diagnosis*. New York: John Wiley and Sons.

Gever, L.N. (1981). Intravenous lipids. *Nursing '81, 11*: 60.

Goldman, C., Jackson, P. (1986). AIDS—Caring for your patient at home. *The Canadian Nurse, 82*(3): 18.

Gramse, C.A. (1983). Diverticular disease. *Nursing '83, 13*(6): 56.

Grant, J.P. (1980). *Handbook of Total Parenteral Nutrition.* Philadelphia: Saunders.

Gresh, C. (1980). Parkinson's disease. *Nursing '80, 10*: 26.

Griffin, C.W., Lockhard, J.S. (1987). Learning to swallow again. *American Journal of Medicine, 87*: 314.

Hahn, K. (1987). Left vs. right: What a difference the side makes in stroke. *Nursing '87, 17* (9): 44.

Hahn, K. (1987). The many signs of renal failure. *Nursing '87, 17*(8): 34.

Haire-Joshu, D., Flavin, K., Clutter, W. (1986). Contrasting Type I and Type II diabetes. *American Journal of Nursing, 86*: 1240.

Haire-Joshu, D., Flavin, K., Santiago, J.V. (1986). Intensive conventional insulin therapy. *American Journal of Nursing, 86*: 1251.

Haire-Joshu, D., Flavin, K. (1986). The pharmacological repertoire. *American Journal of Nursing, 86*: 1244.

Halperin, J.L. (1987). Peripheral vascular disease: Medical evaluation and treatment. *Geriatrics, 42*(11): 47.

Hamilton, H.K. (Ed.). (1984). *Gastrointestinal Disorders.* Springhouse, Penn.: Springhouse.

Hamilton, H.K. (1985). *Immune Disorders.* Springhouse, Penn.: Springhouse.

Hamilton, H.K. (Ed.). (1985). *Neoplastic Disorders.* Springhouse, Penn: Springhouse.

Hamilton, H.K. (Ed.). (1984). *Neurologic Disorders.* Springhouse, Penn.: Springhouse.

Hamilton, H.K. (Ed.). (1984). *Renal and Urologic Disorders.* Springhouse, Penn.: Springhouse.

Hamilton, H.K. (Ed.). (1984). *Respiratory Disorders.* Springhouse, Penn.: Springhouse.

Holden, S., Felde, G. (1987). Nursing care of patients experiencing cisplatin-related peripheral neuropathy. *Oncology Nursing Forum, 14*(1): 13.

Hoole, A.J., Greenberg, R.A., Pickard, C.G., Jr. (1976). *Patient Care Guidelines for Family Nurse Practitioners.* Boston: Little, Brown.

Humphrey, C.J. (1986). *Home Care Handbook.* Norwalk, Conn.: Appleton-Century-Crofts.

Hunt, J.M., Marks-Marvin, D.J. (1986). *Nursing Care Plans.* New York: John Wiley and Sons.

Irwin, B. (1979). Hemodialysis means vascular access . . . *Nursing '79, 9*: 49.

Jaret, P. (1986). Our immune system—The wars within. *National Geographic,* June: 702.

Kane, R.L., Ouslander, J.G., Abrass, I.B. (1984). *Essentials of Clinical Geriatrics.* New York: McGraw-Hill.

Kaplan, L.D., Volberding, P.A., Wofsy, C.B. (1987). Treatment of patients with Acquired Immunodeficiency Syndrome and associated manifestations. *Journal of American Medical Association, 257*(10): 1367.

Kee, J.L., Marshall, S.M. (1988). *Clinical Calculations with Applications to General and Speciality Areas.* Philadelphia: Saunders.

Kelly, M. (1985). *Nursing Care Plans.* Norwalk, Conn.: Appleton-Century-Crofts.

Kim, M.J., McFarland, G.K., McLane, A.M. (Eds.). (1984). *Pocket Guide to Nursing Diagnoses.* St. Louis: Mosby.

King, K.B., Nail, L.M., Kreamer, K., Strohl, R.A., Johnson, J.E. (1985). Patient's description of the experience of receiving radiation therapy. *Oncology Nursing Forum, 12*(4): 55.

Kinley, A.E., Slater, R.J., Yearwood, A.C., et al. (1980). Multiple sclerosis. *American Journal of Nursing, 80*: 273.

Klaus, B.J. (1979). *Protocol's Handbook for Nurse Practitioners*. New York: John Wiley and Sons.

Konstantinides, N.N. (1985). Home parenteral nutrition: A viable alternative for patients with cancer. *Oncology Nursing Forum, 12*(1): 23.

Krachenfels, M.M. (1987). Home tube feedings: Gastrointestinal complications. *Home Health Care Nurse, 5*(1): 41.

Loughlin, K.R., Whitmore, W.F. (1987). Managing prostate disorders in middle age and beyond. *Geriatrics, 42*(7): 45.

Lovvorn, J. (1982). Coronary bypass surgery: Helping patients cope with postop problems. *American Journal of Nursing, 82*: 1073.

MacBryde, C.M., Blacklow, R.S. (1970). *Signs and Symptoms* (5th ed.). Philadelphia: Lippincott.

Mahoney, J. (1978). What you should know about ostomies. *Nursing '78, 8*: 74.

McDonnell, M., Hentgen, J., Holland, N., Levinson, P.W. (1980). MS: Problem oriented nursing care plans. *American Journal of Nursing, 80*: 292.

McGahan-Hutchison, M. (1982). Administration of fat emulsions. *American Journal of Nursing, 82*: 275.

Meader, R. (1979). Learning to live with a new leg. *American Journal of Nursing, 79*: 393.

Meola, D.R., Walker, V. (1987). Responding quickly to tachydysrhythmias. *Nursing '87, 17*(11): 34.

Miaskowski, C.A., Nielson, B. (1985). A cancer nursing assessment tool. *Oncology Nursing Forum, 12*(6): 37.

Miller, M.J. (1983). *Pathophysiology*. New York: Saunders.

Miracle, V.A. (1988). Understanding the different types of MI. *Nursing '88, 18*: 53.

Muir, B.L. (1980). *Pathophysiology*. New York: John Wiley and Sons.

Neal, M.C., Cohen, P.F., Cooper, P.G. (1980). *Nursing Care Planning Guides for Long-term Care*. Pacific Palisades, Calif.: Nurseco.

Northridge, J.S. (1982). Helpful hints for assessing the ostomate. *Nursing '82, 12*: 72.

Nowotny, M.L. (1980). If your patient's joints hurt, the reason may be osteoarthritis. *Nursing '80, 10*: 39.

Ogilvie, C. (1980). *Chamberlain's Symptoms and Signs in Clinical Medicine*. (10th ed.). Liverpool, U.K.: John Wright.

Pajik, M. (1984). Alzheimer's disease. *American Journal of Nursing, 84*: 215.

Performing G.I. Procedures. (1981). Horsham, Penn.: Intermed Communications.

Perloff, D. (1983). Hypertension. *Primary Care, 1*(4): 625.

Peterson, F.X. (1983). Assessing peripheral vascular diseases. *American Journal of Nursing, 83*: 1549.

Phipps, W.J., Long, B.C., Woods, N.F. (1983). *Medical-Surgical Nursing: Concepts and Clinical Practice* (2nd ed.). St. Louis: Mosby.

Plank, C. (1980). MS, AKS, MS, MD—What's the difference? *American Journal of Nursing, 80*: 282.

Popkin, B. (1983). Caring for the AIDS patient—Fearlessly. *Nursing '83, 13*(9): 50.

Price, G. (1980). The challenge to the family. *American Journal of Nursing, 80*: 283.

Procedures. (1983). *Nurse's Reference Library*. Springhouse, Penn.: Intermed Communications.

Prout, B.J., Cooper, J.G. (1983). *An Outline of Clinical Diagnosis*. Great Britain: John Wright.

Reed, S.B. (1982). Giving more than dialysis. *Nursing '82, 12*: 58.

Robinson, J. (Ed.). (1984). *Hypertension*. Springhouse, Penn.: Springhouse.

Robinson, J. (Ed.). (1981). *Implementing Urologic Procedures*. Horsham, Penn.: Intermed Communications.

Robinson, J. (Ed.). (1983). *Managing I.V. Therapy*. Springhouse, Penn.: Intermed Communications.

Robinson, J. (Ed.). (1980). *Providing Respiratory Care*. Horsham, Penn.: Intermed Communications.

Ropka, M.E. (1982). Hiatal hernia. *Nursing '82, 12*: 126.

Saxton, D.F., Pelikan, P.K., Nugent, P.M., Hyland, P.A. (1983). *The Addison-Wesley Manual of Nursing Practice*. Menlo Park, Calif.: Addison-Wesley.

Schroffner, W.G. (1987). The aging thyroid in health and disease. *Geriatrics, 42*(8): 41.

Sebern, M. (1987). Home-team strategies for treating pressure sores. *Nursing '87, 17*(4): 50.

Seiler, W.O., Stähelin, H.B. (1985). Decubitus ulcers: Treatment through five therapeutic principles. *Geriatrics, 40*(9): 30.

Signs and Symptoms. (1986). Springhouse, Penn.: Springhouse.

Skeers, V.B. (1979). How the nurse practitioner manages the rheumatoid arthritis patient. *Nursing '79, 9*: 26.

Slater, R.J., Yearwood, A.C. (1980). MS facts, faith, and hope. *American Journal of Nursing, 80*: 276.

Slusarczyk, S.M., Hicks, F.D. (1983). Helping your patient live with a permanent pacemaker. *Nursing '83, 13*: 58.

Smith, A.M. (1987). Alternatives in AIDS homecare. *AIDS Patient Care, 1*(1): 28.

Snyder, C. (1986). *Oncology Nursing*. Boston: Little, Brown.

Stanford, J.L. (1982). Who profits from coronary artery bypass surgery? *American Journal of Nursing, 82*: 1068.

Starkey, J.F., Jefferson, P.A., Kirby, D.F. (1988). Taking care of percutaneous endoscopic gastrostomy. *American Journal of Nursing, 88*: 19.

Surgeon General's Report. (1986). *Acquired Immune Deficiency Syndrome*. Bethesda: U.S. Department of Health and Human Services.

The Surgical Clinics of North America. (1981). *61*: 3. New York: Saunders.

Sweet, K. (1977). Hiatal hernia. *Nursing '77, 7*: 37.

Teich, C.J., Raia, K. (1984). Teaching strategies for an ambulatory chemotherapy program. *Oncology Nursing Forum, 11*(5): 24.

Thompson, M.A. (1981). Managing the patient with liver disfunction. *Nursing '81, 11*: 101.

Thorpe, C.J., Caprini, J.A. (1980). Gallbladder disease: Current trends and treatment. *American Journal of Nursing, 80*: 2181.

Tilton, C.N., Maloof, M. (1982). Diagnosing the problems in stroke. *American Journal of Nursing, 82*: 596.

Tucker, S.M., Breeding, M.A., Canobbio, M.M., Paquette, E.V., Wells, M.E., Willman, M.E. (1980). *Patient Care Standards* (2nd ed.). St. Louis: Mosby.

U.S. Department of Health and Human Services. (1983). *Teaching Patients Undergoing Cancer Chemotherapy*. Bethesda: Clinical Center Office of Clinical Reports and Inquiries.

Ulrich, S.P., Canale, S.W., Wendell, S.A. (1986). *Nursing Care Planning Guides*. Philadelphia: Saunders.

Walters, J. (1981). Coping with leg amputation. *American Journal of Nursing, 81*: 1349.

Watt, R.C. (1985). The ostomy—Why is it created? *American Journal of Nursing, 85*: 1242.

Webb, P.H. (1979). Neurological deficit after carotid endarterectomy. *American Journal of Nursing, 79*: 654.

Weeks, C.C. (1980). MS: The malignant uncertainty. *American Journal of Nursing, 80*: 289.

Wilson, J., Colley, R. (1979). Meeting patients' nutritional needs with hyperalimentation. *Nursing '79, 9*: 56.

Witt, M.E., McDonald-Lynch, A., Grimmer, D. (1987). Adjuvant radiotherapy to the colorectum: Nursing implications. *Oncology Nursing Forum, 14*(3): 17.

Yearwood, A.C. (1980). Being disabled doesn't mean being handicapped. *American Journal of Nursing, 80*: 299.

■ Index